Older Veterans:

Linking VA and Community Resources

HARVARD UNIVERSITY
DIVISION OF HEALTH POLICY RESEARCH AND EDUCATION

Older Veterans:

Linking VA and Community Resources

Edited by
Terrie Wetle, Ph.D.
John W. Rowe, M.D.

Technical Editing
Catherine A. Olejniczak, M.B.A.

Distributed by
HARVARD UNIVERSITY PRESS
Cambridge, Massachusetts and London, England
1984

ISBN (cloth) 0–674–63275–3

Library of Congress Cataloging in Publication Data
Main entry under title:

Older veterans.

Book grew out of a collaborative project between the Veterans
Administration and the Division of Health Policy Research and
Education at Harvard University.
Includes index.
1. Veterans—Medical care—United States. 2. Aged—Medical-
care—United States. 3. Community health services for the aged—
United States. 4. Medical cooperation—United States. I. Wetle, Ter-
rie Todd, 1946-   . II. Rowe, John W. (John Wallis), 1944-   . III.
United States. Veterans Administration. IV. Harvard University.
Division of Health Policy Research and Education. [DNLM: 1. Health
Services for the Aged—United States. 2. Veterans—United States.
UB 369 044]   UB369.044 1984   355.1'156'0973   84-19244
ISBN 0–674–63275–3

Publication of this book was made possible by funds from the
Research Service of the Veterans Administration.

Printed by
Harvard University Office of the University Publisher

CONTENTS

ABOUT THE AUTHORS

Axel Bang is Vice President for Communications at the Massachusetts Hospital Association. He has staffed long term care activities, conducted surveys on elderly issues, and written several reports on long term care.

Richard W. Besdine, M.D. is Director of Geriatric Fellowship Training, Assistant Professor of Medicine in the Division on Aging at Harvard Medical School, and Director of the Harvard Geriatric Education Center. Dr. Besdine also serves as the Director of Geriatric Medical Education at the Hebrew Rehabilitation Center for Aged; and he is the Director of the Interdisciplinary Geriatric Consultation Service and Associate Physician at Beth Israel Hospital and Brigham and Women's Hospital.

Jay Bonanno, J.D. served as an associate attorney in a general commercial law firm after receiving his law degree from Harvard Law School in 1977. He is currently a fourth year student at Harvard Medical School. While serving as Research Assistant for the Working Group on Health Policy and Aging of the Division of Health Policy Research and Education at Harvard University, he worked on an analysis of Veterans Administration legislation as well as co-authoring an article on Health Maintenance Organization enrollment of Medicare recipients.

Laurence G. Branch, Ph.D. is Associate Professor of Social Medicine and Health Policy at Harvard Medical School, and on the Executive Committee of the Division on Aging at Harvard Medical School. He is an Associate Professor for the Harvard School of Public Health in the Department of Maternal and Child Health and Aging. Dr. Branch also serves as the Associate Director of West Roxbury's Veterans Administration Medical Center, Geriatric Research Education and Clinical Center. Prior to coming to Harvard Medical School, he served as the Program Director at the Center for Survey Research of the University of Massachusetts and the Joint Center for Urban Studies of Massachusetts Institute of Technology and Harvard.

Edward Campion, M.D. is Chief of the Geriatrics Unit at the Massachusetts General Hospital and Director of Geriatric Rehabilitation at the Spaulding Rehabilitation Hospital. He also serves as Assistant Director for Rehabilitation in the Harvard Geriatric Education Center. He is a member of the Task Force on Long Term Care of the Massachusetts Hospital Association and a consultant at the Normative Aging Study of the Veterans Administration in Boston. Dr. Campion is also a member of the Division on Aging of Harvard Medical School.

Nancy R. Cook, D.Sc. is a Research Associate in Medicine (Biostatistics), Brigham and Women's Hospital, Harvard Medical School. Dr. Cook is also an epidemiologist at the East Boston Neighborhood Health Center.

Harry Dunlevy, B.A. is currently enrolled in the John F. Kennedy School of Government and the Harvard School of Dental Medicine and will receive his M.P.P. and D.M.D. in June of 1985.

Linda Evans, Ph.D. is Professor of Sociology at Central Connecticut State University and a Research Affiliate with both the Veterans Administration Normative Aging Study in Boston and the Boston University Gerontology Center. Dr. Evans has served as a division chair for the Society for the Study of Social Problems and authored books and articles about elders' political potential, social control aspects of aging policies and retirement.

Sue Levkoff, Sc.D. has her doctorate in Behavioral Sciences and Geriatrics from the Harvard School of Public Health. She is an Instructor, Department of Social Medicine and Health Policy at Harvard Medical School. Dr. Levkoff is also a Research Associate and a member of the Working Group on Health Policy and Aging of the Division of Health Policy Research and Education at Harvard University.

Margaret Mac Adam, M.S. is the Executive Director of the Massachusetts Association of Home Care Programs/Area Agencies on Aging, Inc. Ms. Mac Adam was formerly the Director of the Massachusetts Long Term Care Channeling Demonstration Program. She is currently completing her doctoral work at Brandeis University.

John Mather, M.D., a medical graduate of the University of London, is a diplomat of the American Board of Otolaryngology. He has served in the U.S. Army at Walter Reed Army Medical Center and in the Bureau of Health Manpower, Public Health Service, as Director, Office of Interdisciplinary Programs prior to joining the Veterans Administration Department of Medicine and Surgery in 1977. He has had successively increased administrative positions in the Veterans Administration Central Office in academic program management and since 1982 has been the Assistant Chief Medical Director for Geriatrics and Extended Care.

Ann Moran, Dr. P.H. is the Executive Officer of the Mental Health Policy Working Group of the Center for Health Policy and Management at the John F. Kennedy School of Government. She is an Instructor in the Department of Social Medicine and Health Policy at Harvard Medical School. Dr. Moran worked in Health Services Research in the Veterans Administration from 1977 to 1984.

James Morse, M.D., a graduate of the Tufts University Medical School, is currently an intern at the University of Virginia Medical Center in Charlottesville, Virginia. He served as a Research Assistant for the Working Group on Health Policy and Aging of the Division of Health Policy Research and Education at Harvard University, and had previously completed a comparative study of mental health care in Ireland and Denmark.

Linda Niessen, D.M.D., M.P.H., M.P.P. is a Dental Geriatric Fellow at the Veterans Administration Outpatient Clinic in Boston and the Bedford Veterans Administration Medical Center, Bedford, Massachusetts. She is a Senior Research Fellow at Harvard School of Dental Medicine and a faculty member of the Harvard Geriatric Education Center. Dr. Niessen also serves as President of the American Association of Women Dentists. She will soon become Director of Geriatric Dental Services at the Perry Point Veterans Administration Medical Center in Perry Point, Maryland.

Diane Piktialis, Ph.D. is Manager of Policy Development and Coordination, Health Programs Development, of Blue Cross and Blue Shield of Massachusetts. She was formerly the Assistant Secretary for Program Planning and Management in the Department of Elder Affairs for the Commonwealth of Massachusetts. Dr. Piktialis is a social work faculty member of Boston University's Metropolitan College. She also serves as a Board Member for the Massachusetts Association against Alzheimer's Disease and Related Disorders.

John W. Rowe, M.D. is Director of the West Roxbury/Brockton Veterans Administration Medical Center, Geriatric Research Education Clinical Center. He is an Associate Professor of Medicine and serves as the Director of the Division on Aging at Harvard Medical School. He is the Chief of the Gerontology Division for the Joint Department of Medicine at Beth Israel and Brigham and Women's Hospitals. He is the Chairman of the Working Group on Aging and Deputy Director of the Division of Health Policy Research and Education at Harvard University.

Paul A. Scherr, Ph.D. is an Instructor in Medicine at Harvard Medical School. Dr. Scherr is also an epidemiologist at the East Boston Neighborhood Health Center. His research includes participation in the East Boston Senior Health Project.

Mark Schlesinger is a Caroline Shields-Walker Fellow at the Division of Health Policy Research and Education of Harvard University. He also serves as Research Coordinator for the Center for Health Policy and Management, John F. Kennedy School of Government. He is a member of the Working Group on Health Policy and Aging, the Mental Health Policy Working Group, and the Working Group on Innovations in Health Policy of the Division of Health Policy Research and Education. He will receive a Ph.D. in economics in 1984.

James O. Taylor, M.D. is Associate Clinical Professor of Medicine, Brigham and Women's Hospital, Harvard Medical School, and Medical Director of the East Boston Neighborhood Health Center. Dr. Taylor is also a member of the Channing Laboratories of Harvard Medical School.

Terrie Wetle, Ph.D. is an Assistant Professor of Medicine at Harvard Medical School, and Associate Director of the Harvard Geriatric Education Center. She also serves as the Executive Officer for the Working Group on Health Policy and Aging. Prior to coming to Harvard, she was the Director of the Program in Long Term Care and an Assistant Professor in the Department of Epidemiology and Public Health, Yale School of Medicine. She has also served as a social policy analyst for the Administration on Aging.

Linda Zangwill, M.S. has a Master of Science from the Department of Health Policy and Management in the Harvard School of Public Health. She has served as a Research Assistant for the Center for Health Policy and Management of the John F. Kennedy School of Government.

PREFACE

This book grows out of a collaborative project between the Veterans Administration and the Division of Health Policy Research and Education at Harvard University, designed to explore improved integration of VA and community resources for serving the elderly. The nation's demographic changes over the next half century will be compressed into two decades for the Veterans Administration. The response of the VA to this challenge will provide models for caring for the growing population of elders, veteran and non-veteran as well.

The VA has assumed a leadership role in the development of geriatric programs. Acute care has been the major focus of special programs addressing illnesses common among the elderly including cancer, cardiovascular disease, diabetes and neuropsychiatric disorders. In addition, the VA has a well established and impressive array of institutional and non-institutional long-term care programs. These include the VA nursing home program, the commmunity nursing home program, the VA domiciliary care program and the VA state nursing home program. Non-institutional services include hospital-based home care, adult day health care and outpatient clinic services. In an important major development, Geriatric Research Education Clinical Centers were established in 1975. These units have attracted and developed staff in gerontology and geriatrics, conducted basic and clinical research, and developed models of care including Geriatric Evaluation Units which are being expanded to many VA Medical Centers and non-VA settings.

By legislative mandate, the focus of the VA is on health care, but it is well recognized that many elderly individuals require a package of health and social services necessitating interaction between the VA and other providers of care. Further, because of the prevalence of multiple health and social problems among elder populations, it is imperative that the various programs serving the elderly coordinate and integrate their efforts.

This project focused on the development of options or strategies for improving care of the older veteran through improved sharing of VA and non-VA resources. Three categories of issues were identified: 1) an overall increase in demand for care, 2) changes in the nature of care required by veterans served, and 3) variations in care demanded related to time and geographic location.

Increase in Demand for Care

The proportion of elders in the veteran population will double in the decade between 1980 and 1990. Expanded demand for care is predicted not only by this growth in the absolute numbers of older veterans, but also by increased utilization which is correlated with advanced age.

Options for improved planning are at the forefront for responding to increased demand. These focus on both central planning as well as regional and local efforts. It is suggested that there be greater coordination of planning efforts among federal agencies, including interagency agreements with the Health Care Financing Administration, Social Security Administration, and the Administration on Aging. These options recognize the impact of non-VA policy decisions on demand for care by elder veterans.

Similarly the VA should increase its involvement in community and regional planning activities, including participation in the work of local HSAs, state health coordinating councils, and Area Agency on Aging advisory councils. This participation is a natural outgrowth of the VA's recently developed district based planning activities (MEDIPP). Such involvements would increase the local VA's knowledge of existing community resources and would identify services with which the VA could supplement its own care package.

Developing new resources is the most obvious response to increased demand. The Veterans Administration can provide increased services by either increasing the VA health care budget or by shifting allocations from other areas. Should such an increase in resources occur, the VA may choose to provide the services directly or through contracts with non-VA agencies to provide services using a model similar to the community nursing home program.

However, there are political limitations to the level of resources which will be made available. Recognizing these limitations, options were developed that would increase the availability of community-based resources for veterans by improving access to such services. A further step in this process would be actual sharing of VA and community-based resources to better serve elders in the community. Such sharing can take a variety of forms, including the pooling of resources or the identification of special capacity or expertise which can be offered into the sharing arrangement. In return for access to non-VA services, the VA might, for example, offer assistance in geriatric education programs or provide health care to certain categories of non-veterans, such as those suffering stroke or spinal cord injury.

Changing eligibility for entitlements is another obvious response to increased demand for services. The question of limiting entitlement among groups of older veterans has been addressed most recently by the Special Medical Advisory Group of the Task Force on the Geriatric Report. A number of options developed in this project include targeting strategies designed to identify those veterans likely to have a greater need for certain services or who benefit most by their provision.

Compensation and payment options address increased demand for service by allowing veterans or their families to purchase needed services from non-VA vendors. Increased compensation for this purpose can be achieved through expansion of the aid and attendance benefit.

A variety of family care options would support the provision of care by families to older veterans. The VA could provide direct financial assistance or tax deductions to families providing care to their elder veteran relatives. Supportive services for family caregivers are likely to improve quality of life of both patient and caregivers and therefore increase willingness to provide such care. Supportive services include counseling, mental health services, personal support, technical assistance and skills development. Services which supplement family care will ease the burden of family caregivers and in many cases delay or avoid institutionalization of the older veteran. These services include home health care, chore services, day hospitals, friendly visitors, and respite care. Cost savings may result when services such as these supplement but do not replace family provider services. As with other options, the VA may choose to deliver these services directly, to develop volunteer programs to assist in their delivery, or to enter into sharing arrangements with community agencies via contracts or pooling of services.

Changes in the Nature of Demand for Services

Old and young veterans differ in the types of diseases they suffer, the presentation of specific illnesses, and the increased need for chronic care. These differences result in changes not only in the amount but in the type of care required as the population ages. The graying of the veteran population will result in the following changes in the nature of care required:

1) increased need for geriatric expertise
2) increased demand for chronic care
3) increased need for continuity of care, and
4) improved response to illness behaviors of older patients.

Geriatric expertise must be rapidly expanded. While the general health care system has been slow to respond to an aging population, the VA has made major efforts to increase the geriatric interest and knowledge of its care providing professionals and has developed substantial capability to train health providers from several disciplines. Options relating to geriatric expertise include expanding the use of the VA as a major training site for future health care professionals. The VA can provide assistance to the community in this critical area, perhaps in return for enhanced access by veterans to collaborative care in community settings.

Improved continuity of care is required by aging populations because of the burden of chronic disease and multiple illnesses. Perhaps the most important factor in continuity of care is appropriate and effective case management. There is general agreement among gerontologists and geriatricians that case management is imperative. Case management which coordinates VA and non-VA services is particularly important for the elder veteran. Again, the VA has a variety of options for expanding case management of this sort.

The VA can serve as case manager for all services, both VA and non-VA, perhaps by developing the previously mentioned options for increased access to community services. The VA on the other hand might choose to contract out for case management services, particularly in those geographic areas which have well-developed programs, such as the Channeling Projects or other demonstration projects.

A somewhat more complex, but nonetheless promising, option is for the VA to cooperate with ongoing case management activities in the community, participating as a partner or in a sharing relationship.

Variations in Demand

The third general category of problems facing the VA involves variation in demand over time and variation in demand from one geographic region to another. Improving capacity to predict variations in demand is important for rational planning and allocation of resources.

The first set of options related to this issue involves strategies for planning. The previously mentioned option of increased involvement of the VA in policy planning and information sharing at the federal level will help in predicting the impact of non-VA actions on demand for VA services. In a like manner, VA involvement in local planning efforts will improve the VA's ability to predict shifts in demand which are specific to certain geographic locations. The VA also can pursue health services research which develops better data and tools for predicting utilization behaviors and patterns.

It is also suggested that the VA increase its flexibility to respond to shifts in demand over time by relying more on contract and sharing arrangements with non-VA providers than on building new physical plants and programs. If the VA chooses a course of developing rigid programs involving a great deal of brick and mortar, new problems will develop down the road as the bulge of World War II veterans passes out of the population.

Responding to the geriatric imperative will strain the current system of care. The challenge faced by the VA provides rich opportunity for major improvements in the care not only of older veterans, but of elders in general. It is hoped that this text will document the VA's leadership role in geriatric care and will suggest new opportunities for better integration of VA and non-VA services, resulting, we hope, in better lives for older people.

Terrie Wetle
John W. Rowe

ACKNOWLEDGEMENTS

The project for which this book is but one product was conceptualized by Dr. Donald Custis, then Chief Medical Director of the Veterans Administration and initiated with Dr. Julius Richmond and Dr. David Hamburg, each of whom has served as the Director of Harvard's Division of Health Policy Research and Education. We are grateful to the Working Group on Health Policy and Aging of the Division of Health Policy Research and Education for providing major contributions regarding the structure of the project in it's formative stages and to the project faculty who prepared background papers and chaired conference workshops.

This project has received substantial assistance from a large number of people within the Veterans Administration and other agencies of federal government, from the aging network, and from academic settings. We are indebted, in particular, to the participants of a conference addressing this topic in the fall of 1983. Their thoughtful reactions to the suggestions developed by project faculty were important in the development of the options described herein.

Individuals from VA central office also provided substantial assistance to the project. We would like to recognize the contribution of the Project Advisory Group who contributed considerable time and effort to conceptualizing the project, to planning the conference and to reviewing the many background papers and option packages. Dr. Richard Adelson and Joy Clay played an active role staffing the advisory group to the project, giving graciously of their time and providing invaluable assistance. The members and consultants of the Project Advisory Group are listed below.

Hollis Boren	Norman Hartnett
Susan Brennan	James Krajeck
Howard Cohn	John Mather
Frank Conrad	Richard Ryan

At the local level, John Fewel of the Veterans Administration earned our gratitude for his administrative assistance and good humor.

We would also like to thank the following VA staff who reviewed chapters. Their comments and suggestions have been most constructive and of substantial aid to the authors.

Robert Abel	Paul Haber	Richard Olson
Mark Adelman	Norman Hartnett	William Page
Lewis Aumack	Norman Hiller	Ann Pizza
William Balfoort	Frank Holden	Marjorie Quandt
Jack Bresler	Gene Hufford	Bill Ramsey
John Castellot, Sr.	Ralph Ibson	Robert Rhyne
Francis Conrad	Thomas Inui	Edward Rose
Daniel Cooney	James Kelly	Andrew Ruoff
Mary Durham	Jim Krajeck	Daniel Schoeps
Carlton Evans	Jerry Krim	Larry Seitz
Jack Ewalt	Michael Lawson	Yasuko Shiraishi
Eugene Fisher	Judith Mabry	Donald Thompson
Kathleen Fitzgerald	John Mather	Lida Verdi
James Fozard	Susan Mather	Phillip Weiler
John Fulton	Jule Moravec	Harold S. Wells
Georgia Georgeson	Thomas Mullon	Eliza Wolff
Peter Goldschmidt	Edwin Olsen	David Worthen
		Charles Yarbrough

The production of the book would not have been possible without the indefatigable assistance of Catherine Olejniczak and Susan Fenwick. And to the many unnamed, but much appreciated, who offered support, assistance and patience, thank you as well.

1. Health and Illness Behaviors in Elder Veterans

Richard W. Besdine, M.D.
Sue E. Levkoff, Sc.D.
Terrie Wetle, Ph.D.

Introduction

The Veterans Administration faces the challenge of planning and developing appropriate services for the increasing numbers of elder veterans. Elder veterans differ from younger cohorts in types of diseases suffered, impact of disease on function, interpretation of and reaction to symptoms, and interactions with health care providers. Because of these unique characteristics, the current VA health care system will experience changes in the needs and demands of the patients it serves. Understanding the special illness characteristics of elders will enable the VA to direct its efforts toward activities which will enhance the delivery of care to elders and promote appropriate use of available resources. The purpose of this chapter is to describe disease and illness in old age and to examine factors which influence illness and service utilization behaviors. Options for improving the match between the needs of elders and the organization of VA health care are presented.

American society is currently witnessing unprecedented changes in its age structure which have important implications for national health care policy. The aged are becoming an ever larger segment of the population. Demo-

graphic estimates predict that by the year 2020, the proportion of people 65 years and older will have increased
from the current 11% to 17% of the population (Health Care
Financing Administration, 1981), and the old-old (85+)
will increase most rapidly. A special characteristic of
elderly populations is their increased use of health services. The prevalence of disease and disability rises
sharply with age and is highest in the very segment of the
elderly population increasing the most rapidly of all, the
old-old. This rapidly growing group of increasingly old
and infirm citizens is making demands on the traditional
health care delivery system that are qualitatively different from any experienced before. Although only 11% of
the population, Americans over age 65 account for 40% of
all acute hospital bed days, use 25% of all prescription
drugs purchased, and account for 30% of our overall $287
billion health expenditures and more than 50% of the $80
billion federal health budget (U.S. DHHS, 1982).

The elderly can be expected to make disproportionate
demands on the nation's health care system well into the
next century due to the higher prevalence of disease and
disability in old age. This disproportionate use of
health resources by elderly Americans, though notable,
should not be regarded as unfair or unjustified. The escalating disease burden coincident with aging produces the
accelerated need for and use of health care. An understanding of the "greying" of America and its consequences
is critical for the successful planning and implementation
of future health care services for the nation's aged.
This understanding depends in part on careful analysis of
the special characteristics of the illness behaviors of
the aged, and how their special needs will require changes
in clinical practice and formal organization of care.

The VA health care system faces a similar demographic
imperative. At present, of the total 28 million veterans,
3.5 million are 65 years of age and older. By the year
1990, this number will nearly triple, exceeding 9 million. Startling changes are also occurring within the
VA's aging population (Special Medical Advisory Group,
1983). At present, the majority of the 3.5 million aging
veterans are the young-old, with the 65 to 74 age bracket
accounting for close to 3 million. By the year 2000,
there will be an appreciable increase in the numbers of
old-old veterans, with the 75-84 year age bracket accounting for 3.5 million veterans, and the 85+ group accounting
for an additional half-million (SMAG, 1983). Although the

2

veteran population over age 65 currently accounts for only 12.5% of all veterans, this segment consumes a disproportionate share of VA services and resources, similar to that consumed by the general population. These demographic projections suggest that the VA will be called upon to serve an increasing older population with its concomitant higher levels of disease and disability. If the VA continues in its present role as the safety net for socially disadvantaged veterans, then it can expect both a massive growth in demand for its services in the coming decades as well as a major shift in the types of services demanded. Changes external to the VA, such as in Medicare and Medicaid entitlements, could enlarge its aged patient population even more dramatically.

An understanding of the aged's illness behavior and help seeking is important to both anticipate the VA's future health care needs as well as to provide appropriate and comprehensive services. Specifically, an understanding is needed of: 1) the presentation of disease in old age, and 2) the social-psychological processes which influence the individual's evaluation of symptoms and responses to illness. Geriatric medicine has shown that there is a unique presentation and distribution of diseases in old age. The growing literature on illness behavior in the general population suggests that a variety of social-psychological processes play an important role in the way individuals perceive, evaluate, and act on their symptoms. Recognition of both the physiological aspects of disease in old age and the psychosocial characteristics of the aged are prerequisites for the VA to design an effective health care delivery system.

The objectives of this chapter are threefold: 1) to describe the state of the art with regard to the illness behavior and help seeking of the aged and to discuss its implications for service delivery; 2) to provide a theoretical framework for examining these behaviors; and 3) to discuss implications for health care policy within the VA medical system and to suggest an agenda for options with regard to health care delivery for the elder veteran.

I. State of the Art: Illness Behavior and Help Seeking

Over the last twenty years, many different approaches to the study of illness behavior and help seeking have emerged. The approach which evolves from the geriatric

3

medicine perspective (Williamson, 1964; Besdine, 1982) provides a rich basis for understanding how the physical processes of aging and disease interact and influence illness behavior. The social-psychological perspective concentrates on the many social and psychological processes which lead an individual to recognize and evaluate a symptom, and to eventually seek care for that symptom (Mechanic, 1983; Becker, 1977; Safer, et al., 1979; Suchman, 1965). Intrinsic to this social-psychological perspective is the observation that health behavior is not determined by physiological factors alone. Different individuals with the same symptom complex may perceive and act on their symptoms in very different ways. It is the purpose of this research effort to combine these approaches in the study of illness behavior and help seeking among the elderly. This blending of perspectives is consistent with the interdisciplinary nature of geriatric medicine and its emphasis on both curing and caring for older patients.

A. Presentation of Disease in Old Age

1. Diseases Specific to Elders

One of the most important differences between young and old individuals relevant to planning health care for the elderly is in the nature of clinical illness itself (Besdine, 1982). Disease in old age has two special features that must be considered in the organization of health services as well as in provision of individual care for the elderly. First, there is a group of disorders, some rare and some common, which usually occur only in aged individuals. These conditions are easily enumerated (Table 1), and comprise a straightforward component of geriatric medicine.

2. Atypical Presentation of Disease

Another group of diseases introduces a complexity with major implications for geriatric care. These are diseases which, though occurring in patients of all ages, behave differently in the elderly. A fundamental principle of geriatric medicine is that virtually any disease with a classic complex of signs or symptoms frequently presents in old age with few or none of the characteristic findings. The classic presentation is often replaced by one or more non-specific problems which may be misidentified as due to aging rather than disease. These non-specific problems are presented in Table 2.

4

Table 1
DISEASES AND DISORDERS USUALLY FOUND ONLY IN THE ELDERLY

1. Diabetic hyperosmolar nonketotic coma
2. Stroke
3. Polymyalgia rheumatica and giant cell arteritis
4. Metabolic bone disease
5. Degenerative joint disease
6. Hip fracture
7. Dementia syndrome
8. Falls
9. Paget's disease
10. Gammopathies
11. Chronic lymphatic leukemia
12. Tuberculosis
13. Herpes zoster
14. Basal cell carcinoma
15. Parkinsonism
16. Angioimmunoblastic lymphadenopathy with dysproteinemia
17. Normal pressure hydrocephalus
18. Pressure sores
19. Accidental hypothermia
20. Urinary incontinence
21. Arteriosclerotic heart disease and its complications
22. Amyloidosis
23. Solid tumor, especially prostate, colon, breast, and lung
24. Carpal tunnel syndrome
25. Hearing and vision impairment
26. Colonic angiodysplasia
27. Autoimmune disease

Table 2
NON-SPECIFIC OR ALTERED PRESENTATION OF DISEASE IN OLD AGE

1. Refusal to eat or drink
2. Falling
3. New incontinence
4. Dizziness
5. Acute confusion
6. New onset or abrupt worsening of dementia
7. Weight loss
8. Failure to thrive

The appearance of any of these findings in an elderly person heralds the onset or worsening of disease and should never be attributed to old age alone. In addition to altered disease presentation and altered clinical course, unpredicted responses and reaction to treatment as well as unexpected outcomes, including recovery, characterize disease in elderly persons. Certain disorders are particularly likely to be obscured in the elderly (Table 3) and should be considered in perplexing clinical situations.

Table 3
DISORDERS LIKELY TO PRESENT NON-SPECIFICALLY IN OLD AGE

1. Depression
2. Drug intoxication
3. Myxedema
4. Alcoholism
5. Myocardial infarction
6. Pulmonary embolism
7. Pneumonia
8. Cancer
9. Surgical abdomen
10. Thyrotoxicosis, masked or apathetic

The underlying cause for these altered characteristics of common diseases in old age has not been definitely identified, but certain observations are relevant. The interaction of disease with the biobehavioral alterations produced by normal aging is one factor exerting powerful influence upon the appearance of disease in elderly persons. Additionally, aging appears to reduce physiologic reserve asymmetrically, making certain organ systems and tissues most vulnerable to the altered homeostasis produced by disease, regardless of the locus of the disorder. Thus, the phenomenon of "weak-link" systems emerges, and locomotion, cognition and continence frequently are disrupted in old persons with new or exacerbated disease occurring in any organ system.

3. Multiple Health Problems

Another characteristic of illness in old age, important in planning geriatric health care and predisposing elderly individuals to functional decline based on late detection of potentially treatable disease, is the common occurrence of illness-clustering in aged patients. Usually called multiple pathology, the existence of several concurrent diseases in an old person who either is not obviously ill or is under treatment for a different problem has a profound negative influence on health and functional independence in old age. A random sample of community-dwelling subjects over 65 years of age found nearly 3.5 important disabilities per person (Williamson, 1964). An earlier study of elderly patients being admitted to hospitals documented six pathological conditions per person (Wilson, et al., 1962). A recent American clinical experience tabulated common problems often coexisting in elderly individuals (Besdine, 1980); these were congestive heart failure, depression, dementia, chronic renal failure, angina pectoris, osteoarthritis/osteoporosis, gait disorders, urinary incontinence, constipation, arterial and venous insufficiency in the legs, diabetes mellitus, chronic pain, sleep disturbance, multiple drug regimens, and anemia.

The number of pathologic conditions in an individual is strongly related to age, often rising to more than a dozen in the very old. If the entire spectrum of multiple pathologic conditions is not identified and carefully considered, virtually any diagnostic or therapeutic initiative is as likely to produce harm as benefit. In the absence of obvious flare-up of one problem, major danger still exists for the patient with multiple pathologies. Korenchevsky (1961) first pointed out the destructive, insidious virulence of unattended multiple pathologies in the uncomplaining elderly patient. Undetected, untreated diseases create ricochetting stress in several organ systems or tissues, producing deterioration of a previously diseased but compensated physiologic function. As each overburdened organ fails, there is created "what rapidly becomes an irreversible concatenation of deteriorations, passing multiple points of no return, leading to infirmity, dependence, and, if uninterrupted, death" (Besdine, 1980, p. 138).

Multiple pathologic conditions thus exert detrimental influence on elderly individuals in at least two important ways. In the first instance, the diagnostic evaluation or treatment of one identified illness interacts adversely with one or several undiagnosed conditions, producing iatrogenic harm. For example, an old man with ankle edema and pulmonary congestion of mild heart failure is given a potent diuretic which rapidly clears a liter of excess fluid from his circulation and improves the identified problem of heart failure. The rippling secondary effects are not beneficial. The abrupt diuresis overwhelms the emptying capacity of his bladder, previously compromised by prostatic enlargement and produces acute urinary retention. The secondary kidney damage and pain of retention produces acute confusion, worsened by early memory loss of Alzheimer's disease. The diuretic raises already high but previously asymptomatic levels of blood sugar and uric acid due to undiagnosed diabetes and gout, respectively. Each of these now becomes symptomatic with impaired consciousness and dehydration of hyperosmolar diabetes, and the exquisitely painful foot of gout.

Another adverse impact of undiagnosed disease interaction can be summarized as disease-disease relationships. An example is the old woman with unreported urinary tract infection producing frequent urgent urination which exceeds the mobility limit of her degenerative osteoarthritis and makes her incontinent. Uncorrected poor vision and urine on the floor cause a fall with fracture of her osteoporotic hip, and secondary decompensation of heart failure. The retrospective identification of previously unidentified disorders that have led to fixed functional losses in a once independent elder is a truly depressing but improvable aspect of geriatric medical care.

4. Chronic Nature of Disease

An additional characteristic of disease in old age is the high prevalence of chronic conditions. The National Center for Health Statistics has recently defined chronic disease as any condition lasting more than three months (NCHS, 1981). Among the population aged 65 years and older, 80% have at least one such chronic disease (Kovar, 1977), and it is estimated that a large number also experience multiple chronic conditions (Besdine, 1982). While some elderly advance to old age with chronic illnesses that were acquired during their earlier years, for many, chronic disease is first experienced in late life, and reacts with the many age-related changes which result in accelerated loss of organ reserve.

Given the lack of population-based epidemiologic studies, it is difficult to estimate the true prevalence of chronic disease among the aged (Evans, 1983). However, mortality statistics do provide information on the link between chronic disease and eventual mortality. Chronic disease accounts for most deaths over age 65 (Siegel,

8

1980). Diseases of the heart account for 44% of all deaths at these ages, and diseases of the heart, malignant neoplasms, and cerebrovascular diseases account for nearly 80% of the leading causes of death among the aged (Table 4).

Table 4
DEATH RATES FOR THE 10 LEADING CAUSES OF DEATH
FOR AGES 65 AND OVER, BY AGE: 1976

Cause of death by rank	65 years and over	65 to 74 years	75 to 84 years	85 years and over
	(Deaths per 100,000)			
All causes	5,428.9	3,127.6	7,331.6	15,486.9
1. Diseases of the heart	2,393.5	1,286.9	3,263.7	7,384.3
2. Malignant neoplasms	979.0	786.3	1,248.6	1,441.5
3. Cerebrovascular diseases	694.6	280.1	1,014.0	2,586.8
4. Influenza and pneumonia	211.1	70.1	289.3	959.2
5. Arteriosclerosis	122.2	25.8	152.5	714.3
6. Diabetes mellitus	108.1	70.0	155.8	219.2
7. Accidents	104.5	62.2	134.5	306.7
Motor vehicle	25.2	21.7	32.3	26.0
All other	79.3	40.4	102.2	280.7
8. Bronchitis, emphysema and asthma	76.8	60.7	101.4	108.5
9. Cirrhosis of the liver	36.5	42.6	29.3	18.0
10. Nephritis and nephrosis	25.0	15.2	34.1	64.6
All other causes	677.5	427.8	908.6	1,683.8

Source: National Center for Health Statistics (U.S. Public Health Service), "Advance Report--Final Mortality Statistics, 1976," Monthly Vital Statistics Report, Vol. 26., No. 12, supplement (2), March 1978; and unpublished data provided by the National Center for Health Statistics.

9

Chronic disease is further responsible for more than 80% of all causes of total disability (Upton, 1977). Disability implies the decreased ability to meet one's own needs, including the functions allowing mobility, cognition, eating, toileting, dressing, hygiene, shopping, cooking, or managing money. Overall, approximately 2.8 million community-dwelling elders have some degree of activity limitation caused by chronic conditions (NCHS, 1983). As is clear from Table 5, the need for the help of another person in basic physical or home management activities increases sharply with age, from roughly 1 in 10 in the 64 to 74 year old category to 4 in 10 among the over 85 age group (NCHS, 1983). The numbers of adults who are generally bed-bound because of chronic conditions also increase dramatically with age (Table 5). Chronic illness, and the substantial burden of functional impairment it brings, exaggerates the multiple losses experienced in other aspects of the elder's life, such as in social or work roles. The presence of chronic conditions and disability thus directly threatens quality of life and independence of the elder person.

Table 5
RATE PER 1,000 ADULTS WHO NEED ASSISTANCE,
BY TYPE OF NEED AND AGE: UNITED STATES, 1979

Type of need	65–74 years	75–84 years	85 years and over
Needs help in 1 or more basic physical activities	52.6	114.0	348.4
Needs help in 1 or more home management activities	57.3	141.8	399.0
Usually stays in bed	11.3	25.6	51.2

Source: NCHS, 1983

The implications of the prevalence of chronic disease among the aged are two-fold. First, it is currently estimated that over 80% of all health care resources in the United States are devoted to chronic diseases (Cluff, 1981). As the population continues to age, chronic disease will become more prevalent and disability a more common occurrence. The management of chronic diseases poses

10

challenges for health care providers. Success requires a sensitive and accurate ability to assess functional status initially and over time. Moreover, health care providers working with the chronically ill elderly must shift their traditional treatment emphasis from cure to efforts aimed at managing the existing condition, improving function, postponing further deterioration and disability, and preventing secondary complications.

B. Illness Behavior and the Social-Psychological Perspective

As suggested in this chapter, research has shown that illness behavior is affected not only by purely physiological disease processes, but also by social-psychological processes. Early research in this area showed that individuals from different ethnic groups vary in their perception of pain, exhibiting very different tolerance thresholds (Zola, 1963). Since these early studies, a number of other factors have been found to be important influences on individual health behaviors, such as the perceived seriousness of symptoms, the extent of disruption of normal activities, the need to deny illness, the availability of alternative explanations and the accessibility of treatment (Mechanic, 1978). It is our hypothesis that the process of aging interacts with many of these social characteristics to influence illness behavior and help seeking.

1. Self-Evaluation of Health

The process by which older people evaluate their health illustrates the importance of the social-psychological dimension to health and illness behavior. While the evaluation of health is significantly related to objective health conditions, individuals are also strongly influenced by social context, or the norms of the reference group of which they consider themselves a part (Neugarten, et al., 1968). For instance, an older person living in the community, whose reference group consists of relatively healthy elders, would evaluate more severely the same conditions that an institutionalized elder would consider less serious. It seems that as people age, their health expectations diminish, regardless of objective health status. This was substantiated in findings by Ferraro (1980) in which 75 year olds reported more physical conditions and disability than the 65-74 year olds, but tended to be more positive in their self-ratings of health.

11

Positive self-evaluation of health may not only lead to the denial of real underlying pathology, it may also lead to a tendency to minimize the seriousness of an illness which is perceived. Old people may attempt to normalize symptoms, by providing explanations for their symptoms which make them more readily acceptable (Clausen and Yarrow, 1955). Someone experiencing a new episode of incontinence may explain away the symptoms as insignificant, "everyone sometimes has trouble getting to a toilet." A spouse may attempt to normalize her husband's erratic behavior in efforts to cope with the onset of his deteriorating mental condition.

When normalization fails to provide an adequate defense, individuals may attempt to make the symptom seem less severe by finding some other reason for its existence, thus recognizing the symptoms but attenuating their seriousness. A person might find a rationale for an episode of incontinence, and place blame on the fact that he has had too much to drink, or a spouse may effectively attenuate the gravity of her husband's erratic behavior if it is confined to their home and not displayed in public places.

In addition to comparing themselves with their age peers, the aged are also greatly influenced in their self-evaluation by their health care providers. Past experiences with the health care system can exert their influence on the elder's evaluation of health. Providers often minimize the seriousness of legitimate complaints elders voice. This process can have devastating consequences, since elders may fail to consult providers on subsequent serious occasions. Although the social processes surrounding the self-evaluation of health have not yet been completely clarified, they nevertheless have important implications for the provision of health care services to the aged. If individuals expect diminished functioning in old age, they may incorrectly minimize the seriousness of their symptoms, and also delay or not seek care for conditions which objectively require treatment. Thus, inappropriate self-evaluation of health can lead to unnecessary morbidity and functional decline.

2. Symptom Reporting

Another critical social process involved in illness behavior relates to the elderly's reporting of physical and psychological symptoms to their health care provid-

12

ers. Research conducted in Scotland as far back as the 1950s found that while older people perceived physical disability, pain, and discomfort quite adequately, they often chose to conceal and not report their symptoms (Williamson, 1964; Anderson, 1966). An iceberg of concealed disease was discovered among Scottish elderly enrolled in the British National Health Service, which appeared to have the necessary features to provide adequate service to the elderly: doctors responsible for each older person's outpatient care, free care, and numerous, accessible doctors' offices. Yet startling numbers of problems hitherto unknown to and untreated by the patient's responsible physician were discovered. Nor were the problems esoteric, requiring sophisticated diagnostic methodology. Frequently encountered disorders included congestive heart failure, correctable hearing and vision deficits, tuberculosis, urinary dysfunction, anemia, chronic bronchitis, claudication, cancers, nutritional deficiencies, uncontrolled diabetes, foot disease hampering mobility, dental disease impeding nutrition, dementia, and depression.

These results from Scotland have been confirmed in more recent studies conducted in the United States. Shanas (1962) found that although the majority of those surveyed had had a health complaint during the month prior to their interview, only a small percentage had either seen or talked to a physician. Brody and Kleban (1981) discovered that over half of both physical and psychological symptoms experienced were not reported to anyone. Other research has found that the elderly fail to adequately report symptoms and conditions because they are lacking in knowledge or are simply misinformed about health and health care (Litman, 1971).

Research evidence suggests that there is a differential in the reporting of certain kinds of symptoms. For example, among the elderly, the embarrassment that accompanies problems with sexual functioning might prevent an old person from reporting these symptoms; while younger people might be more willing to discuss sexual matters. Similarly, the elderly might be more uncomfortable with the reporting of psychological symptoms, like being depressed, sad or anxious. The reporting of these problems is strongly influenced by attitudes held toward mental illness and treatment. The current cohort of elders tends to regard mental illness as a stigma to be avoided and

13

thus may not report symptoms of a psychological nature which might be indicative of mental illness (Cohen, 1976).

The most common explanation offered for symptom tolerance and nonreporting among the aged is the pervasive belief that old age is inextricably associated with illness, functional decline, and feeling sick. Thus, a similar social-psychological process influences the reporting of symptoms as influences the evaluation of health. Old and young, lay and professional, men and women, all believe that to be old is to be ill. Obviously this "ageist" view of health and disease guarantees that older individuals, even when afflicted with the same symptoms that impel the middle-aged sick into the mainstream of the health care system, will not seek care, will suffer in silence the progression of many diseases, and endure the functional losses engendered by untreated illness. That old age in the absence of disease is a time of good health and persisting function has been documented by numerous studies of normal aging (Finch and Hayflick, 1977), but while our society labors in ignorance of gerontologic information, elders will continue expecting decline and dysfunction. A useful geriatric maxim is that sick old people are sick because they are sick, not because they are old. Although decline in numerous physiologic functions characterizes normal human aging, these declines are gradual, and their functional impact is ameliorated by the decades over which they occur and by the remaining, if diminishing, reserve capacities of the individual. Thus, major functional decline, especially if abrupt in an individual already old, is usually attributable to disease, not age.

A second explanation for old people not reporting illness is that a high prevalence of depression, coupled with the many losses common in late life, interferes with the desire to regain vigor. A third block to reporting illness is found to be intellectual loss. Though never normal, the increasing prevalence of cognitive loss with age is doubly dangerous in the detection of disease. Cognitively impaired individuals have a diminished ability to complain and are also evaluated less enthusiastically for associated medical disease or even reversible disease producing the intellectual loss itself (National Institute on Aging Task Force, 1980). A fourth explanation for symptom concealment by elderly patients is fear that something may be found which generates diagnostic or therapeutic interventions that in themselves might produce functional loss and jeopardize independent living. Finally, today's octo-

14

genarians, having grown up when health care systems produced less salubrious interventions, may be reluctant to seek care even in the present.

The abundant documentation that disease is not being reported by the elderly appears to contradict a clinical rule of thumb that identifies hypochondriasis as common among aged patients. Many clinicians caring for elderly patients cite an individual or two who tries their patience and goodwill with endless complaints rooted in trivial or nonexistent illness. Yet when studied, the hypochondriacal, doctor-shopping, old person appears to be one more unverifiable mythical figure in people's ideas about aging (Costa and McCrae, 1980). Not only is hypochondriasis less common among older people, but when elders do complain, important disease is found underlying their complaints substantially more often than in younger, non-hypochondriacal individuals (Stenback, et al., 1978).

II. Overview of Illness Behavior and Help Seeking Model

The development of a new model for the study of the elderly's illness and help seeking behaviors was considered necessary to bridge some of the gaps in our existing understanding of illness behavior. The model proposed hypothesizes that an individual passes through the following sequence of steps upon the onset of a condition: symptom experience, symptom appraisal, decision to seek care, medical care contact, reporting of symptoms, and patient assessment of the medical visit (Figure 1). The framework suggests that individual variations at each step of the model are explained by different combinations of psychosocial and biomedical factors. The major emphasis in this framework is on how aging interacts with these factors at each step of the model. This model is based, in large part, on the decision making models of Suchman (1965) and Safer, et al. (1979), the psychosocial model of Mechanic (1978), and the geriatric medicine perspective of Besdine (1982).

Condition and Symptom Experience

According to this framework, the help seeking process is set in motion with the onset of a physical and/or psychological condition. Individuals may or may not experience symptoms of an underlying condition. The aged often experience non-specific symptoms for diseases which would present with specific symptoms in the general popu-

15

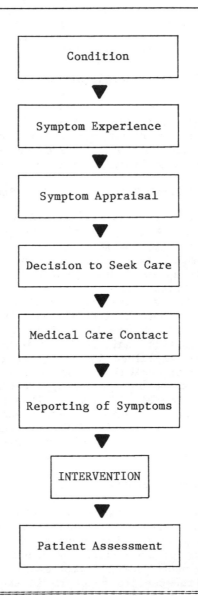

Figure 1
FRAMEWORK FOR ANALYZING ILLNESS BEHAVIOR
AND HELP SEEKING AMONG THE AGED

Condition

Symptom Experience

Symptom Appraisal

Decision to Seek Care

Medical Care Contact

Reporting of Symptoms

INTERVENTION

Patient Assessment

lation. Conditions which present non-specifically in old age as discussed earlier include depression, myocardial infarction, drug intoxication, and pneumonia. The aged also experience delayed presentation of symptoms for many conditions. Breast cancer provides an example of a condition whose "silent interval" between the onset of the disease and the presentation of symptoms is much longer in the aged woman than in her younger counterpart. Another class of diseases are those usually encountered only among the aged. Many of these diseases such as accidental hypothermia and dementia syndrome also present with non-specific symptoms of the underlying disorder.

Symptom Appraisal

In the second step of the model, symptom appraisal, individuals evaluate illness based on the physical experience of their symptoms as well as on a psychosocial dimension. This step further includes a cognitive dimension in which individuals interpret their symptoms placing them in a cause-effect context (Janis and Rodin, 1980). Individual elders can either correctly attribute a symptom to an underlying disease, incorrectly attribute a symptom to normal processes of aging instead of to pathology, or incorrectly attribute a symptom to the wrong disease or disorder.

Biomedical factors, such as the coexistence of multiple pathologies and the extended period of onset of many chronic diseases of old age, make it difficult for the patient and physician to isolate and interpret symptoms. Psychosocial processes, namely the ageism of the elderly themselves, social comparison processes, and the need to deny the stigma of illness often predispose the aged to inaccurate evaluations of their health.

Decision to Seek Care

The next step in the model is the actual decision to seek or not seek help from a formal care provider. Again, biomedical and psychosocial factors help explain variation in the way individuals decide to seek help. Typically, a cue to action is required to trigger the decision to seek care. At times the cue is a biological factor, such as increased pain or functional decline. Individuals actively monitor their symptoms, and often decide to seek care only after experiencing increased pain and discomfort associated with the progression of the underlying condition

17

(Shanas, 1962). At other times, the cue to action is of a psychosocial nature, such as when individuals seek advice and information from a close friend or relative (Brody and Kleban, 1981).

Medical Care Contact

Once the decision to seek care has been made, and the appropriate source of care decided upon, the elder must still decide whether the care is worth the costs (Safer, et al., 1979). Situational barriers may exist which prevent the elder from actually receiving needed health care. The out-of-pocket costs may be too high for elders on fixed incomes. Even when cost is not a problem, physical access to care may present a constraint for the older, less mobile person. The inconvenience in getting to a provider and the difficulty getting an appointment all potentially delay utilization. Having a regular source of care, particularly having a personal physician rather than being a clinic user, has been found to facilitate the elderly's contact with the medical care system (Wan, 1974).

Reporting Symptoms

Even after the elder has successfully negotiated the barriers and made contact with a health care provider, it is still not certain that appropriate care will be received. During the medical care visit, individuals can choose to report or not to report certain symptoms. As suggested earlier, studies have found that the aged under-report symptoms (Brody and Kleban, 1981; Williamson, 1964). Reasons hypothesized for the underreporting include biomedical factors, such as the coexistence of depression and intellectual impairment which may interfere with the ability to recognize and interpret symptoms, and psychosocial factors, such as the presumed unsuitability of medical treatments and fear of pain associated with treatment. Anticipation of functional decline, loss of independence and institutionalization have been found to be especially salient to the elderly's underreporting of symptoms.

Patient Assessment

The last step in this framework is the individual's assessment of the medical visit. Patient experience with a medical care provider and the general health care system influences subsequent evaluation and reporting of symptoms

as well as decisions to seek care. During each medical
encounter, a patient processes new information which is
called upon when the help seeking process is again initiated. Patient assessment of the medical visit is influenced not only by the personal attributes of the patient
but also by characteristics of the provider. The patient
may feel that their reported symptoms were ignored, minimized or not taken seriously, making them less likely to
report similar symptoms at a later time. The intervention
chosen might be interpreted by the elder as inappropriate,
intrusive, painful or frightening, also influencing the
likelihood of seeking care at some other time.

III. Policy Implications

Past research and clinical practice in geriatric medicine suggest that there are many unique characteristics of
disease in old age, as emphasized in this chapter. We
have further demonstrated the influence of various social-
psychological factors on the aged's perception and evaluation of symptoms, and on their help seeking behaviors.
Given the challenge faced by the VA's health care system
to provide comprehensive services to an increasingly aging
population, the current health care system should take into account and respond to the special characteristics,
diseases and illness behaviors of the elderly.

An important feature of the current health care system, both within and outside the VA, is its reactive nature. Our health care system is passive, especially for
elderly people, and lacks prevention-oriented or early
detection efforts. American medical care of the critically ill, elderly hospitalized patient is the best in the
world. Science and technology are most expertly blended
to help the sick. But American hospital beds, health
maintenance organizations (HMOs), physicians' offices,
emergency rooms, and neighborhood health centers all wait
passively for the symptomatic patient to activate the system. For the most part, this passive system of health
care provision is adequate for children, who have parental
advocates, and for young and middle-aged adults who have
the need to work impelling them to seek medical relief of
function-impairing symptoms. But aged persons, without
advocates and usually without jobs, burdened by society's
and their own ageist views of functional loss in the elderly, cannot be relied upon to initiate appropriate
health care for themselves, especially early in the course
of an illness when intervention is most likely to have a

19

favorable outcome. Our health care system relies on the patient to enter the system and initiate care, and that is precisely the one illness behavior most often missing in aged individuals.

Inadequate reporting of illness by the elderly coupled with the passivity of our medical apparatus make it highly probable that disease will be far advanced before the aged patient enters the health care system. During the delay between onset and detection, it is possible for multiple pathologies to interact, harming the patient and producing irrevocable disability in spite of eventual excellent care. For some elderly patients, delay is lengthened because of neglect of a number of nonspecific but serious problems, including immobility, incontinence, and cognitive loss, any or all of which may herald major functional decline.

A second aspect of the current health care system is its very fragmented nature. Particularly in the VA, the fragmentation of service imposed by complex eligibility requirements may impose insurmountable hardships on the provision of long term care. Further, lack of coordination exists between VA and non-VA services. Undoubtedly the lack of coordination both within the VA and between the VA and other health care providers influences the quality of care and resultant health status of older veterans.

A third component of the health care system relates to the health care providers working in the system. Few health care providers have received any formal training in geriatric medicine or public health. Providers bring their own ageist stereotypes to clinical practice in both the VA setting and outside the VA. The stereotypic attitudes of health care providers, when combined with the elderly's own ageist assumptions about disease in old age, may lead to delay in diagnosis and treatment, prolonged disability, long and expensive therapeutic interventions and permanent functional losses. The unique characteristics of illness and disease in the aged require that providers receive specialized training in geriatric medicine and in the psychosocial dimensions of illness behavior.

IV. Policy Options

The preceding discussion has suggested the areas of potential change for care of elder veterans. Five cate-

20

gories of options are presented in this section. They are: A) Education and Training for VA Care Providers, B) Health Promotion/Health Education for Aging Veterans, C) Comprehensive Functional Assessment, D) Surveillance Program for High Risk Elderly Veterans, and E) Research on Disease and Illness Behaviors of Aging Veterans.

A. Education and Training for VA Care Providers

The demographic imperative, both within and outside the VA, argues strongly for more appropriate health professional education regarding care of the elderly. The existence of a body of knowledge specifically relevant to care of the elderly patient has been carefully documented only recently and data documenting normal age-related changes and disease-specific information are accumulating. Dissemination of this geriatric data base to the health professions is critical to respond to the current deficiencies related to geriatric care.

The VA health care system provides a rich opportunity for training in geriatrics. Growing numbers of elder patients encourage VA medical centers (VAMCs) to improve the geriatric knowledge base of current and future care providers. Moreover, the VA system has substantial resources to apply to this effort. Two major categories of educational options can be identified: education of future care providers and in-service training for current providers of care.

1. Education of Future Care Providers

The VA is a major provider of education for health care personnel. VAMCs are clinical training sites for physicians, nurses, dentists, therapists of various types, psychologists, social workers and allied health professionals. Most medical schools have close affiliations with VAMCs, and a large proportion of medical students receive training in VA sites. Thus, the VA has a major opportunity to influence geriatric health care in several ways.

First, the VA can provide a model for comprehensive geriatric care-taking. Students passing through the system will observe, first hand, proper assessment, diagnosis and treatment of multiple problems, management of chronic disease and the development of service plans which are appropriate to the function and resources of the elder pa-

21

tient. Further, the student will have the opportunity to work in interdisciplinary teams, the foundation of good geriatric care. True interdisciplinary care, in which the requisite team members know and respect each other's capabilities and functions, is not currently taught to physicians and therefore denied most patients.

The VA can also become a leader in developing and disseminating the discipline-specific information which relates to geriatric care. Geriatric initiatives such as the Geriatric Research, Education and Clinical Center (GRECC) program provide centers of excellence for such information. VAMCs should work closely with their affiliated medical and other health professions' schools to develop the content of the discipline-specific information.

2. In-Service Training

An equally important aspect of geriatric education is in-service training. Because much of the geriatric data base is new and because relevant geriatric content has not been a major part of medical education, upgrading and updating the information and skills of current providers of care to the elder veteran is imperative. One approach to this effort is through in-service training. The format of such training may vary widely and may include written materials mailed to staff, short presentations on selected topics, or multi-day workshops and learning experiences. The content may range from discipline-specific, disease-specific focused presentations, through experience with interdisciplinary team function.

The VA should expand its current in-service training by developing a package of curricula and materials. One option would be for the VA to work with existing educational and policy centers. One such group of centers, the Geriatric Education Centers recently funded by the Health Resources and Services Administration (DHHS), is intended to improve the content of geriatric education in medical schools, nursing schools and allied health professional schools across the country. Long Term Care Gerontology Centers, supported by the Administration on Aging, also offer resources in certain aspects of geriatric education.

B. Health Promotion/Health Education for Aging Veterans

A major theme throughout this chapter has been the serious consequences of illness behaviors common among the aged. The underreporting of symptoms and conditions, the overly positive evaluation of health, and the tendency to minimize the seriousness of symptoms all combine to produce late detection and at times, irreversible decline. Two approaches may be taken to remedy these problems: one is to change the health care system to better address these behaviors, and the other is to change the behaviors of elders. Health promotion/education efforts directed at elders are one method of changing those health and illness behaviors of elders which are likely to lead to negative consequences.

The VA could offer several health promotion/education experiences to elder veterans, each targeted to specific categories of health and illness behaviors. First, health education efforts could be directed at changing the elder veteran's knowledge, beliefs, and attitudes about disease in old age, with a special focus on early detection of disease. Information on both the symptoms of diseases more common to the aged and on those non-specific symptoms which present differently in older people would be provided. Through a better understanding of the importance of various symptoms, elders would be taught when it is appropriate to seek medical advice. Such activities would be complemented by efforts to debunk the potentially destructive ageist beliefs of elders concerning disease in old age.

A second type of health education/promotion could be directed at providing elder veterans with the knowledge and resources to be actively involved in their own health care. A large proportion of elder veterans have at least one chronic condition which necessitates long term monitoring and care. Thus, many aged face a lifestyle which demands certain adaptations to chronicity and which necessitates active long-term cooperation with health care professionals in a health care plan. Health education/promotion for the chronically impaired can emphasize the stabilization of current levels of health and functioning or the retarding of further decline influencing the elder's ability to maintain functional independence. Specific health education/promotion efforts could be directed, for example, to assist the elderly diabetic to develop the appropriate self-care skills needed for the long term management of his condition.

Health education/promotion activities should include the elder veteran's family whenever possible. Research

23

has shown that simply providing individuals with the knowledge and self-management skills critical for positive health behaviors is often inadequate (Levkoff and Wetle, 1983-84). Individuals must be reinforced in their newly developed positive health activities for these behaviors to persist over time, especially for those with chronic diseases, which often demand long-term involvement with little visible improvement. Health education efforts may use a variety of formats.

One-on-One Education. The most direct form of patient education is explanation to the patient by the primary care provider. It is often the case that physicians, because of conflicting demands, do not take the time necessary to carefully inform patients about their chronic illnesses. Patients are many times confused about the cause of their diseases, the meaning of their many symptoms, the purpose of each medication and the interaction between their own behaviors and their diseases. What may seem obvious to the well trained, experienced formal care provider is likely to be confusing and a mystery to the patient and his family. Compliance with treatment regimens is directly related to understanding the purpose and likely outcome of treatment. Therefore, the better the patient's understanding, the more likely a positive outcome for all involved.

The most obvious approach is for the physician to explain and discuss etiology, prognosis, symptoms and treatment. Unfortunately, the current organization of care and multiple demands on physicians make it difficult for them to take the time to do this. In many cases, nurses, physician's assistants and other health care professionals are the most appropriate personnel to engage in this on-going task. Another format is the use of volunteers. A number of successful projects use volunteers who themselves have experienced the illness or surgery. Examples include the "Reach for Recovery" program for mastectomy patients, as well as colostomy programs and chronic obstructive pulmonary disease programs. The acceptance of this kind of help is high and the programs are effective.

Group Projects. Group formats for health promotion efforts also take a variety of forms. Providers in acute care settings may form groups of inpatients with similar problems to teach about the disease and to answer questions and share information. These groups may have a classroom style, "teacher-students" organization or may be

24

more involved in group process with members of the group teaching and sharing concerns with one another. Similar groups can be organized on an outpatient basis using health care providers in leadership roles.

Just as "peer" counseling has been effective on a one-to-one basis, it has also been used effectively in group settings. Groups of patients and/or their families gather together to share information and provide mutual support. Research evaluating such groups for chronic pulmonary disease demonstrated that patients view these groups as better sources of information for disease management than either their primary care physician or formal educational associations (Jennings, 1980). Professional "back-up" for such groups is important and offers continuing contact with formal care providers.

C. Comprehensive Functional Assessment

There is a substantial burden of functional impairment in the elderly. Diseases producing impaired function are often treatable and curable, but detection is essential. Reliable assessment of functional loss is thus crucial to permit early intervention during active disease. Assessment of functional impairment is also critical for the design, development and allocation of remedial and restorative services for those impaired elderly with progressive chronic disease. Periodic formal assessment is required for rapid response to declines in an elder's independence. Accurate functional assessment and the accompanying provision of compensatory services can serve to decrease further functional impairment and general decline.

To pursue this option, health care providers from a variety of different disciplines must learn comprehensive functional assessment (CFA) in parallel with classic disease-oriented evaluation techniques (Moore, 1978). The value of this CFA is especially relevant in the interdisciplinary setting of geriatric health care. By using functional data each discipline can observe and discuss problems of the old person as they affect life and independence. Use of a common language of functional assessment facilitates true interdisciplinary evaluation and management of elder patients, and avoids discipline-specific jargon which only interferes with communication and coordination of care. An assessment and surveillance instrument would list all functional impairments, assembled side by side with the problem list, which would facilitate

25

careful comparison of diagnosis with lost function. Using the list of functional losses and their severity, items on the problem list could be identified as most likely etiologic of the most troublesome functional impairments for the elderly individual. By addressing problems using this functionally-oriented priority system, the health provider is likely to satisfy the patient/client and, by seeing important gains in independence measured by continuing CFA, reap personal satisfaction as well. Additionally, if interventions produce no benefit, they can be confidently abandoned and new priorities addressed.

To implement CFA the VA should review available assessment instruments to determine those most appropriate for the VA health care system. Once agreement is reached, the assessment instrument chosen should be widely disseminated with instruction as to its appropriate use and applications. Information gathered in these assessments should become a part of the patient's permanent medical record to allow for determination of change over time and to provide documentation of baseline function. Regular up-dating of the assessment information will provide the surveillance function described in Option D.

CFA provides an array of important information which is useful in individual patient care and disease management. It allows for better decision making regarding the appropriateness and effectiveness of treatment. Further, it enhances discharge planning and long term patient care by improving patient placement and planning for home services. Information collected through CFA is also useful for systems planning, by providing objective data regarding function and needed services for populations of elder veterans.

D. Surveillance Program for High Risk Elderly Veterans

This chapter has discussed the risks generated by the passive nature of the current health care system. An active case-finding program which would detect and measure functional impairment could provide better management of current illness and prevent future illness. Decline in function is often the first indicator of new onset or worsening of disease. The purpose of a surveillance program is early detection of such changes in order to diagnose and treat the underlying problems. It is hoped that such early interventions would require less intrusive methods and result in more satisfactory outcomes, such as the avoidance of acute hospitalization or institutionalization. It is necessary to identify those high-risk elders who would most benefit from surveillance. The community-dwelling, high-risk elderly are identifiable by several markers (Palmore, 1976). Those over 75 years of age are three to five times more likely to require assistance due to health impairment compared with 65 to 74 year olds, making advanced age a first reasonable marker. Elderly persons living alone are at greater risk, if only because decline is less likely to be noticed. Persons recently bereaved are at greatly increased risk to become ill and even die in the grieving period and post-bereavement year. Elderly individuals recently discharged from hospitals have a one in four chance of rehospitalization in the following year, marking increased risk. Others who would appear to have increased risk but for whom the risk has not been documented include aged persons with cognitive loss, mobility problems, or incontinence.

Once identified, at-risk elderly would receive a comprehensive assessment and be reassessed periodically, and any decline in function would automatically provoke more formal comprehensive medical assessment by the appropriate facet of the health care system. A surveillance program should involve the older person, close family members, and a specially trained surveillance technician who would be responsible for monitoring the physical, social, and psychological functioning of the at-risk elder. A variety of informal helpers and formal care providers could also be involved in these surveillance activities.

The VA should begin with a demonstration project designed to evaluate the costs and effectiveness of a surveillance program. The demonstration project would refine existing assessment tools to make them most appropriate for the VA health care system and the veterans it serves. Additionally, the VA could encourage physicians to include functional assessments in regular patient visits and to encourage informal care providers to take note of and report functional changes to care providers.

E. Research on Disease and Illness Behaviors of Aging Veterans

While an understanding of the disease processes and illness behaviors in old age has been developing, knowledge in many areas is still rudimentary. There is even less understanding of these processes among certain subgroups of the population, such as veterans. There are abundant opportunities for the VA to support relevant research on these topics. Three areas merit increased emphasis from the VA.

Research on the Underlying Processes of Disease in Old Age. This option begins with continuation and expansion of the current activities in the GRECCs. Increased emphasis could be placed on the management of multiple illnesses and chronic disease in elder patients. Health services research could investigate the management of patients receiving both VA and non-VA services in the community, as companion projects to options suggested in other chapters in this book.

Epidemiology Research on the Prevalence of Disease in the Elderly. Little reliable information exists on the prevalence and incidence of disease in elderly populations. Particularly lacking, are data on the prevalence of chronic disease and levels of functional impairment. Epidemiologic research of this type is particularly fitting for the VA. The availability of a managed system of care and the potential of collecting information on large numbers of elder veterans provides the opportunity for major contributions to the field. Certain specific conditions are particularly relevant for such research including urinary incontinence and dementing illnesses. The dearth of prevalence data on these conditions makes well planned studies of large groups of elders imperative. Data developed in such studies would prove invaluable for care planning and service coordination.

Health Services Research on the Illness and Help Seeking Behaviors of Older Veterans. Further understanding is needed of the psychosocial processes which influence the way individual elders perceive, evaluate and act on their symptoms. Knowledge of the determinants of evaluation of symptoms and underreporting of disease is a prerequisite for the design of intervention strategies to promote early detection and treatment. It is also important to understand the many factors which influence an individual's use of health services. Differences in the use of services for those with and without service-connected disabilities, and differences among those who use VA and non-VA services would be particularly useful for planners and policy makers.

28

REFERENCES

Anderson, R. and Newman, J.F. "Societal and Individual Determinants of Health Services Utilization in the United States." Milbank Memorial Fund Quarterly/ Health and Society, 51, pp. 95-124, 1973.

Anderson, W.F. "The Prevention of Illness in the Elderly: The Rutherglen Experiment in Medicine in Old Age." Proceedings of a conference held at the Royal College of Physicians in London. London: Pitman, 1966.

Becker, M.H. "Correlates of Individual Health-Related Behaviors." Medical Care, 15 (supplement), pp. 27-46, 1977.

Besdine, R.W. "Geriatric Medicine: An Overview." Annual Review of Gerontology and Geriatrics, 1, pp. 135-153, 1980.

Besdine, R.W. "The Data Base of Geriatric Medicine." In Health and Disease in Old Age, Rowe, J.W. and Besdine, R.W. (Eds.). Boston: Little Brown, 1982.

Branch, L., Jette, A., Evashwick, C., Polansky, M., Rowe, G. and Diehr, P. "Toward Understanding Elders' Health Service Utilization." Journal of Community Health, 7(2), pp. 80-92, Winter, 1981.

Brody, E.M. and Kleban, M.H. "Physical and Mental Health Symptoms of Older People: Who Do They Tell?" Journal of the American Geriatrics Society, 29, pp. 442-449, 1981.

Clausen, J. and Yarrow, M.R. (Eds.) "The Impact of Mental Illness on the Family." The Journal of Social Issues, 11 (4), 1955.

Cluff, L.F. "Chronic Disease, Function and Quality of Care." Journal of Chronic Disease, 34, pp. 299-304, 1981.

Cohen, G.D. "Mental Health Services and the Elderly: Needs and Options." American Journal of Psychiatry, 133, pp. 377-383, 1976.

Costa, P.T., Jr. and McCrae, R.R. "Somatic Complaints in Males as a Function of Age and Neuroticism: A Longitudinal Analysis." Journal of Behavioral Medicine, 3, pp. 245-257, 1980.

Coulton, E. and Frost, A.K. "Use of Social and Health Services by the Elderly." Journal of Health and Social Behavior, 23, 1982.

Evans, R. "Health Care Technology and the Inevitability of Resource Allocation and Rations Decisions." Journal of the American Medical Association, 249(15), pp. 2047-2053, 1983.

Ferraro, K. "Self-Ratings of Health among the Old and the Old-Old." Journal of Health and Social Behavior, 21, pp. 377-383, 1980.

Fillenbaum, G. "Social Context and Self-Assessments of Health among the Elderly." Journal of Health and Social Behavior, 20, pp. 45-51, 1979.

Finch, C.E. and Hayflick, L. Handbook of the Biology of Aging. New York: Van Nostrand Reinhold, 1977.

Givens, J.D. "Current Estimates from the Health Interview Survey United States, 1978." Vital and Health Statistics, Series 10, No. 130, Dept. of HEW (PHS) 80-1551. Hyattsville, Maryland: NCHS, 1979.

Health Care Financing Administration. Discussion Paper: Long-Term Care Background and Future Directions. U.S. Government Publication No. (HCFA) 81-20047, Baltimore, MD, 1981.

Janis, I.L. and Rodin, J. "Attribution, Control and Decision-Making: Social Psychology and Health Care." In Health Psychology, Stone, G. (Ed.), pp. 482-522. San Francisco: Jossey-Bass Publishers, 1980.

Jennings, S. "Continuing Care in Chronic Obstructive Pulmonary Disease," Unpublished Master's Thesis, Department of Epidemiology and Public Health, Yale University Medical School, 1980.

Kart, C. "Experiencing Symptoms: Attributions and Misattribution of Illness among the Aged." In Elderly Patients and Their Doctors, Haug, M.R. (Ed.), pp. 70-79. New York: Springer Publishing Company, 1981.

Korenchevsky V. Physiology and Pathological Aging. New York: Basel/Karger, 1961.

Kovar, M.G. "Health of the Elderly and Use of Health Services." Public Health Reports, 92, pp. 9-19, 1977.

Levkoff, S. and Wetle, T. "Adaptation to Transition in Late Adulthood: Implications for Health Education." International Quarterly of Community Health Education, 4(3), pp. 191-199, 1983-84.

Litman, T.J. "Health Care and the Family: A Three Generational Analysis." Medical Care, 9, p. 67, 1971.

Maddox, G.L. "Some Correlates of Differences in Self-Assessment of Health Status among the Elderly." Journal of Gerontology, 17, pp. 180-185, 1962.

Mechanic, D. Medical Sociology (2nd edition). New York: Free Press, 1970.

Mechanic, D. "The Experience and Expression of Distress: The Study of Illness Behavior and Medical Utilization." In Handbook of Health Care and the Health Professions, Mechanic, D. (Ed.), pp. 591-602. Newark: Free Press, 1983.

Mechanic, D., Cleary, P. and Greenley, J. "Distress Syndromes, Illness Behavior, Access to Care and Medical Utilization." Medical Care, 20, pp. 361-372, 1977.

Moore, J.T. "Functional Disability of Geriatric Patients in a Family Medicine Program." Journal of Family Practice, 7, pp. 1159-66, 1978.

National Center for Health Statistics. Jack, S. and Ries, P.: "Current Estimates from the National Health Interview Survey, United States, 1979." Vital and Health Statistics. Series 10-No. 136, DHHS Pub. No. (PHS) 81-1564. Public Health Service. Washington, D.C.: U.S. Government Printing Office. April, 1981.

NCHS Advanced Data. Feller, B.: "Americans Needing Help to Function at Home." No. 92, September 14, 1983.

NCHS Advance Report. "Final Mortality Statistics, 1976." Monthly Vital Statistics Report, Vol. 26, No. 12, Supplement (2) March, 1978.

National Institute on Aging Task Force. "Senility Reconsidered: Treatment Possibilities for Mental Impairment in the Elderly." Journal of the American Medical Association, 244, pp. 259–263, 1980.

Neugarten, G.L., Moore, I.W. and Lowe, J.C. "Age Norms, Age Constraints, and Adult Socialization." In Middle Age and Aging, Neugarten, B.L. (Ed.), pp. 22–28. Chicago: University of Chicago Press, 1968.

Palmore, E. "Total Chance of Institutionalization among the Aged." Gerontologist, 16, pp. 504–507, 1976.

Regier, D.A. and Goldberg, I.D. "The Defacto Mental Health Services System." Archives of General Psychiatry, 35, pp. 685–693, 1978.

Rosenstock, I.M. "The Health Belief Model and Prevention Health Behavior." Health Education Monographs, 2, pp. 354–386, 1974.

Safer, M.A., Tharps, Q.J., Jackson, T.C. and Leventhal, H. "Determinants of Three Stages of Delay in Seeking Care at a Medical Clinic." Medical Care, 17, pp. 11–29, 1979.

Shanas, E. The Health of Older People. Cambridge: Harvard University Press, 1962.

Siegel, J.S. "Recent and Demographic Trends for the Elderly Population and Some Implications for Health Care." In Second Conference of the Epidemiology of Aging, Haynes, S. and Feinleib, M. (Eds.). US Department of Health and Human Services, NIH Publication No. 80–969, pp. 289–314, Washington, D.C., July, 1980.

Special Medical Advisory Group, Task force on the VA Geriatric Plan. Caring for the Older Veteran. May 11, 1983.

Stenback A., Kumpulainen, M. and Vauhkonen, M.L. "Illness and Health Behavior in Septaugenarians." Gerontologist, 33, pp. 57–61, 1978.

Stoller, E.P. "Patterns of Physicians Utilization by the Elderly: A Multivariate Analysis." Medical Care XXII, 1982.

Suchman, E.A. "Stages of Illness and Medical Care." Journal of Health and Social Behavior, 6, pp. 114-128, 1965.

U.S. DHHS, Public Health Service. Health - United States, 1981. Washington, D.C.: U.S. Government Printing Office (PHS 82-1232), 1982.

Upton, A.C. "Pathology." In Handbook of the Biology of Aging, Finch, L.E. and Hayflick, L. (Eds.), pp. 159-186. New York: Van Nostrand Reinhold, 1977.

Wan, T. "Determinants of Physician Utilization: A Casual Analysis." Journal of Health and Social Behavior, 15, pp. 100-108, 1974.

Wan, T. and Odell, B.G. "Factors Affecting the Use of Social Services among the Elderly." Aging and Society, 1, p. 1, 1981.

Williamson, J. "Old People and Their Unreported Needs." The Lancet, 1, pp. 1117-1120, 1964.

Wilson, L.A., Lawson, I.R. and Brass, W. "Multiple Disorders in the Elderly." Lancet, ii, pp. 841-844, 1962.

Zola, I.K. "Problems of Communication, Diagnosis, and Patient Care: The Interplay of Patient, Physician, and Clinic Organization." Journal of Medical Education, 38, pp. 829-838, 1963.

2. An Overview of the Veterans Administration and its Services for Older Veterans

John H. Mather, M.D.

Introduction

Fifty years from now, one of five Americans will be 65 years old or older. The doubling of this portion of the population has been popularly labelled "the graying of America." An understanding of the impact of an aging population, and the basic changes in the social fabric which will result, is only now becoming widespread. For society at large, it is a problem of the future, and tends to be put off while the urgent problems of the present are solved. For one large group in the population, American veterans, the aging phenomenon and the changing needs which accompany it are not matters for future speculation.

Modern medical science has the knowledge and the skills to support older individuals' quality of life and independence beyond anything imagined even fifty years ago. This substantial advancement has not been achieved without cost. The higher prevalence of disease and disability, particularly among those over 75, already accounts for a significant portion of the health care resources expended in this country. The marked increase in use of health care services by older persons reflects both the greater occurrence of disease, particularly chronic disease, in this age group and the fact that such persons

35

often suffer from more than one condition, complicating their treatment and recovery.

The health care needs of an older population cannot be viewed apart from other needs. Declining incomes, marginal retirement benefits, unanticipated medical costs -- all operate to create financial problems for many older people. A commitment to quality of life in the later years -- a commitment the VA has for its eligible veterans -- requires attention to non-medical needs as well.

The Changing Veteran Population

The American population is growing older, but the veteran population is growing older even faster. Since the nation's call on its men and women is greatest in times of conflict, the veteran population tends to cluster in rather narrow age groups representing major conflicts. As one would expect, the largest groups in the current veteran population represent the World War II, Korean Conflict, and Vietnam eras. As these groups age, they accelerate the aging trend in the overall veteran population tremendously. This is predictable, but its predictability does not make it less striking, nor does it lessen its potential for increasing demand on the services the nation has made available to armed services' veterans (Figure 1).

Figure 1
Veteran Population by Period of Service
September 30, 1983

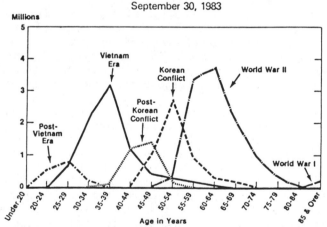

Source: Veterans Administration

36

Figure 2

Number of Veterans Age 65 and Over

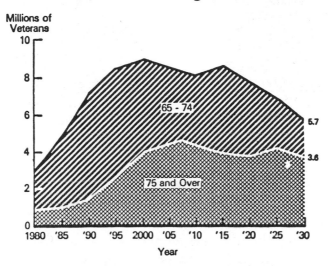

Source: Veterans Administration

The numbers are compelling (Figure 2). As World War
II veterans age, the current four million veterans over 65
years old will swell to seven million by the year 1990 and
triple before the end of the century. Veterans will oc-
cupy a major segment of the elderly male population. By
the year 2000, two out of every three males over the age
of 65 will be veterans (Figure 3). Of even greater
significance will be the numbers of the old-old; the
veterans over the age of 75.

The over 75 year old veteran is the fastest growing
age group in the veteran population. Male veterans 75
years and older are already 46% of the total male population of that age and by 2005 will be close to 70% of the
total. In addition, by the year 2000 there will be over
four million veterans over 75 years old, a number larger
than all veterans over 65 at present (Figure 5).

37

Figure 3
Percent of U.S. Males 65 and Over Who are Veterans

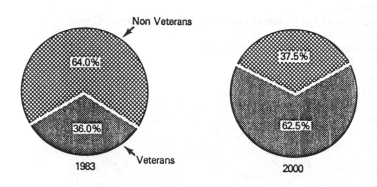

Source: Veterans Administration

Figure 4
Veterans Age 65 and Over
Middle of FY 1983 and Projected to 1990 and 2000

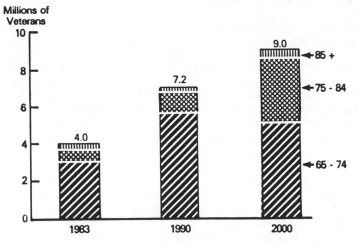

Source: Veterans Administration

Figure 5
COMPARISON OF VETERAN POPULATION BY AGE GROUPS 65-74 AND 75 AND OLDER, 1980-2010

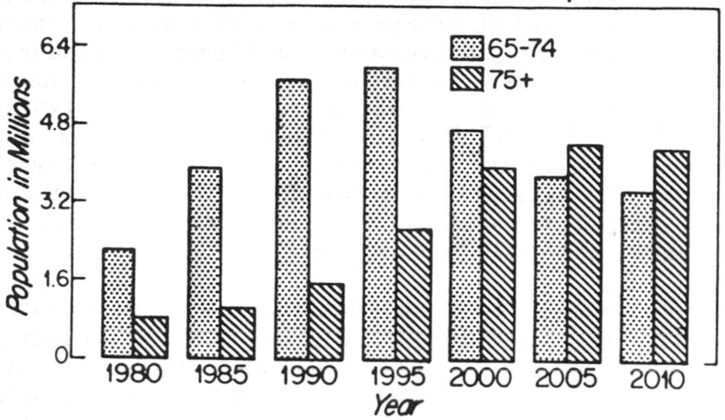

Source: Veterans Administration

Utilization and Eligibility

Our concern for veterans reaching 75 years old is not their numbers alone. Aging is characterized by an increasing risk of acute illness complicated by chronic limitations and socioeconomic problems. Looking just at bed utilization in the VA, this age group uses acute beds at a one and a half times greater rate than veterans 65-74. For nursing home beds, this rate increases to four times the utilization rate of the 65-74 year old group (Table 1). The various medical care programs have adjusted over the past several years to the shift in the age of the veteran population and its needs (Figure 6).

Another issue complicates the situation. In 1970, Public Law 91-500 expanded veteran eligibility. As a result, hospital and nursing home care are available to veterans over 65 years of age regardless of ability to pay. The extent of the older veteran's demand on the VA system for care, therefore, is inextricably tied to the nation's economic condition and health policy. Changing Medicare deductibles or co-insurance and higher eligibility for Medicaid may result in large numbers of veterans unwilling or unable to pay for care in the non-VA sector. The demand on the VA may be even greater. Additional information and analyses of utilization of the VA services and

39

Table 1
AGE-SPECIFIC RATES OF VETERAN SERVICE UTILIZATION
1982

	AVERAGE DAILY PATIENT CENSUS	RATE PER 1,000
NURSING HOMES		
Under 55	2,498.7	(0.1)
55–64	7,021.8	(0.8)
65–74	6,820.9	(2.5)
75+	9,105.2	(9.9)
TOTAL	25,446.6	
ACUTE CARE		
Under 55	10,098.0	(0.6)
55–64	15,906.0	(2.1)
65–74	8,794.0	(3.4)
75+	4,883.0	(5.6)
TOTAL	39,681.0	
PSYCHIATRY		
Under 55	14,826.0	(0.9)
55–64	7,416.0	(1.1)
65–74	3,019.0	(1.3)
75+	1,878.0	(2.7)
TOTAL	27,139.0	
GRAND TOTAL	92,266.6	

Source: Veterans Administration

40

Figure 6

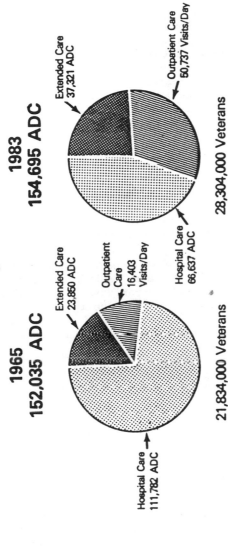

1965
152,035 ADC

1983
154,695 ADC

Hospital Care
111,782 ADC

Extended Care
23,850 ADC

Outpatient
Care
16,403
Visits/Day

Hospital Care
66,637 ADC

Extended Care
37,321 ADC

Outpatient Care
50,737 Visits/Day

21,834,000 Veterans

28,304,000 Veterans

Hospital Care includes VA, non-VA and State Home
Extended Care includes Nursing Home and Domiciliary Care only.

Source: Veterans Administration

41

programs can be found in the Administrator's Annual Reports.

Organization and Missions

The organization of the VA makes it amenable to developing an effective response to the complex medical, social and economic needs of older veterans. The VA consists of three departments: the Department of Medicine and Surgery (DM & S) responsible for the health care needs of the veteran, the Department of Veterans Benefits (DVB) which administers veteran entitlements such as compensation and pension, and the Department of Memorial Affairs which administers the national cemeteries.

There are three major mission areas in the VA: medical care, benefits and services, and memorial affairs. The VA operates the single largest medical care system in the world with 172 medical centers, 226 outpatient clinics, 99 nursing homes, and 16 domiciliaries. The majority of VA hospitals are associated with medical schools, giving the VA access to the most modern approaches to medicine; it also means that approximately half of the doctors in this country receive part of their training in VA medical centers (VAMCs). Also included is an extensive research program of over 4,000 researchers with a budget of over $150 million a year.

The VA's second mission consists of benefits and services. The VA provides a tremendous volume of information on VA services as well as referral to other federal, state and local services. This is achieved through a nationwide system of offices with a network of counselors in every state plus Puerto Rico and the Philippines, and toll-free telephone service extending now to every community in the country. A very effective auxiliary force consisting of local veterans organizations, volunteers and state and county veterans service officers assists in this endeavor. This gives the VA an ability to provide information and assistance well beyond its apparent capacity. A variety of financial assistance programs are administered -- compensation for injury or illness due to military service; pension for impoverished wartime veterans, widows and children; home loan guarantees; education assistance; life insurance; and vocational rehabilitation and job assistance for service disabled veterans.

42

Memorial Affairs maintains a nationwide system of cemeteries and offers financial assistance and memorial markers and flags to commemorate those who have served.

Many are unaware of the magnitude of the VA's mission and its potential to serve. With over 220,000 employees, and with a budget exceeding $25 billion, the VA not only has a tremendous impact on the care and assistance of veterans, but will also have a significant impact on a large part of the aging population in the future.

Department of Medicine and Surgery

Of particular interest is the Department of Medicine and Surgery (DM & S) which has a four-part mission that includes patient care, research, education, and back-up for the Department of Defense.

DM & S has a nationwide system of hospitals -- 172 in number, two-thirds of which are affiliated with the major health sciences teaching centers throughout the country (Table 2). The VA hospital system, to a large degree, reflects the needs of its patients. Faced with the needs of younger veterans after World War II, the VA built an extensive acute care system. This system includes tertiary care facilities supported by a range of smaller primary and secondary general medical and surgical hospitals and major psychiatric care centers.

The VA over the last decade, recognizing the aging of its veteran population, has been increasing its capacity for nursing home care in order to accommodate this age group's extended care needs (Figure 7).

DM & S currently operates 99 nursing home care units within or adjacent to VAMCs. In addition, the VA contracts for an equal number of nursing home beds in the community (9,525). Through the State Home Program, the VA provides grants in aid to states to build or renovate state veteran nursing homes. The VA also provides per diem support to an average of about 15,000 veterans in these state homes.

43

Table 2
VA MEDICAL CARE – FY 1982

	Treated Inpatients	Outpatient Medical Visits
VA OPERATES		
172 Hospitals (80,154 beds)	1,242,544	--
16 Domiciliaries (8,277 beds)	14,535	--
99 Nursing Home Units (9,125 beds)	15,072	--
226 Outpatient Clinics	--	15,861,687
VA CONTRACTS WITH		
Hospitals	29,189	--
Nursing Homes	31,658	--
Private Physicians	--	1,947,290
VA SUPPORTS		
State Hospitals	4,650	--
State Domiciliaries	8,783	--
State Nursing Homes	11,116	--
VA CARES FOR		
Certain Dependents and Survivors (CHAMPVA)	471*	154,169

*Average Daily Census

Source: Veterans Administration

Figure 7

NURSING HOME CARE
Average Daily Census

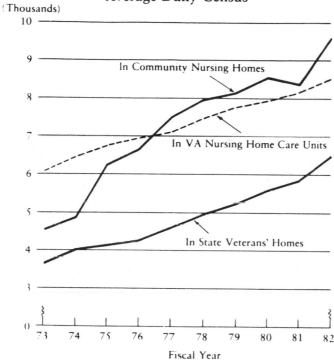

(Thousands)

In Community Nursing Homes

In VA Nursing Home Care Units

In State Veterans' Homes

Fiscal Year

73 74 75 76 77 78 79 80 81 82

Source: Veterans Administration Annual Report, 1982

The VA's lowest level of medical institutional care is the Domiciliary Program operated by the VA, and a state program similar to the state veterans home program. The Domiciliary Program cares for about 22,000 veterans per year (Figure 8).

The VA has also recognized the need to support its institutional program with alternatives that will help support the older veteran in a residential setting. Residential care (a foster home program) has been in existence since the 1950s, and began as a means to deinstitutionalize psychiatric patients who could be maintained in the community. Two newer initiatives, Hospital Based Home

45

Figure 8

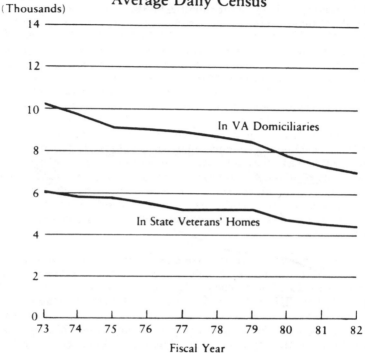

DOMICILIARY CARE
Average Daily Census

(Thousands)

In VA Domiciliaries

In State Veterans' Homes

Fiscal Year

Source: Veterans Administration Annual Report, 1982

Care and Adult Day Health Care, are other programs that provide health services for patients who might otherwise require hospital or nursing home care. A program administered by DVB, Aid & Attendance, provides supplemental income to veterans' pensions that can be used to assist the family with non-medical care to the housebound veteran.

Special Emphases

There are a few selected initiatives that hold promise in achieving certain essential medical care goals in the future:

Geriatric Evaluation Units

The average hospital stay for a veteran 75 years or older is two days more than that of a veteran under 65. Rehospitalization is also more frequent. One reason is that complications due to other medical problems are unmasked during the course of hospitalization. Careful assessment and treatment using a team assessment approach help alleviate the problem. The VA is now operating some 15 Geriatric Evaluation Units incorporating this team emphasis. Based on the definitive scientific evaluation of the Geriatric Evaluation Unit at Sepulveda VAMC, more evaluation units will be created. The results of the VA's study show that rehospitalization and referrals to nursing homes are reduced by the interdisciplinary medical team services provided in the unit.

GRECCs

Another VA initiative was developed to cut across specific disease activities. Realizing that geriatrics and gerontology were not popular among health care professions in the mid 1970s, the VA established eight centers of excellence in geriatrics and gerontology called Geriatric Research, Education and Clinical Centers, or GRECCs. There are now approved plans to establish several more GRECCs in association with their hosting VA facilities to develop programs of research, training and care around one or more medical problems relevant to the process of aging. The learning and research processes in these clinical settings point the way for future care of the aging.

Summary

The Veterans Administration has a mandate to provide high quality health care, human services, and income support to eligible veterans in an efficient and effective manner. This is its primary mission. Secondary, but of great importance, are the Department of Medicine and Surgery's responsibilities for research into the causes and treatment of disease, and its role in the nation's health professions education system. The overall goals of the VA's program for its beneficiaries will not change as a result of the aging of its population. Rather, as the population of eligible veterans ages, their needs will change. The mix of services and facilities required to provide appropriate medical care and benefits programs will also change. What is required is a change in the

47

system's focus and in the way its services are defined, organized, and delivered. These are evolutionary, not revolutionary changes.

3. Legislation Regarding Health Care for the Older Veteran

James B. Bonanno, J.D.

The patchwork of laws relating to veterans which has been enacted by Congress over the past fifty years[1] is consolidated in Title 38 of the U.S. Code. Under Chapters 17 and 81 of Title 38, the Veterans Administration is charged with the establishment and maintenance of a health care system for the benefit of veterans, defined as "persons who have served in the active military, naval or air service, and who were discharged...under conditions other than dishonorable." For the relatively small number of veterans suffering from "injury or disease incurred or aggravated in the line of duty" ("service-connected disability"), special provision is made for care required by such "service-connected disability." For veterans without service-connected disabilities, age- and needs-based criteria for access define a system of entitlements which, in certain ways, parallels Medicare and Medicaid. Especially for this non-service-connected group of veterans, the VA program suffers from some of the same limitations as Medicare and Medicaid as to the non-medical, non-institutional needs for the care of an aging population. However, the lack of deductibles, the relative ease of access and the absence of a "spend-down" requirement for VA hospitalization and nursing home eligibility in the case of veterans 65 years of age and older may combine to make the VA system an attractive alternative to Medicare/Medicaid for the older veteran, particularly in view of the budget cuts and increasing deductibles affecting the latter programs.

Incorporated within Title 38 are a variety of special provisions enabling certain groups of veterans (e.g., veterans of the Spanish-American War and World War I, former prisoners-of-war, and veterans exposed to ionizing radiation) to share in the broader eligibility for certain types of care that is accorded to veterans with greater than 50% service-connected disability.[2] However, this chapter will primarily focus on the more general provisions in Title 38 relevant to the great majority of older veterans (most belonging to the World War II and Korean War cohorts) who neither suffer from service-connected disabilities nor fall into any other special category. Each of the various elements of the VA health care system, as authorized by Title 38 and administered pursuant to VA regulations, will be examined in turn. The chapter will conclude with a discussion of amendments to Title 38 which may be necessary to authorize reforms required to make the VA system more responsive to the needs of an aging population.

I. Hospital Based Inpatient and Outpatient Programs

The VA is authorized and directed under Title 38 to establish and operate hospitals, domiciliaries, outpatient clinics and other medical facilities for the care of veterans [Secs. 5001(a)(1), 5010]. This is to be done in such manner as to "insure timely and complete care" to eligible veterans. [Secs. 5001(a)(1), 5010; see also U.S. v Alperstein, 183 F. Supp 548 (D.C. Fla, 1960), affirmed 291 F 2d 455 (furnishing of hospitalization to eligible veterans is mandatory to the extent of available facilities)]. To this end, the VA is required to operate not less than 90,000 beds in its medical facilities. The 172 VA medical centers (VAMCs) constitute the primary modality through which the VA discharges this obligation. Through the 80,000 beds currently operating in these centers along with the 10,000 in VA nursing homes, the statutory minimum is met. Included in the 80,000 hospital beds are some 10,000 in-hospital, extended care beds for patients with severe, unstable, post-acute or chronic disabilities (e.g., severe respiratory disease) requiring extensive skilled nursing care and frequent physician supervision.

"Within the limits of Veterans Administration facilities," the VA may furnish hospital care to:

- Any veteran with a service-connected disability.
- Any veteran 65 years of age or older.
- Any veteran who is eligible for a state Medicaid
  program, or certifies that he is unable to defray
  the costs of necessary hospital care.
- Certain other special sub-groups of veterans, including those who are receiving VA pensions, are
  former POWs, or are in need of care for conditions possibly related to exposure to herbicides
  while serving in Viet Nam or to ionizing radiation from nuclear testing or detonation.

With regard to service-connected disability, the term
"Veterans Administration facilities" is liberally defined
to include the provision by community hospitals of needed
care which the VA hospitals are unable to provide (Sec.
601(4)(c)). Thus, the VA is authorized to arrange for
treatment of service-connected disabilities in community
hospitals to the extent that such treatment cannot be provided within the VA system itself or other government facilities. In general, no such coverage of community hospital care exists in the case of non-service-connected
disabilities.[3]

Eligibility for outpatient and ambulatory care extends
to the same categories of veterans as inpatient hospital
care (including the over 65 group), "within the limits of
Veterans Administration facilities." Here, too, the extent of VA responsibility is affected by the degree to
which the veteran's disability is service-connected. For
those with a 50% or greater service-connected disability,
all outpatient medical care within the VA system is fully
covered. Similarly, for this group and for a veteran
seeking treatment of any service-connected disability the
VA may cover community based, fee-for-service, ambulatory
medical care if it is unable to provide the care or cannot
do so economically due to distance (Secs. 610(b), 601(4)
(c)).

On the other hand, for veterans whose eligibility for
outpatient care is based only on age or financial need, or
on a less than 50% service-connected disability, outpatient medical care within the VA system is generally
available only where it is:

51

(a) reasonably necessary in preparation for, or (to the extent that facilities are available) to obviate the need of, hospital admission; or

(b) reasonably necessary to complete treatment incident to hospital care (for a period not in excess of twelve months after discharge from in-hospital treatment, except where the [VA] finds that a larger period is required by virtue of the disability being treated). (Sec. 612(f)(1)).[4]

Availability of community, fee-for-service outpatient care is even more limited, and extends only to post-hospital treatment of the sort described in clause (b) above. However, note should be taken of the discretion granted to the VA to waive the 12-month restriction of clause (b), and of the flexible, open-ended nature of the "obviate hospitalization" provision of clause (a). These provisions have already been construed at certain VA facilities to cover continuing outpatient treatment in the VA system for older or indigent veterans with certain non-service-connected disabilities such as diabetes, hypertension, and heart failure (Joint Hearing before Committee on Veterans Affairs, 1979).[5] They could furnish the basis for the VA's further expansion of outpatient programs for elders, particularly in view of the broad delegation of statutory interpretation to the VA which is discussed at greater length at the end of this chapter.

On the other hand, discretionary waiver is not provided for in the case of service-connected disability limitations applied to two particular outpatient programs: the preventive care pilot project (Secs. 661-664), and the dental care program (Sec. 612b). Under the latter of these programs, some non-service-connected conditions may also be covered if VA dental treatment was initiated but not completed while the veteran was an inpatient. Inpatient treatment is available for non-service-connected dental conditions on a less restrictive basis (i.e., for a "compelling medical reason or dental emergency," or to the extent "not needed to furnish services" for service-connected conditions).[6]

II. Institutional, Non-Hospital Extended Care Programs

A. Nursing Home Care

Operating authority and eligibility criteria for the VA's nursing home program generally parallel those for the VA hospital system and are found in the same sections of Title 38 (Secs. 610(a) and 5010). In general, VA nursing home facilities are open to any veteran who is eligible for VA hospital care. Explicit provision is made, "within the limits of Veterans Administration facilities," for veterans 65 years of age or older and veterans "unable to defray the expenses of necessary nursing home care," as well as veterans with service-connected disabilities (Sec. 610(a)). However, as is the case with hospitalization coverage, coverage of non-VA, community nursing care is much more circumscribed for veterans with non-service-connected disabilities. For a veteran who has been hospitalized by the VA for a service-connected disability, community nursing home care may be authorized for an indefinite period, regardless of whether required for a service-connected condition, so long as the cost does not exceed 45%[7] of the cost of continued care in the VA hospital system.[8] In contrast, care in a community nursing home for non-service-connected veterans is limited to six months following a given VA hospitalization episode.[9] However, as was the case with limitations on community hospital coverage, discretion to extend this limit on community nursing home coverage is granted "where warranted... in the judgment of" the VA (Sec. 620).

Current VA regulations indicate that such discretionary extensions of community nursing home care beyond the six-month limitation may be granted "for circumstances of an unusual nature such as when a medical and economic need continues to exist, additional time is required to complete other arrangements for care, or when readmission to a hospital is not deemed professionally advisable, despite terminal deterioration of the veteran's medical condition" (38 CFR Sec. 17.51a).

Although older and indigent veterans are eligible for indefinite care in VA Nursing Home Care Units, a system of priorities set forth in 38 CFR Sec. 17.49 grants priority to veterans with service-connected disabilities. This system of priorities generally applies to VA hospital and nursing home care. However, its primary effect is felt at the nursing home level since it is at this point that serious bed shortages and long waiting lists have developed in recent years.

State nursing home programs for veterans represent an important supplement to the VA system. In recent years, some 25% of nursing home beds devoted to veteran nursing care have been in state veterans homes, with the remaining 75% evenly split between community and VA nursing homes (approximately 10,000 beds each)(Hearing before the Subcommittee on Hospitals and Health Care, 1982). While in many state home programs veterans may be required to contribute toward the cost of their maintenance, these programs may also offer the advantages of institutionalization close to home and acceptance of spouses (Hearing before the Subcommittee on Hospitals and Health Care, 1982). VA support for state veterans homes is based on two grant programs under Title 38. The first is a per diem program which provides reimbursement for the cost of care in state veterans facilities (including domiciliaries and hospitals as well as nursing homes) for veterans who are also eligible for such care in a VA facility (Sec. 641). The second program provides, under the auspices of the VA, federal matching funds up to 65% for the expansion or remodeling of existing state veterans facilities or the construction of new state nursing homes and domiciliaries (Secs. 5032-5033).

B. Domiciliary Care

The VA domiciliaries represent the original programs of the VA and derive from 1866 legislation establishing Soldier's Homes for disabled veterans (Hearing before the Subcommittee on Hospitals and Health Care, 1982). Originally, the homes were converted barracks established with little intent to provide medical or skilled nursing care. Recently plans have been adopted to begin remodelling structures that could be economically altered to conform with contemporary standards of safety and privacy, constructing new facilities and phasing out the remaining structures (VA, 1977). The VA's current policy is to include domiciliary care within the full spectrum of medical care provided to eligible veterans on the rationale that without domiciliary care as a segment of the health care continuum, patients could be forced into higher levels of care or forced to do without needed care. A domiciliary today is meant to provide eligible ambulatory veterans continuing medical care in a therapeutic institutional environment, including rehabilitative assistance and other

54

therapeutic measures. Although a domiciliary provides less intensive care than a hospital or nursing home care unit as measured by the required intervention of a nurse and/or physician, it provides a higher level of care than a residential care setting. Patients need ready access to the specialized services generally available from acute care facilities. The focus of care is in preparing the veteran to function at his or her highest level of independence.

A candidate for admission to a domiciliary exhibits a medical impairment/disability requiring a level of continuing care or rehabilitation in an institutional setting. Generally, because of his or her medical impairment, the patient is mildly to moderately disabled to the extent that he/she requires a structured daily routine and emotional support, or some intervention of a professional nature to carry out living functions or a medical care plan. However, continence and a basic ability to perform activities of daily living are minimal prerequisites for residence in a domiciliary (38 CFR Sec. 17.47(c)). In practice, most domiciliary residents at present fall into two groups: a younger, socially-disaffiliated group (largely chronic alcoholics and discharged psychiatric patients); and an older group requiring a sheltered therapeutic environment for physical reasons, such as chronic disability due to arthritis or stroke residua. At least some patients may require continuing care for an indefinite period, although the ultimate goal is the return of the veteran to independent functioning in the community.

Unlike the hospital, outpatient and nursing home care programs established by Title 38, the domiciliary program is not available to veterans over 65 on the basis of age alone. Rather, "within the limits of Veterans Administration facilities," the VA is authorized to furnish domiciliary care to (1) a veteran discharged for disability incurred in the line of duty who is "suffering from a permanent disability or tuberculosis or neuropsychiatric ailment and is incapacitated from earning a living and has no adequate means of support;" and (2) a veteran who is "in need of domiciliary care and unable to defray the expenses"[10] for such care (Sec. 610(b)). Thus, chronic disability and financial need are required of veterans both with and without service-connected conditions. However, within these broad statutory guidelines, the VA is accorded considerable freedom of action.

III. Non-Institutional Extended Care Programs

A. Home Health Care

Title 38 authorizes the VA to furnish "such home health services as [it] determines to be necessary or appropriate for the effective and economical treatment of a disability" of an eligible veteran (Sec. 612(f)). Explicitly included in this provision is the authority to finance up to $600 worth of disability-necessitated structural alterations and improvements ($2,500 in the case of a service-connected disability).[11] Eligibility criteria generally parallel those for outpatient care as reflected in Sec. 610(a) and outlined in Section I above. The extent to which the restrictions on availability of outpatient care to veterans aged 65 and over with non-service-connected disabilities apply here is not entirely clear from the language of Sec. 612(b). Although the provision appears to similarly limit home health care to pre-hospitalization, post-hospitalization (generally less than 12 months) or "obviation of hospitalization situations." The VA has to date construed Section 612(b) even more restrictively, limiting its availability to the post-hospitalization period.[12] As with outpatient care, the VA retains considerable discretion to define more liberally the scope of this provision to develop viable home health care programs (including, for example, authority to extend post-hospitalization care beyond the 12-month limit). However, a more explicit statutory provision in this connection would be desirable.

One non-institutional extended care program which has been developed by the VA is the Hospital Based Home Care program, currently operational at 30 VAMCs. As a means of helping to maintain homebound patients in the community, home visits are made by hospital based treatment teams consisting of a physician, public health nurse, social worker, rehabilitation therapist, dietician and nursing assistants (VA, 1977). Several of the Geriatric Research, Education and Clinical Centers (GRECCs), set up under P.L. 96-330 to promote medical research and education relating to the problems of older veterans, also contain geriatric assessment centers designed to provide frail elders access to home health and other care or the appropriate institutional placement.[13]

B. Residential Care Home Program

Another development in this area is the gradual reorientation of the VA's Residential Care Home program from community placement for psychiatric patients to community maintenance of impaired older veterans. The type of veteran most likely to benefit is one who is still essentially capable of performing activities of daily living but whose family resources are inadequate to provide the needed supervision and support. Under this program, food, shelter and supervision are financed with the veteran's own resources (often derived from VA compensation or pension) in residential settings inspected and approved by the VA but chosen by the veteran. The veteran receives follow-up visits from VA health care professionals pursuant to Section 612(f) and also utilizes the outpatient facilities of the local VAMC (Hearing before the Subcommittee on Hospitals and Health Care, 1982).

The potential exists for expansion of Hospital Based Home Health Care, Residential Care Home (in the case of less impaired older veterans), and similar programs into an extensive support system providing a non-institutional alternative to the already overburdened VA nursing home network for impaired or terminally ill older patients. The slow pace at which programs such as Hospital Based Home Health Care have been developed is attributable more to budgetary constraints than to issues of VA competence under Title 38. However, as is discussed below, statutory limitations are issues in the development of programs of non-institutional care which are not directly health-related.

IV. Prospects for Developing Needed Programs under Current Law

While it is beyond the scope of this chapter to project the precise health care needs which the VA will be called upon to meet in the coming decade, it is nonetheless clear that the aging of the large cohort of World War II and Korean War veterans will soon place new demands on the VA system. Meeting these demands will require flexibility of response on the part of the VA. As indicated throughout this chapter, the language of Title 38 is broad and does, in fact, allow the VA considerable discretion in determining the precise mix of services provided and in waiving statutory limitations where warranted. Indeed, Congress' exclusive delegation to the VA of the authority

57

to interpret and apply Title 38 (Sec. 211 (a)) makes the VA one of the few federal agencies whose adjudications are not subject to judicial review[14] (National Veterans Legal Services Project, 1983).

To illustrate the VA's considerable room for maneuvering, Title 38 leaves open to the VA several options for dealing with the growing demands being placed on the already overburdened VA nursing home system. Thus, for example, the VA is free to shift beds from acute care to nursing home care within the 90,000 statutory floor, and has in fact done so (Hearing before the Subcommittee on Hospitals and Health, 1982). In addition, subject to the "approval of the President" (Sec. 5010) and (as a practical matter) funding availability, the VA may construct or acquire new nursing home and domiciliary facilities. Expansion of state nursing home and domiciliary facilities could also be encouraged by fully funding and more aggressively promoting the state matching grant program authorized by the statute (Secs. 5031-5033). As an interim measure to meet increased demand, the VA could, for the benefit of the non-service-connected over-65 group, use its discretion to extend the six-month limit. The VA could also invoke its authority under Secs. 5053 and 5054 to enter into cooperative agreements with community providers on the use of community nursing home beds "as in its judgment warranted." Finally, as a means of decreasing pressures for nursing home institutionalization, the VA's home health and other community maintenance programs could be expanded. Increasing the availability of less costly institutional alternatives to nursing homes, such as VA and state domiciliaries, to minimally impaired patients might likewise diminish pressures on the VA nursing home system.

As the discussion above illustrates, the constraints on adaptation of the existing VA programs to the needs of an aging veteran population are, for the most part, budgetary rather than statutory in nature. In the words of the Veterans of Foreign Wars legislative director testifying before the Subcommittee on Hospitals and Health Care of the House Committee on Veterans' Affairs (1982):

> ...There are enough laws presently on the books to take care of our aging veterans. If they [the VA] would fund the GRECC program, the independent living program, the construction program, the

State grant programs, that is all that is needed now (p. 24).

Of a more fundamental nature is the issue of the advisability of restricting the non-service-connected older veteran's access to outpatient medical/dental care and home health care (12-month, post-hospitalization limitation, etc.) while providing unconditional access to VA acute care hospital beds.[15] The analogous Blue Cross/ Blue Shield policy of covering various procedures only if performed on an inpatient basis (even though performable on an outpatient basis) has been criticized as cost ineffective. To be sure, with regard to VA restrictions, the potential for discouraging utilization of less costly, non-institutional alternatives to hospitalization could in the short run be minimized by invocation of the liberal waiver clause of Sec. 612. However, if it were to become general policy to ignore these restrictions, they should be deleted from the statute. In addition, the statutory language governing home health care should be clarified.

Criticism on similar grounds can be made of the VA dental program (the dental outpatient program is much more restrictive than the dental inpatient program or even the medical outpatient program). The same criticism can also be made of providing full eligibility for nursing homes to older veterans while restricting eligibility for less costly alternatives, whether on the basis of financial need (e.g., domiciliaries) or otherwise (e.g., home health care).[16] Indeed, Title 38 provides little coverage of non-institutional care, such as bathing, dressing and meal preparation, which, though not strictly medical in nature, may often be important in maintaining the veteran in the community. Nor does Title 38 allow for access to VA domiciliaries or other facilities by the veteran's spouse, even if the latter is self-paying or covered by Medicare/ Medicaid (no provision for reimbursement by Medicare/Medicaid).[17]

Thus, the VA has examined meals-on-wheels, homemaker and transportation programs, as well as senior centers and congregate housing for veterans and their families. However, it has hesitated to sponsor such programs due to questions of statutory authorization as well as budgetary constraints (VA, 1977). VA-sponsored geriatric day care, provided under the Adult Day Health Care program, has been rationalized as an outpatient treatment program under Sec. 612(f).[18] However here, too, the statutory basis for VA action is ambiguous, and more specific authorization is called for.

In sum, the most pressing problems facing the VA system today are budgetary. However, over the long run, the VA will have to confront many of the same questions as the other major federal health care entitlement programs, Medicare and Medicaid, regarding the degree of government involvement in the provision of non-institutional, non-medical personal care services designed to maintain independent living by elders in the community. To the extent that support of such programs by the VA is found to be desirable in order to maintain independent living arrangements, some revision in Title 38 may be necessary to provide a clearer statutory basis for VA action.

1. P.L. 71-536 establishing the VA was enacted 54 years ago.

2. Title 38 reflects the priority Congress accorded the VA's meeting the needs of the service-connected veteran. The VA's secondary mission under Title 38 is to provide care for non-service-connected veterans, "but only to the extent that facilities are available so as to bring about a patient population size which would promote efficient utilization of resources." Kirkhuff v. Nimmo, 683 F.2d 544 (1982).

3. Non-VA hospital care for non-service-connected disabilities may be authorized in a few specialized cases:
   a) Veterans rated permanently and totally disabled from a service-connected disability.
   b) Adjunct treatment.
   c) Women veterans.
   d) Veterans in Puerto Rico, other territories, Alaska and Hawaii.
   e) Emergent conditions arising during authorized travel.
   f) Emergent conditions arising during care in a VA medical center or other government facilities.

4. Non-VA outpatient care for non-service-connected disabilities may be authorized in a few specialized cases:
   a) Veterans of the Spanish-American War.
   b) Veterans in receipt of pensions with Aid and Attendance or Housebound benefits.
   c) Veterans of World War I or the Mexican border period.
   d) Veterans participating in a VA-approved rehabilitation program.

5. However, the usual VA policy has been to refrain from invoking the "obviate hospitalization" provision to furnish outpatient care on a chronic basis to such patients.

6. Any veteran who has a 100% service-connected disability, was a POW for at least six months, or served in the Spanish-American War, is eligible for any needed dental care, regardless of whether service-connected.

7. 50% "where determined necessary by the Administrator."

8. Such transfers are common where benefit may be derived from local placements in proximity to family and friends. Veterans for whom such community nursing home placements can be arranged generally require a lower level of nursing care than those in VA nursing homes ("severe, chronic disability" as opposed to "moderately severe disability") (VA, 1977, p. 31).

9. It should be noted that even in the case of veterans with a service-connected disability, the six-month limitation on community nursing home care applies if the veteran is admitted directly to the nursing home rather than by transfer from a VA hospital as described above. Thus, apart from this six-month community nursing home stay allowed for service-connected veterans, transfers to community nursing home care are available only to veterans who have been furnished hospital care, regardless of whether they are service-connected or non-service-connected. A similar restriction applies to domiciliary patients. VA Nursing Home Care Unit and domiciliary patients who require this change in level of care are not eligible for such transfers. As a result, veterans in VA Nursing Home Care Units are not able to benefit from a transfer to a community nursing home near their family and residence. Domiciliary patients needing nursing home care are also restricted and must be placed in a VA Nursing Home Care Unit, in some instances requiring a transfer to another VA medical center, or hospitalization. This belies the philosophy and approach of offering true continuum of care levels to veterans as needed. 38 U.S.C. Sec. 620 should be amended to make patients discharged from VA Nursing Home Care Units and VA domiciliaries eligible for direct transfer to any public or private institution which furnishes nursing home care, for care at VA expense.

38 U.S.C. Sec. 620(d) should also be amended to provide that the service-connected veteran in the community who requires nursing home care will be entitled to the same open-ended duration of care as the service-connected veteran who is hospitalized in a VA facility and subsequently requires such care for which he/she was hospitalized.

Three further gaps in the current legislation governing nursing home care for veterans need to be filled. The first relates to the lack of authority for placement of women veterans into community nursing homes at VA expense. Women veterans are entitled to private hospital care in facilities not under the direct jurisdiction of the Administrator when other VA facilities are unable to provide such care because of geographical inaccessibility or inadequate facilities. However, in those cases where the woman veteran is furnished private hospital care, and subsequently requires nursing home care, the VA is without authority to provide it in a community facility. Since admission to a VA facility for subsequent transfer to community nursing home care is unlawful, and transfer to a VA facility under the direct jurisdiction of the Administrator would have occurred if such facility were available, it is necessary to have the authority to place a woman veteran from a private hospital for which the Administrator contracts. 38 U.S.C. Sec. 620(a) should be amended to provide the authority to place women veterans in a contract community nursing home at VA expense following hospitalization in a private facility under the authority of Section 601(4)(c)(iv), of 38 U.S.C.

The second of these gaps relates to the lack of authority for providing emergency hospital care and medical services to veterans in community nursing homes. A VA regulation promulgated pursuant to the VA's general statutory authority, 38 CFR Sec. 17.50b(h), has long provided that such emergency care may be provided a veteran receiving authorized nursing home care in a community facility. In providing specific statutory authority for emergency care in private facilities in certain situations by adding Sec. 601(4)(c)(iii) in Public Law 94-581, Congress unintentionally narrowed the Agency's basis for authorizing such care. In view of the specific language of Sec. 601(4)(c)(iii), there no longer appears to be a statutory basis for the VA regulation. The apparent lack of authority to provide emergency hospital care in private facilities for veterans receiving VA-sponsored nursing home care in facilities distant from VA medical centers could disrupt the Community Nursing Home Care program. Veterans with limited incomes may be extremely reluctant to accept transfers to community nursing homes under these circumstances. Some of the nursing homes may, in turn, become unwilling to accept as a patient a veteran who has no means of financing such care.

An amendment should be made to 38 U.S.C. Sec. 602, which authorizes the VA to furnish private hospital or medical care for treating a medical emergency of a veteran receiving medical services in a VA health care facility to provide a statutory basis for the VA regulation which purports to authorize such care.

The third of these gaps relates to the lack of authority for outpatient treatment for non-service-connected veterans discharged from VA Nursing Home Care Units and VA domiciliaries. Under Chapter 17 of Title 38 U.S.C., the VA may furnish treatment on an outpatient basis for any disability to complete treatment initiated during VA hospitalization. Veterans discharged from other modes of care in VA facilities -- VA Nursing Home Care Units (NHCUs) and domiciliaries -- have no comparable entitlement. Since these patients, when discharged, are generally not eligible to obtain necessary medical care on an outpatient basis, many remain institutionalized longer than necessary, often for very prolonged periods. Lack of access to assured VA care becomes a powerful disincentive to return home or to an alternative independent living arrangement such as Hospital Based Home Care. This gap in the scheme of eligibility for needed health care stands in marked contrast to a philosophy which stresses rehabilitation, independence, and return to community living.

New authority to make veterans discharged from VA NHCUs and domiciliaries eligible for medical services for any disability treated during such institutional care can meet several key needs. Not only would such authority help veterans make the transition from institutional to community placement, but it would as a by-product result in a better utilization rate of facilities for which demand presently exceeds supply.

38 U.S.C. Sec. 612(f)(1)(B) should be amended to include those veterans discharged from VA nursing home or domiciliary care in the program of medical services provided on an outpatient or ambulatory basis.

10. 38 CFR 17.48(B) defines this to mean with "no adequate means of support," specifying a ceiling of "an income

64

of $415 or more per month from any source." This specific guideline differs from certification by the veteran of inability to defray the cost of hospital or nursing home care.

Moreover, since age is made a basis for eligibility independent of financial need for hospital or nursing home care but not domiciliary care, a dichotomy is created whereby aging veterans do not have comparable access to all three levels of medical care.

The increasing age of World War II veterans will create an increasing demand for medical care. The availability of, and equal access to, all three levels of care may make it possible for some veterans to receive appropriate institutional care in a domiciliary rather than at a higher level such as a nursing home or hospital. This would make it possible to stretch available funds to provide care for a greater number of veterans.

38 U.S.C. Sec. 610(b) should be amended to align the domiciliary care eligibility of older veterans having non-service-connected disabilities with the hospital or nursing home care eligibility of this group.

11. This is a lifetime total grant under the Home Improvement and Structural Alterations Program set up by the VA.

12. Such an interpretation of Section 612(f) seems unduly narrow in view of the language of the provision, which reads as follows:

> The Administrator, within the limits of Veterans Administration facilities, may furnish medical services for any disability on an outpatient or ambulatory basis: 1) to any veteran eligible for hospital care under section 610 of this Title (A) where such services are reasonably necessary in preparation for, or (to the extent that facilities are available) to obviate the need of, hospital admission, or (B) where such a veteran has been furnished hospital care and such medical services are reasonably necessary to complete treatment incident to such hospital care (for a period not in excess of

65

twelve months after discharge from in-hospital treatment, except where the Administrator finds that a longer period is required by virtue of the disability being treated); and 2) to any veteran who has a service-connected disability rated at 50% or more; and 3) to any veteran who is a former prisoner of war. The Administrator may also furnish to any such veteran such home health services as the Administrator determines to be necessary or appropriate for the effective and economical treatment of a disability of a veteran (including only such improvements and structural alterations the cost of which does not exceed $600...).

13. This program began in Fiscal Year 1975 and authorization for appropriations will, unless renewed, expire at the end of FY 1984. Currently, there are eight GRECCs at various locations across the country. The GRECCs were intended to attract outstanding professionals to teach and conduct basic and clinical research on aging, to provide education in geriatrics, and to experiment with alternative means of providing care to the aged. GRECC activities have been directed towards utilizing existing resources to provide geriatric care and to integrate clinical research and trained health care providers in geriatrics and gerontology into the VA system. Each Center typically emphasizes one area of research relevant to aging.

14. Section 211(a) notwithstanding, the courts have begun to "pierce the veil" of VA immunity in constitutional or procedural challenges to VA determinations (National Veterans Legal Services Project, 1983).

15. Here, too, resource limitations have played as important a role as statutory constraints in limiting access. In recent years, demand for outpatient care in excess of available facilities has forced restrictions on acceptance of new outpatients in accordance with the priority categories outlined in Sec. 612(i). Both the statutory constraints on outpatient care eligibility and the rationing by priority categories under Sec. 612 have been utilized to control the level of expenditures for veterans' medical care.

16. There is also a general restriction on VA reimbursement for travel expenses relating to treatment for non-service-connected disabilities unless a "poverty oath" is taken (Sec. 111). This may likewise be criticized as deterring utilization of medical care until disability is far advanced.

17. Title 38 does allow VA facilities to provide mental health services to members of the veteran's immediate family, legal guardian, or person with whom he/she will be living, when essential to the treatment of a hospitalized veteran.

18. Adult Day Health Care programs provide to veterans, in a congregate setting during normal working hours, health care services including medical, nursing, rehabilitative, social, recreational and educational programs. Mid-day meals and transportation to and from the Center are usually provided. The provision of these services enables patients to be maintained at home in a supportive environment rather than be institutionalized in a nursing home or hospital.

There is no current legislation which provides specific authority for the VA to establish and operate an Adult Day Health Care (ADHC) Program. There is only limited legislative authority for ADHC-like services under Section 612(f)(1)(B) (in the case of non-service-connected veterans) and Section 612(f)(2) (in the case of service-connected veterans). Veterans who require such care for 50% or more service-connected disabilities may thus receive it as long as determined medically necessary for this condition. However, for non-service-connected veterans this means in the current VA view that ADHC can be provided only following a period of hospitalization, under specific medical prescription and for a period of time not to exceed one year. The VA has to date been reluctant to extend ADHC to non-service-connected veterans under Section 612(f)(1)(A), on the basis of obviating the need for hospital admission.

REFERENCES

Hearing before the Subcommittee on Hospitals and Health Care, House Committee on Veterans' Affairs. "Oversight of the VA's Extended Care and Geriatric Programs." 97th Congress, 2nd Session, July 14, 1982.

Joint Hearing before Committee on Veterans Affairs. "Oversight on Admission to VA Medical Care Facilities." 96th Congress, 1st Session, October 25, 1979.

National Veterans Legal Services Project. "Developments in Veterans Law in 1982." Clearinghouse Review, 16(8), p. 825, January, 1983.

U.S. Veterans Administration. The Aging Veteran: Present and Future Medical Needs. Washington, D.C., October, 1977.

4. Transition of VA Acute Care Hospitals into Acute and Long Term Care*

Axel Bang
James H. Morse, M.D.
Edward W. Campion, M.D.

Introduction

The purpose of this chapter is to examine the role of the acute care hospital in the development, management and delivery of acute and long term care. The chapter is divided into four sections. In the first section, "The Graying of the Population," changing trends in patient mix and their effects on hospital utilization and costs are presented. The implications of these changes on future patterns of care are discussed as well as the multiple barriers to change which currently exist in the second section, "Pressures upon the System." Characteristics of the national and VA nursing home systems and their effect on the acute care hospital are the topics of the third section, "Nursing Homes and the Health System." The fourth section, "The Challenge for Hospitals," describes the rationale for hospitals' entry into long term care and the advantages of doing so in terms of cost effectiveness

* This chapter is an adaptation of an article entitled "Why Acute-Care Hospitals Must Undertake Long-Term Care" by Edward W. Campion, M.D., Axel Bang and Maurice I. May, M.S.H.A. which originally appeared in the New England Journal of Medicine, Vol. 308, No. 2, Jan. 13, 1983.

and improved medical training. In addition, several proposals are offered as to how the VA could provide comprehensive long term care to its increasing numbers of elderly veterans.

This chapter is not intended to be the final statement on the role of acute care hospitals in acute and long term care. Rather it is designed to provide information around which discussion of the issues can revolve and through which policy proposals may evolve; it is a broad outline of the problems with a few suggestions as to how these problems might be approached by both the VA and non-VA systems. Importantly, in making these proposals, it is not the intent of the authors to advocate the substitution of long term care at the expense of short term care but merely to recognize those changes which are existent and to define the issues raised by those changes. Finally, to the extent that VA health care interacts with and is dependent on U.S. health care, an attempt to view the VA within the larger context of the national health care system can only be a valuable and productive exercise.

The Graying of the Population

From 1970 to 1980 the elderly population (those over age 65) grew by 27.3% in the United States. The population over age 85 -- 22% of whom are institutionalized -- grew by 48%. This "graying of America" promises to continue and will radically change the future patient mix and utilization patterns in acute care hospitals. At present, the elderly account for 38% of patient days in acute care hospitals and 35% of net revenues (The Hospital Research and Educational Trust, 1982). With the elderly group projected to grow from 11% of the population today to 20% of the population by 2030, these utilization and cost figures will increase substantially. Within the over 65 age group, those over the age of 75 will grow as a percentage of the total, and the 65-74 age group will decline. This is important because of hospital utilization patterns. In 1979, for example, people aged 65-74 used 3300 inpatient days per 1000 population while the 75-85 age group used 5600 days per 1000 population and those over 85 used 7500 days per 1000. In comparison, the average for the under 65 population during this time was only 811 inpatient days per 1000 (The Hospital Research and Educational Trust, 1982).

These long-range population, utilization, and cost trends for the nation as a whole will be reflected in the VA more quickly and with greater intensity. The 3.5 million elderly veterans presently eligible for VA services will increase to approximately 9 million by the year 2000. Already, between 1970 and 1980, the number of veterans over 85 increased an astounding 1200%. Current projections indicate that by 1990 the number of veterans falling within the age groups of 65-74 and 75-84 will have increased by 153% and 170%, respectively, in comparison to 1980 levels (Table 1). Because most Americans who achieve the status of veteran do so during periods of armed conflict, the distribution of veterans according to age does not mirror the distribution of males in the population-at-large. In fact, due largely to the World War II cohort, the percentage of the total veteran population aged 65-74 is larger than for the nation as a whole. In addition, the aged veteran accounts for substantial and increasing portions of the total days of care provided in VA acute care facilities. During FY 1982, veterans 65 and older, making up 12% of the total veteran population, utilized 32% of the total number of days of care provided by VA hospitals (VA Annual Report, 1982). Similarly, the hospital utilization rate for elderly veterans has shown a steady and progressive rise over the last several years (Table 2).

Pressures upon the System

Although the patient mix has changed, patterns of care have not. Hospitals have continued to increase the intensity of services to a point that has become distinctly uncomfortable economically and politically. Acute care hospitals are only beginning to broaden their philosophy of care to address the long term medical, rehabilitation, and social needs of the elderly. There are multiple barriers to hospitals' shifting into long term care, not only in reimbursement but also in the traditional patterns of teaching and practicing medicine in acute care institutions. Despite these barriers, acute care hospitals must move into the field of long term care. Such a move will result in improved delivery of health care to the elderly and in more efficient use of health resources.

Already, acute care hospitals are feeling the effects of economic difficulties suffered by the traditional providers of long term care such as chronic care hospitals, mental health hospitals, nursing homes, and home health

71

TABLE 1
SELECTED DATA FROM THE 1980 U.S.
CENSUS OF POPULATION[1,5]
AND THE VETERANS ADMINISTRATION [2,3,4]

VETERAN POPULATION[1]
(in 000s)

AGE	1970	1980	% change	1990[4]	% change
0–14	--	--	--	--	--
15–64	25,647	25,670	+.09	19,909	-22.4
65–74	1,070	2,220	+107.5	5,621	+153.2
75–84	910	490	-46.1	1,326	+170.6
85+	20	260	+1200.0	208	-20.0
65+	2,000	2,970	+48.5	7,155	+140.9
TOTAL	27,647[2]	28,640[3]	+3.6	27,064	-5.5

TABLE 1 (Continued)
SELECTED DATA FROM THE 1980 U.S.
CENSUS OF POPULATION[1,5]
AND THE VETERANS ADMINISTRATION [2,3,4]

	U.S. POPULATION[1] (in 000s)				
AGE	1970	1980	% change	1990[5]	% change
0-14	57,900	51,282	-11.4		
15-64	125,247	149,678	+19.5		
65-74	12,435	15,578	+25.2	17,800	+14.3
75-84	6,119	7,727	+26.3	9,100	+17.8
85+	1,511	2,240	+48.2	2,900	+29.5
65+	20,066	25,544	+27.3	29,800	+16.7
TOTAL	203,212	226,505	+11.5	243,000	+7.5

[1]1980 Decennial Census, U.S. Census Bureau, 1980.
[2]The Aging Veteran: Present and Future Medical Needs,
Veterans Administration, October, 1977, pg. II.
[3]Veteran Population, Office of Reports and Statistics,
Veterans Administration, 1970.
[4]Veteran Population Projections, by Age and Period of
Service, Selected Years, 1984-2030. Office of Reports
and Statistics, Statistical Policy and Research Service,
Research Division (711), Veterans Administration, April
29, 1983 in VA Geriatric Plan, Part 1. The Challenge,
Veterans Administration, July 22, 1983 (draft).
[5]Additional census data.

TABLE 2

DAYS OF CARE FOR THE ELDERLY (65+ years)
AS A PERCENTAGE OF TOTAL DAYS OF CARE
FOR ALL PATIENTS IN ACUTE CARE HOSPITALS
U.S.[1] AND V.A.[2]

% Days of Care for Elderly

	1975	1976	1977	1978	1979	1980	Total % Change
U.S.	33.8	34.9	35.3	36.4	37.0	38.4	+4.6
V.A.	29.3	28.3	29.8	29.9	31.7	31.7	+2.4

1 Data from utilization of short-stay hospitals from Vital and Health
  Statistics, U.S. Department of Health and Human Services, Washington,
  D.C.: 1975-80.

2 VA Annual Reports, 1975-1980.

agencies. The result is a growing number of chronically ill elderly who do not seem to fit into any level of care.

These elderly are becoming the "boat people" of the health care delivery system. Many remain inappropriately placed in hospitals while awaiting placement in nursing homes. Within the VA system, it has been estimated that at least 8.6% of the acute care hospital population or approximately 6000 patients would be more appropriately (and inexpensively) served by placement in an extended care facility such as a nursing home (VA Office of Program Analysis and Development, 1982).

This placement bottleneck can be attributed to the virtual freeze on nursing home construction across the country and to the large number of patients with needs greater than nursing homes can meet (GAO, July 15, 1982). The shortage of nursing home beds is tied to problems that pervade the elderly housing market and the home health care system. Although it is estimated that 15-40% of the elderly in nursing home facilities could be more appropriately cared for in private homes (Portnoi, 1979), most no longer have a home, are entirely alone in the world, or are ineligible for home care services. In its 1977 report, the National Academy of Science noted that the residents of VA nursing homes have in common with a national sample of nursing home patients the characteristics of poverty, advanced age and absence of family care providers (National Academy of Science, 1977).

This estimation of such a high degree of inappropriate admissions, however, is being challenged by recent evidence that nursing home patients today are more seriously ill and in need of more services than in years past (GAO, July 15, 1982).

Home health care has traditionally been a low priority of Medicaid and Medicare, receiving less than 2% of those budgets. It remains a low priority, though change is slowly occurring. The fastest growth rate in Medicaid expenditures in the past five years, for example, has been in home care, not nursing home care (Muse and Sawyer, 1982). Also, many states are taking advantage of a Medicaid waiver under the 1981 Omnibus Reconciliation Act to offer community based home care services as an alternative to nursing home care.

75

Within the VA's Department of Medicine and Surgery, home health care programs have a small but expanding role. Of the approximately $1.4 billion allocated for outpatient care in FY '82, only $9 million or less than 1% of the total outpatient budget was marked for Hospital Based Home Care (HBHC) programs (VA Annual Report, 1982). In 1982, while over 60,000 veterans were treated in long term care facilities, only 6500 were treated by home care teams (VA, Report of the Geriatrics and Gerontology Advisory Committee, 1983). Although plans call for an expansion in the number of these programs from 42 to 72 by 1986, the majority of smaller, non-affiliated VAMCs will still be unable to offer home care services to their clients. Expansion of this program under its present arrangement of hospital based multidisciplinary teams operating within a 15–30 mile radius of local VA hospitals will exclude many needy veterans on the basis of geography alone. In addition, if home health care is to become a priority of the VA, it will be necessary to study in depth the interactive effects of entitlements, eligibility and reimbursement incentives that presently favor institutional rather than non-institutional care. One possible option is for the VA to contract with the 7000 non-VA hospitals or other health organizations in the non-VA system to provide home care. In considering alternatives in home care, it is important to understand that these services may not reduce the cost of care as noted in a recent GAO report entitled The Elderly Should Benefit from Expanded Home Health Care But Increasing These Services Will Not Insure Cost Reductions (GAO, December 7, 1982).

Recognizing these pressures, the American Hospital Association in 1981 established an Office on Aging and Long Term Care to help hospitals face the challenge of adapting to meet the needs of their older patients and others with chronic conditions. This AHA office has held conferences, published books and articles on aging, developed a directory of services for elderly patients, and co-sponsored (with the Robert Wood Johnson Foundation) pilot programs across the country encouraging acute care hospitals to launch long term care projects.

Likewise, the VA established the Geriatric Research, Education and Clinical Center program (GRECC) in 1974 to study how to respond to the medical, psychological and social needs of the increasing number of older veterans. A principal conclusion of the VA Geriatrics and Gerontology Advisory Committee (GGAC) in its April, 1983 report was that the VA needs to "accelerate reallocation of acute care resources from areas which are declining in need to the development of resources for delivery of chronic care" (p. 5).

Nursing Homes and the Health System

Since the advent of Medicare and Medicaid in 1965, the nursing home has become the centerpiece in the long term care system in the United States. There are 1.3 nursing home beds for every acute care bed in the United States. In contrast, only 25% of the VA system's beds (or 27,000 of the total of 112,000 beds) are for long term care patients (National Academy of Science, 1977, p. 209). In addition to its own beds, however, the VA system pays for 10,000 veterans in community nursing homes, 7000 veterans in state nursing homes, and 5000 veterans in state domiciliary housing (Table 3). Taking into consideration all available extended care beds, there is 0.73 long term care bed for every acute care bed in the VA (VA Office of Reports and Statistics, September, 1983).

TABLE 3
Extended Care Beds in VA[1]

Type	Number
VA Nursing Home	9,414
Community Nursing Home	10,212
State Nursing Homes	6,919
VA Domiciliaries	8,201
State Domiciliaries	4,489
State Hospitals	541
Intermediate Care Beds	10,605
TOTAL	50,381

[1]Extended care bed statistics compiled from the VA Office of Reports and Statistics, Summary of Medical Programs, 1983 (some figures represent the average daily census).

Eighty-six percent of U.S. nursing home residents are over 65, and about 25% of all elderly Americans will spend part of their life in a nursing home (GAO, November 26, 1979). The growth in nursing homes has been accompanied by increasing concern about their impact on residents. Once in a nursing home, the elderly generally become physically, emotionally and economically dependent on the home for the rest of their lives. Recent data from VA nursing home studies reveal that only four out of every ten nursing home patients are discharged to independent living situations (VA Office of Reports and Statistics, September, 1983). After only a few months in the nursing home, most residents have used up personal savings, are impoverished and entirely dependent on Medicaid. Depending upon the state, up to 75% of nursing home beds are occupied by patients receiving Medicaid. Discharge is usually impossible for these people even if their health improves, since they have no means of support in the outside community. Coordinating successful community discharges for these vulnerable persons is a complex, time-consuming and risky task. Moreover, at present there are no financial incentives for nursing homes to do so. Knowing this, the majority of nursing home staff do not emphasize -- and cannot afford to emphasize -- rehabilitation and community placement.

Nursing homes have also become a repository for psychiatric patients, drastically changing the nature of care in many homes. The National Institute of Mental Health estimates that 750,000 nursing home residents have either recognizable mental illnesses or conditions commonly referred to as senility (GAO, September 16, 1982, p. 5). Mental illness is the primary diagnosis for about 33% of those patients. An estimated 21% of all elderly persons with mental disorders are in nursing homes (GAO, September 16, 1982, p. 6). That so many mentally ill elderly are in nursing homes can be attributed to several larger societal pressures: a) deinstitutionalization of individuals from state mental institutions accompanied by a reduction in the total number of inpatient psychiatric beds, b) the fact that many elderly have developed debilitating physical ailments in addition to their mental problems, and c) the availability of federal reimbursement for long term care through Medicare and Medicaid (GAO, September 16, 1982).

The influx of psychiatric patients has caused a similar burden for VA nursing home facilities in which a large share (43%) of the patients have mental disorders (VA Office of Reports and Statistics, October, 1982). Of the

78

estimated 51,000 patients with primary psychiatric diagnoses in VA facilities in October, 1975, only half were in psychiatric beds (National Academy of Science, 1977). The others were mainly in extended care beds. To compound the situation for nursing home facilities, in the decade preceeding 1975, beds designated as psychiatric declined from 49% to 32% of the VA operating beds (National Academy of Science, 1977).

The need for more nursing home beds is apparent, despite the difficulties of financing and access. The number of elderly patients backed up in hospitals awaiting placement is one indicator. One VA report estimates that "in the judgement of VA health care professionals, one of every 4 inpatients in a VA hospital could be discharged if outside resources were available" (VA Office of Program Planning and Evaluation, 1983, p. 28). Presumably, a significant proportion of these patients are awaiting nursing home placement. The VA's GGAC estimates a need for 70,000 VA supported nursing home beds by the year 2000. Nationally, however, there is an effective freeze on nursing home construction, coupled with restrictive Medicaid reimbursement. With 40% of the VA's nursing home population cared for through contracts with community homes, this freeze assumes particular significance.

The shortage of nursing home beds is not the only cause of back up of patients in acute care hospitals. Economic incentives of nursing homes discourage accepting those elderly patients who require more attention ("heavy care" patients). Patients who require minimal care and less staff attention are more attractive economically. An astonishing absence of physician involvement in nursing homes further discourages acceptance of patients who require extensive care and are dependent on Medicaid.

Broad societal changes contribute to the pressures to institutionalize the elderly. Increasing numbers of women are joining the work force, reducing the number of women available to care for elderly relatives at home. Family size is declining and mobility in the work force has created a geographic separation of children from parents, making care logistically difficult. Increases in the divorce rate and in the number of single parent families have further complicated family ties and therefore willingness of family members to care for elders. Moreover, progressive inflation has eroded the savings and pensions of the elderly, diminishing their capacity to remain economically independent in the community. The potential poverty of the elderly veteran is of primary concern because the VA system serves as a "safety net," with those veterans who earn less than $4,000 four or five times as likely to use VA services than those who earn $10,000 or more (VA, Report of the GGAC, 1983).

While there are parallels in providing nursing home care to veterans and non-veterans, there are also differences. The most obvious is that a majority of patients in VA homes are men, whereas non-VA nursing home patients are predominantly women. Another difference between the two systems is that VA nursing homes are likely to be physically connected to VA medical centers (VAMCs), whereas most non-VA nursing homes are freestanding. VA nursing homes are generally more expensive than community nursing homes. For example, at the Bedford VA in Massachusetts, a nursing home bed is calculated to cost $90 per day versus $60 per day for a contract community nursing home bed. The reason for this cost difference is unclear. Do VA nursing home patients have greater needs? Is it because the VA homes have higher staffing ratios, because patients have easier access to medical treatment in adjoining hospitals, or because VA homes offer more extensive and expensive social and recreational programs?

Placement in a nursing home of service-connected elderly veterans despite poverty status may not be as difficult as for Medicaid patients, primarily because VA contracts with community nursing homes usually guarantee a higher per diem than Medicaid. The VA's higher rate stems from its intention to pay an all-inclusive rate. In terms of coverage, non-service-connected veterans are limited to six months of coverage in community homes. Most service-connected veterans have no time limit on coverage.

The Challenge for Hospitals

The hospital remains the primary point of contact for meeting the acute health care needs of the elderly. It is virtually the only community institution that is open 24 hours a day, 7 days a week, to provide emergency care, and social and rehabilitation services. This is important to the elderly, who are admitted three times more frequently, stay twice as long and use five times more inpatient days than other adults (see Table 4). Elderly patients are readmitted more frequently than other age groups in the course of a year, and a small percentage of elders ac-

TABLE 4

A COMPARISON OF V.A.[1] AND U.S.[2] HOSPITAL UTILIZATION BY AGE

	Admissions Per 1000 Population	Average Length of Stay in Days		In-patient Days Per 1000 Population
	U.S.	U.S.	V.A.	U.S.
Total Pop.	166	7.1	15.4	1,185
Adults 19-64	136	5.9	15.1	811
Adults 65+	400	10.4	16.2	4,149

[1]V.A. data from Geriatrics and Gerontology Advisory Committee, Table 4, p. 28.
[2]U.S. data from the Hospital Research and Educational Trust, 1982.

counts for a disproportionately large number of patient days. For the country as a whole, data from the Health Care Financing Administration indicate that 70% of annual expenditures are used for care for a mere 8.8% of Medicare beneficiaries (Iglehart, 1982). Comparing the elderly and non-elderly use of hospitals in the VA system, the results are not as dramatic. Lengths of stay are very long for both the under-65 (15.1 days) and for the over-65 (16.2 days) groups (see Table 4). What is important to note is that the number of patient days for the over-65 and over-75 groups in the VA system are expected to increase three- and five-fold, respectively, by the year 2000, while use by the under-65 group is expected to decrease (VA, Report of the GGAC, 1983).

Despite the large numbers of elderly patients in acute care hospitals, few of these institutions have a comprehensive geriatric program geared to meet the long term medical, rehabilitative, and social needs that are linked to acute illness. To provide quality geriatric care, hospitals must make a clear commitment to long term care for the chronically ill elderly patient. It appears that no one else will or can.

If hospitals are to provide more long term care services, fundamental changes in the hospital environment and in reimbursement must be made. The rapid turnover of patients in acute care hospitals is unsettling to older persons, who need stability, patience and friendship. Hospital staff have not been trained to care for the long term needs of the elderly. In the acute care hospital environment, rampant testing and technical procedures can result in the "overmedicalization" of patients and can exacerbate the problem of escalating health care costs. An option for acute care hospitals is to develop long term care units specifically for such elderly patients. Medicare "cost allocation" regulations, however, provide disincentives to hospitals for operating such units. If the costs of long term care could be isolated from overhead for acute care, a long term care unit would be economically viable. A recent federal regulation that permits selected hospitals to operate "swing beds" for chronic care is a step in this direction.

The VA system already has models to study the cost and quality issues of converting acute care beds into long term care beds. There are 10,565 "intermediate" (chronic) care beds and 9,239 nursing home beds which are, in effect, long term care units in the VAMCs. However, the creation of extended care units from existing beds is not without problems. For example, the quality of care in the intermediate care units is reportedly less satisfactory compared to that in VA nursing home units (National Academy of Science, 1977, p. 216), and hospital based nursing homes in the VA system are about twice as expensive as community based homes (GAO, September 30, 1982).

Acute care hospitals must reorient their patterns of care to emphasize continuous rather than episodic care of elders. Unlike other providers, hospitals can offer comprehensive case management of patients, from home care to acute care, thus ensuring continuity of services. Pilot projects, such as the Urban Medical Group in Boston, have shown that a comprehensive approach to caring for the chronically ill elderly can be cost effective (Master, et al., 1980).

In the VA system, however, there may be serious logistical problems implementing such a program nationwide. There are only 172 VAMCs in the U.S., many of them clustered along the Eastern seaboard. Conversely, there are approximately 7,000 non-VA hospitals in the U.S. One option for the VA would be to contract with hospitals or community groups to provide geriatric team care for the elderly in their homes and in local hospitals. The VA could use its present system of contracting with community nursing homes as a model. Another option involves the lending of VA managers and facilities to community programs for the development of care programs for both veteran and non-veteran elderly. The Day Ambulatory Service for Health (DASH) and Desert Area Wellness Network (DAWN) of Loma Linda, California are only two examples of proposed services which would utilize this approach.

Hospitals could most readily provide the physician care needed to eliminate the costly shuttle from nursing home to acute care facility. Moreover, hospitals with long term care beds would have a tremendous incentive to use those beds preferentially for patients requiring long term care, particularly those inappropriately and expensively occupying acute care beds. In the VA system, this would be true only if changes were made to the present system of payment, in which average daily census by service center (regardless of the severity of illness of patients) is the key determinant in revenues. Under the present system of reimbursement in the VA system, if a chronic patient is occupying an acute bed, the VAMC is paid the rate for an acute patient. If the VA system is about to experience an upsurge in chronic patients, a better method of balancing actual costs generated by patients with revenues should be studied. Experiments by the VA with diagnostic-related groups (DRGs) for acute care patients and consumption-related groups (CRGs) for long term care patients are in this direction.

Using existing funding sources, hospitals could develop a full array of institutional and community services for the elderly: congregate housing; nursing home, day, home health, foster, hospice, and "respite" care (which offers a short term relief for those providing care at home); meals on wheels; and health education and screening. Some of these services, such as nursing home, day and home health care, are supported by Medicaid; a smaller number are reimbursable by Medicare. To limit their liability and protect themselves financially, some hospitals are reorganizing their corporate structures and creating holding companies to oversee such programs.

The financial risks of providing community and long term care are less than hospitals fear. Nationally, private entrepreneurs manage to find the $24.2 billion nursing home industry profitable, though largely by attracting private payers, who contribute $10.6 billion to the industry (Waldo and Gibson, 1982). With effective management, quality nursing home care is certainly possible. Hospitals can also take unique advantage of economies of scale. In addition, acute care hospitals can reap additional economic benefits from a more efficient use of acute care beds while providing the continuity of medical care needed by elderly veterans.

Hospitals are becoming increasingly aware of the long term care system. In fact, their economic survival may depend upon it. As cost control efforts put the pinch on nursing homes, the acute care hospitals will feel the squeeze. Severely impaired, hard-to-place elderly patients account for most "administratively necessary days" for which hospitals have been paid less than the full per diem rate. The growing numbers of such patients threaten the financial viability of some hospitals. Growing numbers of these patients in the VAMCs may force a reallocation of acute and long term care beds, with attendant changes in medical service budgets, personnel and physical plant.

The financial benefits deriving from long term care will become particularly appealing to acute care hospitals if the trend toward prospective reimbursement continues. On October 1, 1983, Medicare began reimbursing all hospitals on a DRG-based prospective system. Some states, such as Massachusetts, have an "all payer" prospective reimbursement system which encompasses Blue Cross, Medicaid, and commercial insurers as well as Medicare. The VA, as mentioned, is already experimenting with DRGs and CRGs. With hospitals held directly liable for cost control, comprehensive management of the patient requiring extensive care in a long term unit or at home can become cost effective. For example, the physician's home visit currently appears to be costly and inefficient. However, as part of a comprehensive system of health care for the elderly, home visits would be recognized as an effective means of providing high quality, low technology care that can prevent expensive institutionalization. Hospitals have the knowledge and incentives to direct such resources to the elderly who are truly at risk for costly hospitalization.

At present acute care hospitals are wandering into long term care with no clear strategy (Eisdorfer, 1981; Kane & Kane, 1978). Some have established close ties with local nursing homes by providing in-service education, consultation, and even medical coverage. A few hospitals have actually become long term care facilities, entirely or in part. Others have developed close administrative ties to local nursing homes as a means of gaining influence in decisions concerning bed use and patient transfers. A few large hospitals have simply purchased nursing homes and now run them. The objective of all these activities by acute care hospitals is to gain greater access to long term care beds.

Difficult access to long term care creates dangerous pressures on administrators and physicians to manipulate the utilization review process or even patient care in order to keep patients defined as acutely ill and thereby covered by Medicare. This may be equally true in the VA system, where VAMCs are reimbursed according to census and unused budgeted dollars must be returned to the central office.

Exposed to the severely impaired elderly patients found in teaching hospitals, residents and medical students may acquire a distorted and pessimistic view of aging, entirely losing sight of the fact that 95% of the elderly reside at home. Approximately 40% of the trainees in relevant medical specialties and a total of 100,000 students in the health professions obtain all or part of their training in VAMCs (VA Annual Report, 1982). This point is of particular importance because the rapid increase in elderly veterans will make the VA system a model for society at large, preparing young health care providers for the needs of an aging society. Concern has been expressed by some that the attractiveness of VAMCs as medical school affiliates and as training sites for students and residents will decrease as the proportion of elder patients increases. This concern is based in part on recognition of negative attitudes toward elder patients in general. However, a number of factors ameliorate these concerns. First, there is some evidence of changing attitudes among care providers as geriatric information and sophistication improve. Secondly, as medical schools improve the geriatric curriculum content, enthusiasm for geriatric patients also improves. Finally, as VA facilities become recognized as centers of excellence in geriatric research, training and clinical care – the interest in participation of the various specialties is likely to increase. In fact, the VAMCs may wish to publicize this unique role as teaching centers in aging to insure that close ties are kept with medical schools and teaching hospitals and that quality of care in the VA system is maintained.

If acute care hospitals assume responsibility for long term care, they must do far more to prevent institutionalization of elders at risk. This means moving decisively into community geriatric care, which is currently a tangled array of medical, social, and economic services badly in need of coordination. Hospitals have painfully learned that problems in any of these community services can result in increased numbers of hospital admissions, long term institutionalization, and increased costs.

A more effective preventive approach will move hospitals far from their traditional roles and into comprehensive community screening and delivery of services. The homebound and severely impaired elderly are the group that private practitioners and group practices now find most difficult to care for because of the numerous social needs, logistic difficulties, and low financial reimbursement. Hospitals and their affiliated community clinics are best equipped to care for such patients, coordinating the complex services and providing round-the-clock social and medical support. At present, not even prepaid health maintenance organizations (HMOs) carry strong incentives to prevent nursing home institutionalization, since, like most other health insurers, HMOs do not cover long term nursing home care. The costs of such care fall to the individual members and are therefore outside the utilization strategies of the HMO plan. It is important to note, however, that cooperative pilot projects between HMOs and Medicare, such as the Fallon Community Health Plan in Worcester, Massachusetts, have halved inpatient use by the elderly. Strategies for a truly comprehensive "social health maintenance organization" are only now being developed (Ruchlin, et al., 1982). Demonstrations of total care for the homebound elderly are underway in experimental federal programs, such as the one at St. Vincent's Hospital in New York City (Bricker, 1982). Given its experience and a pre-existing network of long term care facilities and support services, the VA's ability to adopt the comprehensive care strategies of HMOs may well exceed that of private sector hospitals.

Hospitals should not lose sight of the fact that long term care will be one of the greatest growth areas in health care over the coming decades (Russell, 1981). The budgets of nursing homes are projected to reach $76 billion within this decade (Freeland, et al., 1980). New explorations in federalizing Medicaid and shifting Medicare resources toward long term care suggest that future control of total federal allocations for health care may be gained primarily at the expense of the acute care sector (Somers, 1982). If hospitals remain concerned solely with acute care, they may soon be delivering extraordinarily expensive care to a very small fraction of the population. If they do not begin to move into long term care, acute care hospitals may also find themselves at the mercy of the growing and tightly organized for-profit nursing home chains.

The resources, power, research skill, and versatility of acute care hospitals are crucially needed by the growing and changing long term care system. The greatest resistance to hospitals' moving in this direction comes from those who fear that hospitals will "medicalize" the long term care system, bringing expensive, high technology procedures into what should remain a simpler, low technology system. This suspicion concerning acute hospitals reflects a problem in their identity, which has become so tied to technologic interventions that they have difficul-

87

ty recognizing long term care as an important and valued challenge. The demographic and economic realities of an aging society may force a form of identity crisis on acute care hospitals. That process could be painful, but it could also put hospitals in closer touch with their own historical mission of supporting and caring for the elderly and chronically ill.

REFERENCES

Bricker, P.W. Nine Years of Long Term Home Health Care, 1973-1981. New York: St. Vincent's Hospital and Medical Center, 1982.

Campion, E.W., Bang, A. and May, M. "Why Acute-Care Hospitals Must Undertake Long-Term Care." New England Journal of Medicine, 308, pp. 71-75, January 13, 1983.

Eisdorfer, C. "Care of the Aged: The Barriers of Tradition." Annals of Internal Medicine, 94, pp. 256-60, 1981.

Freeland, M., Calat, G. and Schendler, C.E. "Projections of National Health Expenditures, 1980, 1985 and 1990." Health Care Financing Review, 1(3), pp. 1-27, 1980.

Government Accounting Office. The Elderly Remain in Need of Mental Health Services. HRD-82-112. Washington, D.C., September 16, 1982.

Government Accounting Office Report. The Elderly Should Benefit from Expanded Home Health Care But Increasing These Services Will Not Insure Cost Reductions. IPE83-1. Washington, D.C., December 7, 1982.

Government Accounting Office Report. VA Should Consider Less Costly Alternatives Before Constructing New Housing Homes. HRD-82-114. Washington, D.C., September 30, 1982.

Government Accounting Office Report. IPE-82-4. Washington, D.C., July 15, 1982.

Government Accounting Office Report. PAD-80-12. Washington, D.C., November 26, 1979.

The Hospital Research and Educational Trust, American Hospital Association. "Hospitals and Older Adults: Current Actions and Future Trends." In Series on Aging, from Office on Aging and Long Term Care, 1982.

Iglehart, J.K. "Report on the Duke University Medical Center Private Sector Conference." New England Journal of Medicine, 307, pp. 68-71, 1982.

89

Kane, M.L. and Kane, R.A. "Care of the Aged: Old Problems in Need of New Solutions." Science, 200, pp. 913-9, 1978.

Master, R.J., Feltin, M., Jainchill, J., et al. "A Continuum of Care for the Inner City: Assessment of Its Benefits for Boston's Elderly and High-Risk Populations." New England Journal of Medicine, 302, pp. 1434-40, 1980.

Muse, D.N. and Sawyer, D. Medicare and Medicaid Data Book 1981. U.S. Department of Health and Human Services, Washington, D.C., pp. 31-35, 1982.

National Academy of Science. Health Care for American Veterans, report of the Committee on Health Care Resources in the Veterans Administration, Assembly of Life Sciences, National Research Council. Washington, D.C., May, 1977.

Portnoi, V.A. "A Health Care System for the Elderly." New England Journal of Medicine, 300, pp. 87-90, 1979.

Ruchlin, H.S., Morris, J.N. and Eggert, G.M. "Management and Financing Long Term Care Services: A New Approach to a Chronic Problem." New England Journal of Medicine, 306, pp. 101-5, 1982.

Russell, L.B. "An Aging Population and the Use of Medical Care." Medical Care, 19, pp. 633-43, 1981.

Schwartz, J. American Hospital Association Brief, No. 41. Demographic Trends and Hospital Utilization: The Elderly Population. March 17, 1982.

Somers, A. "Long Term Care for the Elderly and Disabled: A New Health Priority." New England Journal of Medicine, 307, pp. 221-6, July 22, 1982.

U.S. Veterans Administration, Administrator of Veterans Affairs. Annual Report, 1982. Washington, D.C., June, 1983.

U.S. Veterans Administration. The Aging Veteran: Present and Future Medical Needs. Washington, D.C., October, 1977.

U.S. Veterans Administration. Health Care of the Aging Veteran: A Report of the Geriatrics and Gerontology Advisory Committee. Washington, D.C., April, 1983.

U.S. Veterans Administration, Office of Program Analysis and Development, Health System Information Service, Data Application and Planning Support. Nursing Home Care Needs of Veterans in 1990: A Quantitative and Social Assessment. 0-361-487/3531, Washington, D.C., USGPO, 1982.

U.S. Veterans Administration, Office of Program Planning and Evaluation. Hospital Based Home Care Program Evaluation. Washington, D.C., July, 1983.

U.S. Veterans Administration, Office of Reports and Statistics. Statistical Brief: A Comparison of Selected Characteristics of VA Nursing Home Patients and National Nursing Home Patients. SB 70-82-4, Washington, D.C., October, 1982.

U.S. Veterans Administration, Office of Reports and Statistics. Summary of Medical Programs. Washington, D.C., September, 1982.

U.S. Veterans Administration, Office of Reports and Statistics. Summary of Medical Programs. Washington, D.C., September, 1983.

Waldo, D.R. and Gibson, R.M. "National Health Expenditures, 1981." Health Care Financing Review, 4(1), pp. 1-35, September, 1982.

5. Experiments and Demonstrations in Sharing and Coordination

Diane S. Piktialis, Ph.D.
Margaret A. Mac Adam, M.S.

Introduction

A major concern of the Veterans Administration is how to provide for the long term care needs of a large number of aged veterans. While this "geriatric imperative" presents a relatively recent challenge for the VA, public policy makers concerned with the needs of the non-veteran aging population have been grappling with how to provide for the long term care needs of the general elderly population for more than a decade. A variety of demonstration projects have been funded by the federal government to examine different organizational arrangements for providing long term care and an impressive array of literature examines financing, organization, and delivery of long term care services. As a result of this long-standing interest, federal legislation and funding have enabled the development of a wide array of institutional, community based, and in-home long term care services which are available to individuals eligible for public assistance. These programs are funded through a combination of Medicare, Medicaid, Social Service Block Grants, Older Americans Act appropriations, and a combination of state and local funding.

These two parallel service systems share a commonality of interest, namely how best to provide long term care for the aged. As with other policy chapters in this book, this chapter attempts to bring together issues related to both the needs of the aged veteran and the needs of the general elderly population. Until now, the interrelationships of these overlapping populations have not been fully examined by policy makers. If the VA is to play a leadership role in addressing the problems of the aged veteran, and provide high quality care for veterans in the least restrictive environment, coordination with all long term care providers and funding sources is imperative.

This chapter focuses on findings from many non-VA demonstrations conducted over the past decade. Early experiments in single service programs, such as adult day health, are discussed first. Demonstrations which tested models of community-wide coordinated care systems will then be described. The third section analyzes new models for long term care such as the Channeling Program and the Social Health Maintenance Organization, which build upon earlier experiments and feature innovative concepts like capitation. The final section will outline possible strategies for VA coordination with the community long term care system.

The challenge to provide for the long term care needs of a rapidly aging veteran population presents an opportunity for the VA to play a leadership role in developing a model national system for long term care. It also provides the chance to prepare providers in the health professions for delivery of geriatric health care through advanced research, education, and training in gerontology and geriatrics.

THE NON-VA LONG TERM CARE SERVICE SYSTEM

Over the past decade, the United States has experienced a heightened interest in problems and policy issues involved in the provision of long term care to the elderly. The piecemeal development of long term care programs led to a "non-system" of long term care plagued by inefficiences and coordination problems. Each public program provided funding for different services, to be provided under different regulations with different eligibility requirements for individuals in need of long term care services. The primary elements of that system included four separate public assistance programs: Medicare, Medi-caid, Title XX and the Older Americans Act (See Appendix A for a description of these programs).

By the early 1970s, increased attention was being focused on several problems in the long term care system. Among these problems were the increasing expenditures for long term care and the excessive utilization of institution based care. Other inefficiencies included lack of coordination of services, lack of availability of needed community services, and poor matching of client needs and services provided. These problems led to a public commitment to develop options for changing the existing forms of financing and organization of long term care service delivery.

LONG TERM CARE DEMONSTRATIONS

Experiments[1] in providing alternatives to institutional care and mechanisms for coordinating community care became the major strategy of the Health Care Financing Administration (HCFA) to address the problems presented by growing numbers of elders needing service. Both single service demonstrations and community wide coordination projects were funded and evaluated. The latter type of demonstration was designed to provide a coordinated system of health and social services. Coordination of care was an important component in these experiments since, unlike nursing homes which are primarily funded by Medicaid, non-institutional long term care services are funded by many agencies at the federal, state, and local levels. The intent of the demonstrations was to develop alternatives that would be more appropriate and cost effective. In addition to providing alternative long term care delivery systems, these early demonstrations also attempted to provide data on a number of other questions: 1) could community based services be targeted to those certifiable for nursing home care or those "at risk of institutionalization," 2) were expanded community based benefit packages cost effective -- that is, less costly than institutional forms of care, 3) could utilization of community based

---

[1] The terms demonstration and experiment will be used interchangeably to refer to demonstration projects designed to test new options for providing long term care.

services forestall and/or substitute for institutional care, and 4) could non-institutional alternatives have a positive impact on patient or client outcomes?

The early long term care demonstrations were not research projects, per se, rather they were demonstrations of how to develop non-institutional services and keep frail elderly people at home. Those that are described in this chapter were chosen because they represent those projects which had an evaluation component and therefore which collected data for analysis. Because these early programs were not designated as research projects, the findings have frequently been criticized on methodological grounds. However, they do provide the basis upon which most of the long term care literature and service delivery systems have been established.

SINGLE SERVICE DEMONSTRATIONS

Several long term care policy issues were first addressed by early single service demonstrations conducted under the authority of Section 222 (B) of the 1972 Amendments to the Social Security Act. The policy issues of interest in these experiments were serving the elderly in need of health and social services, demonstrating the effectiveness of alternatives to institutionalization, containing costs and developing an alternative public policy.

As a means of containing costs and providing alternative means of delivering long term care services, two experiments were conducted. One assessed the impact of homemaker services on clients discharged from acute care facilities who required post hospital services. The less intensive services were to be offered as alternatives in addition to regular benefits under Medicare (Part A). The second experiment would offer adult day care to clients in need of continuing care under Medicare (Part B). At about the same time, other adult day care demonstration programs developed independently of the Section 222 experiments, most notably On Lok in San Francisco. The following discussion of single service demonstrations will begin with the adult day health care experiments.

I. Adult Day Health Care Experiments

Adult day health care programs generally offer a range of psychiatric, health, and/or social services. Among

96

adult day health service centers, there is considerable
variation in the relative focus on health as opposed to
social services. Weissert (1978) has examined these differences to conceptualize some of the variables by which
the two types can be categorized. However, most considerations of adult day health care as a long term care benefit have emphasized programs predominantly oriented toward
health-rehabilitation. A definition of this health model
of day care was drafted and incorporated into the Section
222 legislation which authorized examination of adult day
health service programs as an alternative to institutional
long term care. That definition follows:

> "Day Care" is a program of services provided un-
> der health leadership in an ambulatory care set-
> ting for adults who do not require 24 hour insti-
> tutional care and yet, due to physical and/or
> mental impairment, are not capable of full-time
> independent living. Participants in the day care
> program are referred to the program by their at-
> tending physician or by some other appropriate
> source such as an institutional discharge plan-
> ning program, a welfare agency, etc. The essen-
> tial elements of a day care program are directed
> toward meeting the health maintenance and resto-
> ration needs of participants. However, there are
> socialization elements in the program which, by
> overcoming the isolation so often associated with
> illness in the aged and disabled, are considered
> vital for the purposes of fostering and maintain-
> ing the maximum possible state of health and
> well-being (U.S. Congress, 1976, pp. 8-9).

While experiments in adult day health care did not address policy issues related to changing the service delivery system, they did examine the potential for adult day
care programs as an alternative to institutional placement. The target group of concern was individuals receiving nursing home care because of a lack of service availability in the community. In their review of the literature, Stasson and Holakan (1981) identify a number of advantages of adult day health that have been advanced by
gerontologists. These potential advantages include:

1) Day care might postpone institutionalization by
    providing preventive care.

2) Day care may substitute for nursing home care by providing older people with an array of services including respite care for families and other informal supporters.

3) Day care may substitute for convalescent care in a nursing home following a period of hospitalization.

4) Day care may provide an alternative in areas where availability of community based and in-home services are in short supply.

5) Day care might allow an elderly person to maintain a community residence and current social relationships.

6) Depending on how frequently an individual used day health care, this alternative might prove less costly than nursing home care.

A review of several day care programs follows, along with a brief discussion of evaluation findings.

On Lok

While On Lok has expanded and broadened its orientation and operation since its inception in 1972, it began with a day health center emphasis in response to an Administration on Aging (AOA) request for proposals for an Adult Day Center. Prior to that (1971-1972), On Lok had received a series of grants from the National Institutes of Health to develop a service organization. AOA funding lasted for three years, 1972-1975, and enabled the development of day health operating and service capacity. In addition, the On Lok Senior Health Services program received state Title XIX monies earmarked for day health center projects. The expanded On Lok efforts during subsequent phases of development are described elsewhere. The findings of early evaluation of the adult day health center experiments are detailed below.

Program description. While the On Lok day care experiment developed in incremental stages and under several funding sources, the program was characterized by the following basic components. On Lok provided an array of health and social services to elderly Chinese in the North Beach section of San Francisco. Most of the project participants were elderly males who spoke little English and who were frequently living alone on incomes below $3,600 per year. Compared to the national nursing home population, On Lok clients were dissimilar in terms of both eth-

98

nicity and sex distribution, being predominantly Chinese and male.

Criteria for admission to the day health center included: required post-operative care or rehabilitation or at least one acute or chronic medical condition that required treatment. Based on assessment of participants' functional and cognitive abilities, about 5% were considered sufficiently impaired to require nursing home care. Although the majority of clients could take care of themselves with assistance from others, most were dependent on assistance in activities of daily living such as bathing, dressing, toileting, and household tasks such as laundry.

Program evaluation. From 1974 to 1978 On Lok underwent three different evaluations. While each methodological approach had different strengths and weaknesses, the findings are summarized below.

1. The first evaluation of On Lok was based on data gathered on 94 clients over a six-month period in 1974. Analysis of the program's impact on participants was based on measurement of four indicators: medical or health status, functional capacity, cognitive function, and level of care required. This evaluation found marked improvement in medical status which may have been partly a function of most participants having been admitted to the program after hospitalization. Some improvement in functional status was also found. No change was found in the mean rating of cognitive status of the group nor was there change in level of care required.

When compared to a matched community comparison group, there was some improvement in function in the day care group. Day care costs were found to be less expensive than care in a skilled nursing facility and more expensive than care in an intermediate care facility. Evidence also indicated that many On Lok clients would not have entered nursing homes, yet day care filled an unmet need for the less severely impaired. Thus, services provided by On Lok in its early years met needs that otherwise would have been unmet, yet because it did not provide an alternative or substitute for nursing home care, it added to the total systems cost for long term care.

2. A second evaluation also considered the impact of day care on service utilization, on clients, and on costs. The major service utilization impact was the reduction of days spent in a skilled nursing facility by 90% for individuals qualifying for adult day health care. When measuring perceived client impact, researchers found day care clients were satisfied with their health, the services they received, their physical and social environment, and life in general. Day care participants were most satisfied with the health care they received.

The cost analysis found that service costs were similar for both the day care and the control groups. When considering total government costs, it appeared that day care costs were lower than those of care in a skilled nursing facility, but higher than the costs of caring for individuals in board and care homes or maintaining them in their own homes.

3. The third evaluation conducted by the state of California found that 87% of On Lok participants in the third year of the project were not institutionalized in either a hospital or long term care facility. Costs for adult day health were determined to average $25.62 per day. When compared to California Medicaid costs, per capita costs for day health participants were lower than for nursing home clients. However, as noted earlier, the research did not demonstrate that individuals participating in the adult day health program would have been institutionalized if the day care program had not been developed.

The evaluation report did conclude that the On Lok day care program was successful. "It clearly showed that persons judged eligible for ICF and SNF as well as those persons at risk of institutionalization, can be cared for in a more humane and less costly way without enduring the trauma of disruption of lifestyle and family relationships which accompanies long term institutionalization" (Von Behren, 1978, p. 86).

Summary. From a policy perspective, On Lok was successful in the areas of patient care and program operations. It was successful in providing services to a frail elderly population and filled a service gap in community services. This program's success was instrumental in the state-wide development of adult day care as a part of the California Medicaid program.

100

Despite the program's successes, the research did not demonstrate that adult day care would reduce overall public expenditures on long term care. This is because adult day care services, though less costly than nursing home care, did not substitute for institutional care, thus there were increased overall costs to the system. In spite of the lack of definitive conclusions on nursing home substitution or cost, the program did provide an appropriate service to a population in need.

Section 222 Day Care Experiments

Experiments in providing day care and homemaker services were conducted under authority of Section 222 of the 1972 Amendments to the Social Security Act. This section will describe only the policy issues and findings of the day care experiments while the next section will discuss, in greater detail, the results of the homemaker demonstrations.

The Section 222 Day Care experiments were carried out under the auspices of the National Center for Health Services Research with funding by Medicare. There were four demonstration sites across the country: San Francisco, California; White Plains, New York; Syracuse, New York; and Lexington, Kentucky. All four programs provided a medical model of adult day health care, though both health and social services were provided. Thirteen services were required at all sites. These were:

Nursing	Social Services
Patient Activities	Nutrition Services
Personal Care	Transportation
Meals	Speech Therapy
Physical Therapy	Hearing Examinations
Eye Examinations	Occupational Therapy
Podiatry	

The relative utilization of these services, however, varied across sites and in the opinion of some analysts, significantly changed the intervention so as to render general conclusions about costs and client outcomes somewhat difficult.

The major policy issue of concern in the 222 projects was whether Medicare should cover adult day health and/or homemaker services. In other words, would availability of these services assist in containing costs, demonstrating

101

the effectiveness of non-institutional alternatives, and assist in the development of an alternative public policy?

In order to receive services under the demonstration, clients had to be Medicare eligible and satisfy a number of other eligibility criteria (U.S. DHHS, HCFA, January, 1981). Referrals were solicited from physicians, hospitals, and community agencies. Clients who were eligible were assessed by a clinical team the composition of which varied across sites. Assessments were performed on both the experimental and control groups. The assessment considered client health, clinical needs, and functional status. Once a care plan was developed and signed off by the client's physician, services were provided for a period of one year from the date of admission and the client was reassessed periodically during the course of that year. Assignment to a control group did not occur until after a care plan was developed.

Research and evaluation design. An experimental design was used to study the project with half of the eligibles assigned to experimental groups and half to control groups which did not receive day care services. Data were collected on 384 participants.

A number of factors was felt to affect the research design and hence the research findings. First, although an evaluation contractor was selected, data collection was the responsibility of each site. Because each site had a slightly different data collection system based on the information system already in place, somewhat different data were collected from each site. For example, changes in functional status were not reported uniformly across providers. A second problem stemmed from the different population characteristics across sites. Finally, as noted earlier, the interventions were not comparable in the different sites because of differences in the mix of services provided at each site. Despite these differences, data were pooled for the analysis, which may hide some program outcomes.

Utilization. Across sites, the study found that individuals who had recently been hospitalized used day care services most frequently. However, findings did not indicate that day care was a substitute for either hospital or nursing home care. Hospital utilization rates did not vary between the experimental and control groups. When examining the overall use of skilled nursing facilities by both groups, evaluators found that day care acted more as an additional benefit under Medicare rather than as a substitute for institutional care. In those instances in which day care services functioned as an alternative, it was as a substitute for short term nursing home stays, not for long term institutionalization.

Costs. Overall, the study found that for the project participants, day care was not less costly than other services in the existing system. Although day care reduced the average use of existing Medicare services by $543 annually, adding the additional day costs ($52 per day; $3,235 per year) raised the annual net Medicare cost 71% even though clients were not institutionalized ($6,501 for experimental group vs $3,809 for control group). One important limitation in this cost comparison is the inclusion of exclusively Medicare costs. Thus, assessment of the impact of day care services on total system costs was not possible.

Outcomes. Members of the experimental group had lower death rates than the control group. Patients who received services experienced improvements or maintained physical functioning and social activity, though these differences were not statistically significant.

The results of the Section 222 day care experiments suggested a need to examine more fully the appropriate mix of services to be provided in a day care program.

Summary of Day Care Experiments

As indicated in the On Lok and Section 222 experiments, it was found that most day care participants would not have received care in a nursing home if the day care program had not been available. This finding is common to other day care experiments (Stasson and Holakan, 1981). Evaluators suggested that day care may be able to substitute for inpatient services for some subgroups of the population. Frequency of attendance and mix of services provided are also important in determining the scope of substitution. Although day care services may substitute for institutional care in some instances, the majority of participants who used these services in early demonstrations would not have entered a nursing home. Thus, total system costs of providing day care can apparently increase. On the other hand, day care generally has a positive effect on participants' outcomes.

II. In-Home Services

Some experts have suggested that inappropriate nursing home placements and overall expenditures for long term care could be reduced through the provision of in-home services. Shortened lengths of hospital stays and reduced chance of readmission are purported benefits. While most admit that provision of in-home services would probably increase total costs because they would most likely be provided to some elderly people who would not otherwise have been institutionalized, substitution may occur depending on the type of population toward which services are targeted. Others claim home care services can have a positive impact by preventing illness or deterioration in functional capacity thereby preventing or delaying the need for long term institutional care. While the literature on in-home services by no means answers these questions definitively, the results of at least one major study of in-home services, the Section 222 Homemaker demonstrations, will be presented. This study was chosen because it was designed as a service program to substitute for long term institutional care.

Section 222 Homemaker Experiments

Findings from a study of Section 222 experiments to demonstrate the possible effects of adding homemaker services to benefits under the Medicare program have been reported by Weissert, Wan, and Liveratos (1980). As with the day care demonstrations, four sites were developed: San Francisco, California; Los Angeles, California; Providence, Rhode Island; and Lexington, Kentucky. Eligibility and assignment to an experimental and control group operated similarly to the day care sites. Homemaker services were provided to participants for a period of a year. Allowable activities under this service included home management, such as cooking, cleaning, laundry, and related tasks; personal care, such as assistance in bathing, dressing, eating, walking, etc.; supportive services which included activities outside the home such as walking; and health management services.

104

The evaluation of these projects suffered similar methodological problems as those noted in relation to the day care experiments. Researchers found great variation by site in the number of hours of service used by each client as well as substantial variation in the cost per unit of service across sites. The research also found that homemaker services did not significantly affect institutionalization rates and concluded that these services did not substitute for nursing home care nor was the population using homemaker services likely to have used nursing homes at all. With respect to client outcomes, however, the study found that homemaker recipients had a lower death rate than the control group and that a greater proportion of the experimental group experienced improvement in functional capacity compared to the control group. Improved or maintained levels of functioning were also found in client satisfaction, mental functioning, and social activity in the experimental group.

Cost analysis found that the average cost of Medicare services, excluding homemaker services, was greater for the experimental group than for the control group. It was hypothesized that homemakers could have contributed to greater use of health services since homemakers could act as a monitor of clients' health. Costs of services provided by funding sources other than Medicare were not included in the analysis.

Thus, these experiments found that expanded homemaker services would not decrease total costs since these services functioned as an additional service and not as a substitute for institutionalization. In spite of increased cost, however, homemaker services also seemed to have positive impact upon patient functioning by reducing mortality rates and improving life satisfaction, mental functioning, and social activity.

COMMUNITY-WIDE COORDINATION PROJECTS

This section of the chapter will describe the early long term care coordination experiments and discuss the findings of their evaluations. The assumption behind this first group of projects was that community-wide, coordinated care projects could better address long term care policy issues than single service strategies (Stasson and Holakan, 1981). Consequently, the focus of the projects was less on the direct services provided than on the effects of providing client management services improving both the coordination of care and the likelihood of appropriate placement (Stasson and Holakan, 1981). While discussion of all the early experiments is beyond the scope of this chapter, we have attempted to include the most noteworthy and representative and those most frequently discussed in the long term care literature because they included some evaluation component to assess outcomes.

Triage – Connecticut

Project Triage was initiated by the state of Connecticut in February, 1974. Triage was a single entry, service coordination effort for Medicare eligible elderly in a small seven-town area in central Connecticut. Federal funding for research and Section 222 waiver authority began in 1975. As in all Section 222 projects, services were funded by Medicare. When the project stopped taking clients in April, 1978, its active case load was 1517. Another 2106 were on a waiting list. During its five years as a demonstration, Triage served approximately 2128 clients.

Program description. The Triage project involved a channeling or single entry point agency concept with comprehensive coverage of health and social services for the elderly. Triage provided:

1) service coordination including client assessment and periodic reassessment, ordering services, and referral to other service providers;
2) follow-up and monitoring including periodic review of care plans, contact with the client, and review of claims for services rendered; and
3) direct services.

In order to provide appropriate services, Triage developed new services where needed. Services available to clients, in addition to traditional Medicare benefits included:

Home Health Aides   Home Delivered Meals
Homemaker Services   Chore Services
Nursing and Physician Visits   Companion Services
Psychological and Family   Dental Care
   Counseling

106

Medicare waivers removed traditional Medicare requirements for coinsurance and deductibles. The waivers also eliminated many restrictions placed on home health care such as the three-day prior hospitalization requirement, the 100 visit limit, the homebound requirement, and the skilled nursing definition.

Unlike other single entry point demonstrations, Triage did not target services to those individuals most at risk of institutionalization. All elderly people in the target area were eligibile to receive assessment and services. The use of the assessment function to regulate service provision was the major test of cost effectiveness. The intention was to reduce overall utilization by providing interventions or preventive services that would postpone rapid deterioration. Clients enrolled on a first-come, first-served basis, with neither income nor health status as criterion for eligibility.

Triage contracted with local providers for most services and providers operated under Medicare Part B regulations. All provider contracts specified that for Triage clients, only services authorized by Triage would be reimbursed.

The clients served by Triage were similar to the nation's elderly population in age, marital status and living arrangements. The client group was not as old or as predominantly female as the nursing home population.

Program evaluation. For evaluation purposes, a comparison group of 195 individuals from another county were matched with 307 Triage clients. The focus of the analysis was on the difference between the two groups on per capita expenditures, the rate of institutionalization within each group, and the effectiveness of services received.

Many reports on Triage and other early demonstration projects point out the methodological problems inherent in the quasi-experimental research and evaluation design. In Triage, for example, it is difficult to judge the comparability of the experimental and control groups (Stasson and Holakan, 1981). Keeping in mind these limitations, research findings are presented below.

Service utilization and cost. While the absence of an appropriate control group precludes definitive conclusions, analysis of the available data suggests that a Triage type program would be more expensive, requiring greater expenditures than the existing health care system. The data also indicate that substitution of non-institutional services for institutional care did not occur. The per capita costs for a Triage client were 8-32% higher than those in the comparison group. However, the Triage service population was somewhat more impaired than the control group which might contribute to the cost difference. Expanded benefits for many services might also have increased utilization. Finally, the cost-savings in the Triage model were a function of reducing per capita health care costs by preventing the need for costly services sometime in the future. Short term findings could not adequately test whether this objective was met.

Client outcomes. While methodological issues also make it difficult to identify outcomes of the Triage intervention, some tentative conclusions about client outcomes are possible. Fewer Triage clients experienced increased functional dependence than the control group. A greater number of clients in Triage showed improved mental status functioning over time. Overall, preliminary findings suggest that the Triage project may have achieved improved health status for their clients, though at increased overall costs to the government.

ACCESS - Monroe County, New York

Program description. ACCESS (the Monroe County Long Term Care Program in upstate New York) was designed as a single entry point for all long term care services on a county-wide basis. Clients entered the program through a central unit which received referrals from both the community and acute care hospitals. Program components included a comprehensive assessment of all clients applying for long term care services, and development of a service plan for all clients for whom home care was considered an option. ACCESS did not provide direct patient services. To be eligible for ACCESS, an individual had to be a resident of Monroe County, 18 years of age or older, and need either in-home or institutional long term care services. Control of service utilization of the Medicaid population was accomplished by requiring all Medicaid eligible clients to be referred to ACCESS. Medicaid clients were assessed free of charge.

ACCESS had strong information, outreach, and public relations components that were considered a part of the intervention. Individuals referred to ACCESS were screened during intake to determine if they met a set of predetermined "criteria." If eligible, the individual was then assessed. If not, the person was referred to other service providers. Eligible clients received a comprehensive assessment by a case manager either in the home or in a hospital setting. A care plan was developed based on this assessment. The care plan was then analyzed to determine if it would cost less than 75% of the cost of institutional care. If the cost exceeded the limit, Medicaid approval was required before the plan could be implemented. Non-Medicaid clients could also have care plans developed, though these clients had to arrange for payment of recommended services on their own. Families and clients were also involved in the development of the care plan.

After the care plan was finalized and approved, ACCESS case managers arranged for services. Services not reimbursable under Medicaid (e.g., home maintenance, housing and moving assistance, chore services, transportation, respite care, and friendly visiting) were provided under waivers of Medicaid regulations. The ACCESS program also provided follow-up and monitoring to Medicaid recipients receiving care in the community and Medicaid recipients in institutions.

In the initial 14 months of the project, ACCESS received 3434 referrals: 1735 from community resources, and 1699 from hospitals. Of these, 2492 received assessments.

Program evaluation. The evaluation design, originally concerned with issues of cost utilization and the effectiveness of ACCESS, changed over time to focus primarily on long term care cost-related issues. The experimental design was a case study approach documenting cost and institutional occupancy rates before and after the intervention. Because the intervention was system-wide, random assignment of clients to experimental and control groups was not feasible, nor were project evaluators able to secure funding for a "matched sample" evaluation approach. These data constraints limit the definitiveness of the findings which were based on a comparison of levels of and changes in Medicaid expenditures for Monroe County and six comparison counties. A second part of the evaluation included analysis of impact on acute care back-up and the third was an analysis of differences in rates of change in per capita Medicaid expenditures in the respective counties.

Findings. The research data indicate that Medicaid days in skilled nursing and health related facilities declined but that back-up days for Medicaid patients in acute hospitals increased. It is difficult to identify causes of decline in overall nursing home days in that available nursing home beds were increasingly scarce. Private pay patient demand could account for this reduction in Medicaid nursing home days as could availability of alternative community based services for Medicaid recipients. However, because the study design could not control for differences in counties, definitive conclusions were not possible.

Data on the overall level of expenditures were more easily comparable, and the comparisons showed that costs of long term care services were not lower in Monroe County than in comparison counties.

Measurement of changes in patient outcomes, in terms of mortality, functional status, or patient satisfaction was beyond the scope of the evaluation.

Alternative Health Services Project - Georgia

The Georgia Alternative Health Services Project (AHS) was established to test the cost effectiveness of comprehensive, community based long term care services as an alternative to nursing home care for the Medicaid eligible elderly. Medicaid eligible clients were offered three service alternatives: adult rehabilitation, in-home and supportive services, and alternative living services. In addition to the above services, clients were assessed by a multidisciplinary team and service providers were designated as case coordinators and were responsible for developing a care plan and arranging for services. The case coordinator either directly provided services or contracted with other providers for service delivery. The original assessment team assumed and maintained the role of case manager, monitoring the client's progress, recommending changes in the care plan, and deciding when to terminate service. Care plans were limited by guidelines that quantified service costs, which could not exceed $500 per client per month. The target population included Med-

110

icaid eligible persons 50 years of age or older who were either in a nursing home or certified as eligible for nursing home care. The project evaluation was based on random assignment of project participants to an experimental or control group. Participants in the control group received services already available in the community.

The project began in July, 1976, and by the end of the second operational year, there were approximately 1200 clients in the project's service and control groups.

When compared to the national nursing home population, the AHS group was younger, had more blacks, had a similar sex distribution, and had approximately the same number of individuals living alone. Information on health status, mental functioning, and social support systems was not available for comparison purposes.

Program evaluation. The evaluation was based on an experimental design in which 75% of the clients appropriate for the project were assigned to the experimental group to receive the case coordination and full service components of AHS. Twenty-five percent of the eligible clients were assigned to a control group. The control group could not receive AHS services, but they could receive nursing home care or any other services regularly available in the community. The findings summarized below were based on a December, 1979, client case load by which time 1016 clients had been assigned to the experimental group and 320 to the control group.

Service utilization. Analysis of preliminary data indicated that AHS was a potential substitute for Medicaid home health care and a substitute for a combination of home health and nursing home care. When comparing data on nursing home use, the utilization of nursing home and Medicaid home health services was 6% lower for the client group in the AHS program than for the controls. Also, Medicaid costs for the AHS intervention, nursing home and home health costs were 58% lower for the experimental group than the cost for the combination of nursing and home health services provided to the control group.

For most project participants, AHS did not substitute for institutional placement, but rather served as an additional source of care. Only 13% of the experimental group did not receive project services. While all control group members were certified as appropriate for nursing home

111

care, fully 69% did not receive any long term care services. Other factors, such as limited service availability, may have contributed to this finding though the evidence is not conclusive.

At the time of the evaluation, the project was considering adding a mandatory nursing home preadmission screening program which was expected to change the rate and extent of substitution for nursing home care.

Cost. Average monthly total Medicaid costs were lower for the AHS service recipients than for the control group members ($208 vs $591). However, the data did not include costs not reimbursed directly by the Medicaid program such as Medicare, Title XX, SSI, etc., costs to the client, or informal support systems for maintenance in the community. The addition of these costs would possibly increase the cost of maintaining an AHS client in the community compared to the controls. Thus, the findings did not support any definitive conclusion about whether it is less costly to keep someone in the community with an intervention such as AHS than to use the existing service system.

Client outcome. No statistically significant differences were found in client outcomes as measured by activities of daily living, instrumental activities of daily living, mental status and morale. However, project participants had a reduced mortality rate during the first year when compared with control group members (13% vs 25%).

Community Based Care Systems for the Functionally Disabled in the State of Washington

Like many other long term care demonstrations, the Community Based Care project in the state of Washington was based on the concept of a single entry agency for long term care. A three-year demonstration project, funded through a Section 1115 grant from the Health Care Financing Administration (HCFA), was established to provide an organization for the provision of health and social services to the physically disabled and aged persons at high risk of institutionalization in a community setting. Services included those authorized under Titles XIX and XX. High risk was defined as an individual so impaired as to probably require institutional placement within the next six months or an individual in a nursing home who could return to community living with the assistance of an array of health and social services.

The intervention included development of a Community Services Unit (CSU) which provided a client with needs assessment, care plan development, and coordinated arrangement for the necessary services with providers in the community. Two CSUs delivered services to approximately 793 clients for 22 months.

Program description. The CSU served as the single entry point for elders residing in the community and offered residential services for individuals at high risk of institutional placement and eligible for SSI, Title XIX, Title XX, or other social services. Clients were self-referred or referred by family members, physicians, and other health providers from community agencies.

The CSU teams were comprised of a project nurse, a social worker, a medical consultant community worker, and a case worker. The project nurse was responsible for all decisions about nursing home placement. Each CSU site supervisor was responsible for developing and maintaining a network of community service providers.

The CSU had prime responsibility for service planning and coordination for each client. Upon referral to the CSU, each client was assessed by an interdisciplinary team which evaluated the need for services and was responsible for arranging an appropriate package of institutional and non-institutional services. Teams also provided case management by monitoring clients and reviewing "high risk" clients monthly.

Due to Title XIX and Title XX waivers, the following wide range of services was available for care planning:

Congregate Care
Adult Family Homes
Adult Day Care
Congregate Meals
Sheltered Workshops
Visiting Nurse Service
Home Health Aide
Chore Services
Home Delivered Meals

Reassurance
Senior Volunteer Companion
Housekeeping
Meal Preparation
Yard and Home Maintenance
Personal Care
Winterization and
    Household Repairs
Housing Referral
    Information

113

Cost considerations were an integral part of care planning and service allocation. The team was discouraged from developing a care plan to maintain an individual in the community that exceeded the cost of institutional placement unless a short term community placement was likely to lead to less costly nursing home care over the long term. Only "high risk" clients received assessments and project services through the CSU. Other clients received services from the existing system. A further intent of this project was to evaluate the overall demand for services among the "high risk" population. With the exception of mental functioning, the project participants exhibited an impairment level that was not substantially different from that of the population residing in institutions.

Project evaluation. The program evaluation included a quasi-experimental design. Client experience in the two CSU sites was compared to a sample of recipients in a comparison county chosen to provide a comparison group for the 15-month experimental phase of the project. The evaluation reported on service utilization (both nursing home and community based care), total systems costs, and the cost of nursing home versus community based care. Evaluation of client outcomes was not reported.

Service utilization. Nursing home utilization declined in the two demonstration sites during the course of the project, reducing overall utilization by the Medicaid population. Analysis showed a growth in provision of community based services for most services during the project period. This was most evident for chore services.

Cost. The project evaluation concluded that in spite of the decrease in use of nursing homes by the Medicaid population, total systems costs increased in both experimental sites. The project experienced an unequivocal increase in the demand for community services by persons living in the community. Considered individually, community based care was shown to be less costly than care in a nursing home. The cost of case management in the demonstration represented 40% of the total cost of community based care. Overall, public expenditures on community based care were less costly because project participants did not receive the full range of health and social services provided in an institution.

114

The Wisconsin Community Care Organization

The Wisconsin Community Care Organization Project (CCO) was a HCFA 1115 waiver, research and demonstration project which operated from 1975-1980. The project was designed to implement an organizational structure for a comprehensive community based program to provide coordinated in-home and community services to functionally disabled individuals. The demonstration tested whether this organizational structure could delay or prevent institutionalization, deliver services at less cost than an equivalent level of institutional service, and whether these alternative services could produce positive outcomes in client functioning and quality of life. The project was implemented in three counties and was accompanied by a well-developed evaluation.

Program description. The CCO units were established at three sites throughout the state, each of which operated independently. For example, the sites differed in terms of target population, services developed, and coordinating mechanisms utilized. The Milwaukee site admitted the most disabled clients who were eligible for Medicaid. Milwaukee also used case management as a formalized coordination mechanism. Client pathways at the three sites differed somewhat in detail, although each provided client intake, assessment, care planning, ordering services, and reassessment.

In order to hold local agencies responsible for the scope and amount of services they were providing prior to the development of the CCO project, the LaCrosse and Milwaukee sites built a "maintenance of effort requirement" into their contracts with providers. By allowing each agency already involved with a case to maintain a certain degree of power in that case including case planning development, the effectiveness of the CCO project was diminished by the maintenance of effort requirement. Existing patterns of fragmented service delivery were maintained.

Although the project was originally intended to target services to individuals who would have required institutional care if they did not receive in-home services, and despite using an assessment instrument designed as a screening device, the actual clients who participated in the program were not at high risk of being placed in institutions even though they had very real unmet service needs.

115

Finally, the project experienced strong opposition to a vigorous evaluation with random assignment of clients. It was not until the second site, Milwaukee, was chosen that it became possible to institute a truly experimental design with random assignment. For this reason, only the findings from the Milwaukee site will be discussed.

The Milwaukee site. During the course of the demonstration, a total of 1143 clients were served at the Milwaukee site. Of these, only 417 were randomly assigned to the experimental and control groups. All clients were eligible for Medicaid.

Comparison of the experimental and control groups prior to the interventions indicated there were no statistically significant differences between the groups in the following areas: proportion of elderly and disabled, sex, marital status, year of birth and race. Some differences between the groups (though not statistically significant) indicate that the experimental group may have been at greater risk of nursing home placement.

Cost. Because of the maintenance of effort criteria, most project participants received both CCO and non-CCO services. Because utilization data were only available on CCO services, total service use was probably underestimated. About half the clients received one or two services, while 75% of the remaining received three or four services. The most frequently used services were: homemaker, home delivered meals, transportation, and personal care.

The evaluation included analysis of Medicaid utilization and cost data collected through the state's Medicaid MIS system. These data indicated that CCO services substituted for traditional Medicaid services particularly in the areas of hospital and home health care, and that total Medicaid costs of providing services through the demonstration did not increase total system costs. Some analysts have concluded, however, that data and targeting problems make the cost effectiveness analysis inconclusive (U.S. DHHS, Project Share, 1981). Also, non-CCO costs were not counted, nor were other Medicaid costs such as SSI payments or food stamps.

Utilization. Medicaid data for nursing home utilization indicated that members of the control group spent more days in hospitals and nursing homes than CCO recipi-

116

ents (14.3 vs 2.95 hospital days and 37.8 vs 29.2 nursing home days). Only 2-3% of nursing home referrals were de-institutionalized indicating that the ability of a project such as this to take individuals out of a nursing home and maintain them in the community is doubtful. The ability to prevent institutionalization was statistically insignificant.

Client outcomes. As noted earlier, evaluation of client outcomes was limited. Disability score comparisons suggested that there was no statistically significant difference between experimental and control groups in the area of physical functioning.

Summary of Community-Wide Coordinated Care Programs

This section has reviewed five long term care demonstrations to provide coordinated long term care services. While the projects varied greatly in terms of program organization, the findings can be summarized with respect to several important policy questions identified in the Urban Institute's working paper: Long Term Care Demonstration Project: A Review of Recent Evaluations (Stasson and Holakan, 1981). The questions are:

1) What were methodological problems with the research and evaluation aspects of these projects?

2) Does use of community based, coordinated programs reduce utilization of institutional services such as nursing home and hospital care?

3) What are the costs of these experiments?

4) Do communty-wide programs increase or decrease overall system costs?

5) Are outcomes of clients receiving services through non-institutional outcomes improved?

Table 1 summarizes the findings of these five experiments in coordination. Overall, these demonstrations indicate that attempts to coordinate care on a community-wide basis did effect the organization of long term care service delivery. While total systems costs increased, policy makers concluded that several desirable social outcomes were significant. These included the provision of

117

Table 1

REPORTED OUTCOMES OF FIVE COMMUNITY COORDINATION EXPERIMENTS

	Institutional Utilization	Costs of Service Coordination	Overall System Costs	Client Outcomes
TRIAGE	Increased	No definitive conclusions	Increased	Less functional dependence/Improved health status/ Improved mental status
ACCESS	Decreased	No definitive conclusions	Reduced	Not reported
GEORGIA	Decreased	No definitive conclusions	Increased	Reduced mortality rates; no other statistically significant differences
WASH. STATE	Decreased	No definitive conclusions	Increased	Not reported
WISCONSIN	No difference	No definitive conclusions	No difference	No statistically different outcomes reported

more appropriate services, the ability to serve more people with unmet needs, and improved methods of allocating services.

Summary of Findings Relating to the Cost and Service Effectiveness of the Early Long Term Care Demonstrations

This section of the chapter has reviewed a number of the critical studies and demonstrations in long term care. Analysis has focused on early experiments in community-wide coordinated care programs and some review of single service experiments was provided. While the limitations in many of the research and evaluation designs were noted, these demonstrations provided a great deal of information to public policy makers concerned with critical questions about long term care benefits for in-home and community based services. Issues for which much information was gathered included the cost effectiveness of non-institutional care, whether non-institutional care substitutes for nursing home care, whether community based alternatives in and of themselves are more or less expensive than nursing home care, and finally, whether community based services can improve client outcomes.

Here, the research findings will be summarized and also conclusions will be discussed of a recent GAO report (Comptroller General, 1982) and of a Department of Health and Human Services report (U.S. DHHS, HCFA, January, 1981), both of which attempted to analyze the implications of these various experiments for future long term care public policy.

Substitution for nursing home care. From the review of the most prominent demonstrations in community-wide care, day care, and in-home services programs, experts have concluded that there is only limited evidence that community based services substitute for nursing home care. Only one project, however, reported increased use of skilled nursing facilities and other services for project participants. Overall, evidence indicates that coordinated community based services could serve as substitutes for nursing home care for some persons which suggests the need for more focused targeting efforts to serve individuals who otherwise would have entered nursing homes. Evidence from the early organized care demonstrations generally indicate that the persons served were not as im-

119

paired as the nursing home population, though they were more disabled than the general elderly population. Even programs designed to serve the prospective nursing home population, such as Georgia and Washington state, were not particularly successful in targeting services. These demonstrations also pointed out the importance of a person's marital status and living arrangement on the amount and type of service used. Persons living alone and without a spouse frequently lacked sufficient resources to remain in the community even with supportive services.

Similarly, the GAO and DHHS reports found that expanded community based services did not always substitute for nursing home or hospital use. Both reports indicated the need to better identify high risk populations in need of service in order to delay or prevent institutionalization. Early studies showed wide variability in the effectiveness of targeting efforts, lack of clear cut definitions of risk factors, and insufficiently clear guidelines "relating level of functioning or other client characteristics to service need and service setting" (U.S. DHHS, HCFA, January, 1981, p. 35). Of particular importance, is the need to identify those patients who can be treated at a lower cost in the community and those whose disability level is such that it will be more expensive to maintain that person at home or in the community.

Cost of community based long term care service packages. Findings of the early demonstrations showed that while these coordinated service packages substituted for institutional care in some cases, overall cost reductions from using these less costly services did not occur. Only two evaluations indicated that programs did not increase overall costs. Cost comparisons were also frequently limited to consideration of only those costs associated with the community programs not total public subsidy of a client including programs such as SSI or food stamps. Finally, study conclusions took note of the fact that the programs served many more persons than were likely to be placed in nursing homes, thus adding to, not substituting for, services in the system. While these findings do not apply to all projects, it does appear that the early community based programs increased rather than decreased total costs. Again, a major reason for this was the unwillingness or inability to target services to persons who were most likely to be in nursing homes at the time of the demonstration or in the near future. Table 2 summarizes reported effects of demonstrations on costs.

```
═══════════════════════════════════════════════════════════════════
                            Table 2
        REPORTED EFFECTS OF LONG TERM CARE DEMONSTRATIONS ON COSTS
```

	Nursing Home Costs	Hospital Costs	Total Costs (a)
Studies using control group			
Georgia (1982)	No difference	No difference	Increased (b)
Georgia (1981)	No difference	Increased (b)	Increased (b)
Wisconsin (1980)	No difference	Reduced (b)	No difference
Section 222 Day Care			Probably increased
Section 222 Homemaker			Increased
Studies using comparison group			
Triage (1981)	Increased		Increased
ACCESS (1980)			Reduced
Washington (1980)			Increased
On Lok (1977)			No difference

(a) Total costs are the sum of all expenditures measured by the researchers in
    each study and are not necessarily the sum of nursing home and hospital
    costs.
(b) Statistically significant

Adapted from GAO report The Elderly Should Benefit from Expanded Home Health
Care But Increasing these Services Will Not Insure Cost Reductions (Comptroller General, 1982, p. 30).

It is important to qualify this finding by noting that demonstration projects frequently experienced start-up problems such as finding clients and lacked operating efficiency. Clearly, these problems should be considered in judging overall costs.

Both the DHHS and the GAO studies suggested, however, that because of future growth and demand, the total financial burden for long term care is certain to increase in the future. The GAO report went further noting that because of growing public support for non-institutional long term care services, the critical policy issue is likely not to be a question of whether community based long term care is less expensive than institutional care, but rather how these services should be organized for maximum efficiency and effectiveness (Comptroller General, 1982).

Effect of case management on system fragmentation. In summarizing results of findings on this question, the DHHS concluded in 1980 that the effectiveness of the case management component of both state programs and on-going demonstrations had not been systematically evaluated. Great variability in case management systems and their costs were identified as an underlying problem in drawing definitive conclusions about case management's effectiveness. Variation in scope of responsibility, degree of authority and influence, and organizational arrangements were to become central concerns in developing the second generation of demonstrations known as channeling projects. These will be described in the next section of this chapter.

Patient outcomes. The early demonstrations also measured effectiveness in terms of client outcomes. Important variables in this analysis included mortality rates, functional capacity, physical and mental status, and degree of life satisfaction.

Many studies reported decreased mortality rates for individuals receiving coordinated community based services. Improved functional capacity was not found, though many projects indicated improved medical status, mental functioning, and level of satisfaction.

On balance, experts conclude that expanded coverage of community based services seemed to have a favorable impact on patient outcomes in the areas of lower mortality rates and increased life satisfaction, but differences in functional capacity were not discernable.

122

In summary, evaluations of early demonstrations indicated that community based long term care was a viable alternative for many individuals. At the same time, they also concluded that community based services were frequently an add-on to institutional forms of care thereby creating demand in a larger population. Severe methodological problems made interpretation of results difficult. Hence, the need for new demonstrations with better research designs was imperative. Assuming the desirability of and public pressure for non-institutional long term care options, the second generation of demonstrations focus on the following program design issues:

1) Targeting - As noted in the Urban Institute, Comptroller General (GAO), and DHHS reports, improvement in targeting community based services is one of the most difficult design problems facing non-institutional long term care programs, particularly since cost containment continues to be a goal.

2) Cost Control - Since cost containment is a program goal, development of broader and more flexible benefit packages needs to be accompanied by mechanisms to control and limit the potential cost of non-institutional long term care alternatives.

3) Case Management - Specific research on the cost and effectiveness of case management as a coordination strategy was needed.

SECOND GENERATION LONG TERM CARE DEMONSTRATION PROJECTS

While findings of the early demonstrations indicated that coordinated, community based, long term care could provide a single entry point and an enriched package of service to prevent institutionalization, other policy issues remained unanswered. A new series of demonstrations have been developed to test new organizational arrangements to address these issues. These new research initiatives are concerned with use of reimbursement to control costs and with the impact of community based services on families and other informal supporters. Some also reflect a concern about targeting services better in order to control costs. In order to provide better understanding of these problems, the demonstrations described in this section include a number of additional program elements being tested for the first time. Since cost issues were paramount, most received no funding other than

123

waivers under Medicare, Medicaid, and the Title XX program and most include some type of capitation model. Some also have a specific targeting approach. Others address what some experts consider another shortcoming of the earlier demonstrations, namely, the exclusive focus on long term care.

One of the elements common to all the second generation demonstrations is the effort to change prevailing financial incentives. These demonstrations attempt to provide long term care services under a fixed budget arrangement. The underlying assumption is that providers who are reimbursed on a cost basis to provide services to frail populations entitled to open-ended services will prescribe and provide larger quantities of service. Since services provided are frequently similar to those that are a part of normal living, consumers may also have a tendency to demand large amounts of service. For these reasons, financial controls are now considered essential to long term care service delivery. According to Diamond and Berman (1981), policy analysts have viewed fixed budgets or capitation models as the means to achieve the following three objectives:

1) curtail the sharply increasing costs borne by federal programs for nursing home care;
2) facilitate case management and improved resource allocation in the long term care sector; and
3) introduce improved management systems and controls among long term care providers.

The organizations described in the early demonstrations are frequently referred to as channeling agencies because they provided a single entry point for long term care. However, this terminology really came into widespread use following implementation of a second generation experiment which will be the first discussed in this section, the National Long Term Care Channeling Demonstration.

National Long Term Care Channeling Demonstration

In 1980, the DHHS funded ten states under the National Long Term Care Channeling Demonstration Program. One of the purposes of this national demonstration effort was to explicitly analyze the effectiveness of case management, particularly in reducing fragmentation of services. It was intended to provide research on the cost of alternatives to institutionalization and on their effectiveness

124

in reducing system fragmentation and enhancing family supports without substituting costly formal services. The program introduced more rigor into the research and evaluation of case management services than did previous demonstrations.

Overview. The National Long Term Care Channeling Demonstration is a federally funded research project whose goal is to maximize and direct long term care resources at a community level in ways that will contain overall system costs. The project, funded by the U.S. DHHS through monies from the HCFA and the AOA, will attempt to examine the effectiveness of case management as a technique to mobilize the spectrum of community supports and services for frail elderly clients. The project tests a simple and a complex model. Local channeling sites began operation in 1982 and will run through 1985. Data collection will be conducted by a national evaluator and will, for the first time, be comparable across sites. The primary goal of the project is to test whether "a managed system of long term care can be established, operated and produce results more favorable than the present arrangements for long term care" (Callahan, 1982). The desired results are:

- Improved targeting for those in greatest need
- Improved estimates of the nature of the need/demand
- Improved knowledge of the impact of different levels of care
- Improved client outcomes
- Better matching of client needs and services
- Less costly utilization of services
- Reduction of overall system of costs

In addition, the goals of the project include promotion of the use of the least restrictive environment and the development of state agency as well as local coordinating mechanisms for service development and control.

State plan. One of the primary tasks of the planning year was preparation of a State Long Term Care Plan for long term care services that would change or modify currently established systems. This requirement set forth in the Request for Proposal provided a major opportunity to establish a coordinated state planning and management system for long term care services that was intended to last long beyond the demonstration period. Since this chapter is more focused on patient-level demonstrations, no analysis will be provided of these state plans. However, the chapter in this book, "Mechanisms of Access and Coordination," more fully discusses these state level planning initiatives as a possible strategy for the VA.

Sites. As noted earlier, ten states were chosen to participate in the Channeling Demonstration Program to test the effectiveness of a strengthened case management model. Channeling refers to coordinated case management services. The core activities are: outreach/case finding; screening; assessment, case management reassessment and services audit; and program review. Five of the states are testing a "basic" channeling model, which will consist of a single entry point for case management as well as uniform client screening, assessment, care planning, service delivery, and case monitoring. These states (Texas, Maine, New Jersey, Maryland, and Kentucky) are developing a comprehensive case management model for the first time. The other five states were selected to participate in the "complex" channeling model. Each of these states (Massachusetts, New York, Florida, Ohio and Pennsylvania) already has an existing network of community based services from which to build the more "complex" channeling features.

Program design. The complex model includes all of the components of the basic model as well as several additional features which strengthen the case management role. These additional components are:

1. The case manager has authority over the amount, scope, and duration of non-institutional health and social services.
2. Funds for services are pooled and capped at a level which will be 60% of the cost of institutional skilled nursing care in the demonstration area.
3. Non-institutional services are available to Medicare clients whose incomes are above the Medicaid eligibility level. These services are available through the use of Medicare service waivers. Medicare waivered services include adult day health, foster care, transportation, in-home services, and skilled home health as well as other services.

126

In summary, "the intervention consists of the following:

1. An outreach component to identify and attract the target group;
2. A comprehensive assessment of each client to determine needs and service requirements;
3. Development of a care plan and arrangements with providers to carry it out;
4. Case management to actually assist the client in doing his or her part to assure the implementation of the plan;
5. Creation of service options to assure that high cost options are not used unnecessarily;
6. Change of provider incentives by providing funding for alternative services (service waivers);
7. Reducing inappropriate use of high cost alternatives by making early intervention possible (eligibility waivers);
8. Monitoring and quality control of provider services;
9. Data information systems to give full cost and utilization picture, e.g., case mix, client costs, system costs, utilization;
10. Cost controls through appropriate utilization, efficiency improvements, and capped funding;
11. Creation of an organization that is accountable for what happens both to the total client and for the total costs" (Callahan, 1982).

Using an experimental design, potential clients are screened for appropriateness and then randomly assigned to a treatment or control group. The target population for the project is the very frail elderly adult who could not continue to live in the community without some services or support. Both treatment and control groups are given an in-depth initial assessment interview as well as follow-up assessments. Services audit and program review functions are required for each site.

The case manager serves as the focal point for the coordination of services provided by a variety of agencies. Interagency agreements with such major community service providers as home health agencies, senior centers, mental and physical health programs, homemaker, chore, day care, etc., are used to spell out referral procedures for channeling clients, service protocols, and the role of the case manager. These types of agreements strengthen the case manager's ability to coordinate the implementation of the care plan and to monitor its on-going effectiveness in meeting client needs. The expansion of service availability and the facilitation of access to the services strengthen the tools with which the case manager, the client, and the client's family have to work. It is expected that this channeling model will overcome many barriers to more efficient service delivery to those most in need.

Research/evaluation design. The National Long Term Care Channeling Demonstration has an experimental design in which potential clients are screened for appropriateness and then randomly assigned to a treatment or control group. There will be a pre-post test design. Both groups will be tracked over a three-year period and evaluated every six months in terms of cost of services, utilization, and outcomes. The national evaluation will be conducted by Mathematic Policy Research, Inc., in Princeton, New Jersey. Part of the national evaluation will also include a "process evaluation" identifying organizational issues at the site level in both the development and operation of the demonstration. Although results are not yet available in that sites have been operational for approximately one year, the rigor of the evaluation design and data collection methods should yield definitive information particularly regarding case management as an intervention. As a result of the data collection efforts of the national evaluators, a great deal of new information about client service needs, client functional ability, and the costs of care of the frail elderly is expected to emerge from the channeling demonstrations nation-wide.

Medicare and Health Maintenance Organizations

Prior to the enactment of the 1972 Amendments to the Social Security Act, Medicare beneficiaries enrolled in Health Maintenance Organizations (HMOs) could only receive services covered under Part B of Medicare on a prepaid basis. However, a different method of reimbursement was possible with the enactment of Section 1876 which was implemented through final regulations published in late 1976.

Section 1876 allowed two methods of reimbursement to HMOs, both of which involved a single capitation for services covered under Parts A and B of Medicare. A mature HMO was able to enter either type of contract. A cost

128

contract only allowed reimbursement for reasonable cost. A risk-based contract allowed reasonable costs based on a comparison of reasonable costs and an average cost of providing services in the fee-for-service sector in the same areas as the HMO, adjusted for demographic characteristics of Medicare beneficiaries enrolled in HMOs. Under a risk contract, the Medicare enrollee is "locked in" to the HMO, meaning that the beneficiary must receive all services through the HMO in order for them to be reimbursed. The HMO is financially at risk for covered services. In 1980, Medicare had several capitation demonstration projects in operation.

While the HMO demonstrations cover only acute care services, the model of managed care they apply to acute care service delivery has suggested "methods for controlling long term care through improved case management" (Diamond and Berman, 1981, p. 187). For example, HMOs have reduced hospitalization rates and thus incurred some cost savings from decreased institutional care by more efficient management of patient care and allocation of services.

Program design. HMO Medicare capitation projects are characterized by voluntary enrollment, a defined set of services, prospective prepayment, fixed capitation rates, and single entry into a managed care system. They emphasize health maintenance and early detection and prevention of chronic conditions. HMOs also attempt to enroll a representative cross-section of the population to protect against adverse selection and offer centralized services.

Evidence of the effectiveness of managed care in an HMO setting. While the data available on the performance of the eight capitation demonstration sites are limited, preliminary evaluation indicates the organizational structure and financial incentives work together to control cost and increase effectiveness (Jurgovan and Blair, 1982). In several earlier studies of HMOs with cost contracts, comparisons have been made with non-HMO control groups. Every HMO studied showed evidence of lower hospital admission rates and lower lengths of stay than comparable non-HMO Medicare beneficiaries. HMOs also showed increased use of ambulatory services and home health care. Overall, moderate systems savings were achieved for most HMOs since savings in institutional care more than offset higher use of physician services and home health care (Diamond and Berman, 1981).

Of particular interest to the VA is a study conducted by Weil (1976) showing that HMOs which owned and operated their own hospitals, nursing homes, and home health services, showed the most marked shift from institutional care to use of home health and ambulatory services.

In sum, HMOs offer effectively managed health care systems in that they directly control institutional admissions, discharges, and costs and ordinarily manage patient's transfers to less intensive care settings.

Social/Health Maintenance Organization

Many experts, including some within the federal government, have considered the feasibility of the social/health maintenance organization (S/HMO) as a single entry, prepaid, long term care delivery system and efforts are now underway to test its feasibility in several demonstration sites.

A major problem with the long term care demonstrations discussed earlier is that they did not link acute care and long term care so as to provide incentives to encourage the substitution of appropriate, less expensive alternatives for hospitalization (Diamond and Berman, 1981).

Evidence from managed care system approaches to acute care delivery such as the HMO demonstration just discussed suggested the potential of a method for long term care cost containment which combines a fixed budget or capitation with strengthened case management. By expanding the HMO model to include long term care services, experts have proposed that the HMO's ability to contain costs would be improved in several ways. According to Diamond and Berman (1981, p. 187), this type of entity could provide "a coordinated and comprehensive services package; incentives discouraging institutionalization and encouraging community and home-based care; and net savings to the system due to the substitution of appropriate, less expensive treatment strategies."

Several S/HMO sites are now being developed under the leadership of the Florence Heller School at Brandeis University to test the feasibility of this health system reform. Based on the preliminary evidence of the effectiveness of comprehensive medical care in the recent Medicare demonstration projects, selected features of the medical

130

model HMO, namely, locally centralized case management capacities, will be combined with the personal care organization's locally centralized control of essential long term care services. Through this integration, the S/HMO "builds upon the widely held belief that more comprehensive, integrated, and managed systems of health care can result in significant cost savings in contrast to the current separation of acute and chronic care fee-for-service programs which discourage the efficient use of alternatives" (Diamond, et al., 1983, p. 148).

The S/HMO is a system which manages health and long term care services. Under this model, a single provider organization at the local level assumes responsibility for providing a full range of acute inpatient, ambulatory, personal care, and home care services under a prospectively determined, fixed capitation rate. The S/HMO will exhibit a strong shift toward centralized patient management controlling entry, patient assessment, certification, and case management including referral, advocacy, and follow-up. Individuals in the designated service area are enrolled voluntarily and are "locked in" to receiving all services through that single provider. One hypothesis to be tested in the S/HMO demonstration is whether preventive health care can delay or postpone deterioration that frequently accompanies old age.

Financing will be through pooling of various funding sources such as Medicare, Medicaid, and other sources such as Older Americans Act funds. The S/HMO entity will be at risk with third party payers for costs incurred above a predetermined capitation. Services will either be provided directly or contracted for with local providers or a combination of both. Four sites are in the early stages of development to field test the S/HMO under a demonstration project funded by the HCFA.

Because the various sources of funding will be pooled, the S/HMO will have flexibility in designing the service package and should reduce considerable amounts of paperwork for providers.

Since the S/HMO will enroll a broad cross section of the elderly, it is expected that only a small percentage of enrollees will use long term care services in any given year.

The elderly individual will pay a monthly premium probably equal to current out-of-pocket costs in the fee-for-service sector and in return will have access to a far greater range of health and social services and centralized case management. It is expected that combination of a capitation through prepayment financing, a comprehensive benefit package that provides both acute and long term care, and a single provider entity to assume organizational responsibility will achieve cost effectiveness.

Though this new model for delivery of services to the elderly holds great promise for integrating health and social services in a single model that is also cost effective, data from the demonstration sites will not be available until sometime in 1984 at the earliest.

Summary. While various demonstrations described in this section differ slightly, all have the following program design and financing features: 1) single entry point, 2) strengthened case management, 3) a fixed budget or capitation, and 4) single stream or pooled funding. The Channeling program is targeted only to the frail elderly. The S/HMO will target long term care services to a small group of frail elders that represents a subset of a larger enrolled population. The larger enrolled population will represent a cross section of the elderly. The S/HMO encompasses both acute and long term care. While these demonstrations appear to offer new, more effective models for long term care coordination, no substantial data exist upon which to evaluate outcomes for clients or for overall costs.

In the next section, however, specific strategies will be outlined through which the VA can better coordinate with the community based long term care service system using some of the mechanisms developed in the previously discussed demonstrations. These strategies include patient management mechanisms that could be implemented to more effectively use existing VA resources and to maximize non-VA resources to provide care for the aging veteran. The conceptualization of these strategies is largely based on findings from the earlier long term care demonstration studies as well as on concepts more recently developed by policy analysts and reflected in the second generation of long term care demonstrations. The strategies emphasize building on the already existing strengths of the VA system.

STRATEGIES FOR THE VA:
COORDINATION BETWEEN VA and NON-VA MODELS

Before examining some of the strategies the VA might pursue for community collaboration, it is useful to first delineate what the VA system of care currently provides and to compare that to the non-VA system.

CURRENT VA INVOLVEMENT IN LONG TERM CARE

In recent years, the VA has begun to focus a considerable share of its resources toward geriatric and extended care programs, some of them experimental. These include institutional and non-institutional services.

Institutional Extended Care Programs

The programs comprising the institutional spectrum of care in the VA include the following:

- VA Nursing Home Care — for patients usually requiring prolonged nursing supervision and rehabilitation services.

- Community Nursing Home Care — under contract for veterans requiring skilled or intermediate nursing care to assist in the transition from hospital to the community.

- VA Domiciliary Care — provides necessary professional and medical services for eligible, disabled veterans who are ambulatory, and do not require institutionalization.

- State Veterans Homes — provide direct hospital, nursing home, and domiciliary care to eligible veterans through grant programs to states or through providing a per diem rate for veterans in those homes.

- GRECC — a Catalyst Program — In addition to the programs described above, the GRECC Program (Geriatric Research, Education and Clinical Centers) functions as a catalyst in geriatrics at VA medical centers (VAMCs). Designed to attract and develop superior staff in the field of gerontology and geriatrics, this program helps to advance

133

and integrate research and educational activities into the VA system.

Non-Institutional Care Programs

A variety of non-institutional services are provided to veterans through the following programs:

- Hospital Based Home Care - provides chronically-ill veterans with services in their own homes through VA treatment teams.

- Adult Day Health Care - provides a wide range of health care services including medical, rehabilitative, social and recreational services to veterans in congregate settings. Several demonstrations are currently in operation in the VA system.

- Residential Care Home Program - (formerly known as Personal Care Home) provides residential care to veterans who are not capable of independent living because of health conditions, but who are not frail enough to require nursing home or institutional care. This is the largest of the extended care programs with 12,800 veterans in placement.

Program Developments in Extended Care

In the past several years the VA's Department of Medicine and Surgery has undertaken to establish new alternatives for extended care. These include:

- Discharge/Community Placement/Aftercare - Social work case management projects which consist of joint activities and developments with community agencies regarding health and social support networks for aging veterans have begun in several areas.

- Geriatric Evaluation Units - A comprehensive diagnostic, treatment, and discharge planning process for multiply-impaired hospital patients is provided. Objectives of the units include better management of chronic illness and reduction of improper placement in long term care institutions. Twelve Geriatric Evaluation Units are now operational.

- Hospice - In 1978, a pilot hospice program was developed to examine care of terminally ill cancer patients.

- Respite Care - Services to relieve the spouse and family caregivers of the burden of caring for a dependent elderly person at home have been piloted in the Palo Alto VAMC. This approach has strengthened the link between the VA, the veteran, and the caregiver and has reinforced the critical role that the spouse plays in providing care in the community.

The increasing number and diversity of non-institutional extended care programs in the VA parallels that in the nation and provides sound beginnings for long term care.

COMPARISON OF VA AND NON-VA LONG TERM CARE SERVICE SYSTEMS

There are many differences between the VA extended care programs and the non-VA service system. First, long term care services for the general elderly population are more evenly distributed geographically across the nation, whereas VA services tend to be concentrated around VAMCs. (It should be noted that the VA does provide community nursing home care and residential care in 6,300 facilities, many of them at great distances from a VAMC.) Second, the non-VA system has become somewhat less dependent on institutional forms of care over the past decade as resources have been concentrated on developing alternative forms of care. Third, most public long term care programs have evolved targeting mechanisms that are being used to provide services based on the appropriateness of need which are quite different than the criteria that now characterize the VA's eligibility regulations. Finally, many community based long term care systems have developed some form of care management component to control overall growth in costs through controls on utilization.

On the other hand, the VA service system has greater potential to provide continuity of care for patients as they move along the continuum of care by integrating all program levels. Community based programs sometimes cannot

135

provide continuity of care because the acute and long term care systems are frequently only partially integrated. The VA thus provides "a broadly based clinical program extending from hospital through extended care to the home and ambulatory care, a large and experienced educational system..." and is "...the natural clinical resource of the universities which are just beginning to respond to the problem" (U.S. Congress, 1978, p. 49).

In spite of these many differences, the literature reflects a convergence of principles and goals for a long term care model system. These goals include availability, accessibility and appropriateness of services, continuity of care, quality of care and cost containment.

Given the similarity in the goals of both systems to meet the needs of a growing proportion of elderly citizens in this country who will progressively require a range of health and social services for long term chronic illness, coordination among different health providers, the VA and non-VA, and among funding sources should be encouraged.

OPTIONS FOR VA AND NON-VA COOPERATION AND COORDINATION

The key question in developing coordination mechanisms with the community is how to coordinate services for people with multiple entitlements and multiple needs. Four areas of specific concern to the VA will be addressed in the strategies identified for closer coordination between the community and the VA service systems. These are related to the VA's planning, service delivery, client eligibility, and payment functions. Changes from the current system are likely to require additional financing and/or alterations in the methods of paying for services. One set of options is presented which uses the VA payment function and may be pursued, alone or in combination with other alternatives. Change in service delivery is another major consideration. How should long term care services be provided by the VA? Should the VA be the community focal point for long term care? Is the VA properly organized to fill this role? If not, what kind of organizational structures are needed? Client eligibility is a third variable in any overall long term care strategy. The key question here is whether current eligibility guidelines for veterans are appropriate and suitable for developing cooperative arrangements with the community based long term care system.

136

Assumptions

The set of options described below is based on the following assumptions:

1. Present mechanisms of health care financing will continue.
2. The socio-economic characteristics of veterans who will apply to the VA for long term care services will not change significantly.
3. The veteran population will remain essentially male.
4. The community system should be included in analysis of the total resources available.

Principles for Coordination

The following principles were used in developing the various options for community cooperation available to the VA:

1. Long term care services are already being provided to non-veterans and veterans at the community level. Any VA plan should build upon the local long term care delivery system so as to maximize available resources.
2. Any option for service delivery must have provision for a coordinating mechanism, such as case management, as a necessary management function for the coordination of the continuum of services.
3. Efforts at coordinating long term care should take place at the local level to take into account community differences and because this is usually where the older veteran receives services.
4. Expansion of community based services, either through the VA or the non-VA system, should be justified on its own merits and not only as a cost saving alternative to costly institutional care.

These principles provide a solid foundation for a system that could make best use of VA and community resources.

The following section identifies potential planning, service delivery, eligibility and financing options based on the assumptions and principles discussed above.

PLANNING STRATEGIES

VA leadership in coordination of community services. The VA could assume the lead role in the coordination of community services for the entire elderly population through playing a leadership role in community planning. In those areas where the existing long term care system is fragmented, the VA could act as a catalyst to bring together the major actors in the community to join with the VA in developing a comprehensive plan for coordination among community providers and between these community providers and the VA system. The foundation for the expanded role of the VA in long term care planning could be the linkage between the plans of the medical districts and those of the states. Each state is required to prepare a State Health Plan which inventories resources and targets unmet needs for priority action. In the past, VA resources and needs have usually not been included in the health plans prepared by the states. In another chapter in this book entitled, "Mechanisms of Access and Coordination," there is a detailed discussion of this topic which relates these elements of planning to the Medical District Initiated Program Planning process (MEDIPP).

Coordinated planning with non-VA providers at the state and local level. This option is similar to the first in that it is primarily a planning strategy. The major difference is that the VA would play a role equal to each of the other parties involved in coordinated long term care planning either at the state or local level. This type of planning strategy was part of the overall system requirements for the National Long Term Care Channeling Project.

Maintain current arrangements. The VA could decide not to change current planning practices, thereby maintaining the current situation of two independent, uncoordinated planning functions.

SERVICE DELIVERY STRATEGIES

VA service delivery strategies can be identified by looking at possible variations of two program elements: case management and resource sharing. This analysis yields the following service strategies options:

138

Program Element	Options
Case Management Role	• VA as case manager • VA cooperates with community case manager • VA contracts for case management
Resource Sharing	• VA develops new resources • VA accesses community resources • VA and community share resources • VA and community pool resources • VA controls both VA and community resources

Brief descriptions of the various models these combinations employ follow.

1. Case Management Options

VA as case manager. Under this option, the VA would take the lead as broker and primary case manager. The VA might play this role in the following circumstances: 1) when the VA is the primary provider, 2) for veterans regardless of whether the veteran requires services from VA or non-VA providers, or 3) under a VA/non-VA program of pooled resources. This kind of model which would closely approximate the S/HMO could begin with the expansion of the GRECC and Geriatric Evaluation Unit approaches in selected VAMCs.

This model would be most appropriate in areas where the VAMC is readily available to users or easily accessible by public transportation and in communities in which the VA is more service rich than the non-VA long term care system. Changes in current VA organization would be needed. In addition to clinical and diagnostic interventions, the VA would need to develop long term care assessment instruments and the protocols to screen, assess, plan care, monitor, and reassess clients. A shift from a medical model to a more social model of long term care would be more appropriate for patients placed at home or in another non-institutional setting. Finally, depending on the resource mechanism used, interagency agreements would need to be developed to specify protocols for referral to non-

139

VA programs for which veterans may be eligible or to establish criteria by which an individual becomes eligible for pooled resources.

At a minimum, the VA needs to develop a case management function within the VA system. One possible model that would build on existing medical and social care strengths would be one that links the roles of the GRECCs and VA social workers. The GRECCs now provide models for geriatric evaluation, clinical research and education within the VA. Also, within the present VA system social workers function as case managers for a wide range of "at risk" patients that include the frail elderly. The chapter, "Mechanisms of Access and Coordination," recommends expansion of the GRECCs as models for geriatric evaluation within the VA, including adoption of this model throughout the VA system. Following a geriatric evaluation, VA social workers could be designated as case managers responsible for care planning, client tracking and coordination of the full range of community health, welfare and social support services for the veteran. This model would enhance the social workers' opportunities for sharing expertise and for expanding the range of community services available to veterans and non-veterans.

While the social work service alone does not maintain the case management role, the social work service at each VAMC carries a primary responsibility for accessing, integrating and coordinating VA and community resources for the ill and disabled. Moreover, the development of the social work case management program and assignment of social workers in each medical district to function as a community service coordinator does provide an infrastructure upon which a multidisciplinary long term care case management function could be built.

VA cooperates in case management with non-VA providers. This option calls for joint involvement of both service systems that would be limited to collaboration during the case management process, following which the veteran would receive the care recommended by the assessment team from either the VA or non-VA providers. This type of multidisciplinary team approach to assessment and care planning was a prominent feature of many HCFA long term care demonstrations. The same concept can apply to more limited situations such as VA and non-VA collaboration in pre-admission nursing home screening programs.

140

VA contracts for case management. The VA also has the
option to contract with one or more providers in the community to provide the case management for veterans in need
of long term care services. In areas where effective case
management programs are in place, this model should be
given serious consideration.

One issue of concern to the VA is where the case manager should be located regardless of whether the person is
a VA employee or paid by the VA on contract. If the VA
wants a strong relationship between the case manager and
the VAMC, then the case manager should be located at the
VAMC. This placement would also facilitate continuity of
care for the aging veteran. However, in areas where the
VAMC is not easily accessible or where the VA already has
interagency agreements with community agencies such as the
Area Agencies on Aging, the case manager could be located
at an established community focal point for long term care.

A second issue to be considered is whether the case
management function should include a mandatory screen for
all veterans applying for VA nursing home benefits. Nursing home pre-admission programs have shown this to be cost
effective and efficacious in areas where there is an array
of community services available.

A final note of caution should be made with respect to
case management options. While the issues of access and
coordination presented in the chapter, "Mechanisms of Access and Coordination," outline the reasons why coordination is essential in the provision of long term care, the
demonstrations previously cited indicate certain problem
areas that should be addressed in developing an effective
case management function. First, case management must include careful screening to identify the desired target
populations. It must include complete assessment and comprehensive care and services management. Finally, the
literature suggests case management should be coupled with
a financial cap on the cost of individual service plans so
that costs for non-institutional long term care will not
exceed those of institutional care for a similar population. The ability of the VA to integrate acute and long
term care services for the elderly and the VA's past success in designing the extended care programs to improve
hospital utilization, place the VA in a strong position to
overcome many of the problems that have plagued earlier
case management and coordination demonstrations.

2. Resource Development and Sharing Options

VA develops long term care resources. Since the VA
should not duplicate existing community services for which
veterans are eligible, program development efforts should
be concentrated on filling gaps in the existing continuum
of long term care services. The VA could assist in development of alternatives to institutionalization either by
funding alternatives within the VA, such as geriatric day
care or respite care, or by assisting in providing start-
up funding to local non-VA service providers. One consideration in locating such services at VAMCs would be an
assessment of suitable space and population served. In
those cases where the VA decides it would be best to fund
community based providers, grant programs such as those
now used to fund the State Veterans Homes could be developed.

VA accesses community resources. One likely scenario
under this option would be the development of interagency
agreements as a basis of referral to non-VA programs for
which veterans may be eligible. This approach requires no
capital outlay to the VA and precedence has been set for
major initiatives of this type. While the VA does not
share in care management or in providing care, this type
of arrangement will enable older veterans to benefit from
resources available in the community.

For example, several years ago, the VA and the AOA
signed an interagency agreement committing the local VAMCs
and Veterans Benefits Offices to develop information and
referral programs with the AOA's Area Agencies on Aging
(AAAs). In those areas where the VA and AAAs have worked
well together, veterans in the community have benefited
from better services. Through this type of information
and referral program, AAAs can identify and guide veterans
toward VA services. At the same time, it can provide the
client access to many important non-VA programs. For example, many AAAs can enable older veterans to receive
benefits and VA health care they may not have received
otherwise. Many AAA staff currently provide service management and care planning that can be used to link the
veteran to AAA in-home services. In other areas, AAAs
have been able to prevent individuals from being inappropriately placed in institutions through multidisciplinary
nursing home preadmission assessments.

VA and community share resources. One variation of this option could be the sharing of VA acute care resources for non-veterans in exchange for veterans' use of community based long term care services. In this model, the VA would not require extensive capital expenditures and would not duplicate services already available to the veteran. From a patient or case management perspective, however, the VA might lose control of the continuity of veterans' care. A program design component to address this problem in such an arrangement is the development of a multidisciplinary team including both VA and community professionals to review clients receiving services from both systems. As in the case of other service delivery options mentioned, the VA's contribution might include training and education for non-VA providers or access to non-aging programs for which the VA has known expertise such as the Spinal Cord Injury Program.

The interagency agreement between the VA and AAAs previously described provides an example of this type of sharing. In return for AAAs providing service to veterans, service by the VA to the AAAs took many forms. One example is Veterans' Benefits Training Seminars that were provided for AAA intake counselors in several areas.

Another area in which collaboration can take place is between VA home service workers and community care providers. The Hospital Based Home Care Program provides the home-bound veteran with visits by members of a multidisciplinary treatment team. It may sometimes be the case that the veteran approached the VA for service after home health care benefits under Medicare expired. In these cases, patient care and management would be greatly enhanced by case conferencing, transfer procedures, and other collaborative arrangements.

The VA might also offer training and education to community care providers and access to VA trained personnel in geriatrics and gerontology.

Pilot efforts currently in place by the VA to increase collaborative efforts such as the VA Cooperative Health Manpower Education Program should be expanded.

VA and community pool resources. A fourth possibility for resource sharing is an arrangement in which services and/or funding for services are pooled. This type of pooling mechanism was briefly described as a major compo-

143

nent of the National Long Term Care Channeling Program in which the case manager was allowed access to and authority over the complete array of long term care services. In a pooling arrangement, the funding sources give up a portion of control over resource utilization, in return for lifting of restrictions on the allocation of resources to which they have access. Benefits of a pooled approach to funding and providing long term care services include a reduction in duplication and fragmentation thereby increasing service coordination. If this option is pursued, it should be considered along with a cap in resources that could go to individual care plans.

VA controls both VA and community resources. In this option, the VA would become the focal point of long term care in a given community having control of resource allocation to both clients and providers. As noted in the option on the VA as case manager, this type of arrangement is likely to be viable only in areas where the VAMCs are easily accessible, where the community is service poor, and where the VA could be organized to manage the complete continuum of long term care services.

Assessing the Long Term Care Environment

Because of the substantial geographic variability in both the VA and non-VA long term care systems, any effort to develop coordination models that are sensitive to regional differences in needs and resources will require a careful assessment of the long term care environment before any specific strategy is developed. Several criteria are relevant in assessing the respective abilities of different types of providers to perform the necessary patient management functions in long term care. These include: provider incentives, management capacity, groups served, incentives for recipient to use provider, scope of coordination, comprehensiveness, continuity of care, and appropriateness of care (Piktialis and Callahan, 1982).

It is also important to note that at the local level, the long term care delivery system is comprised of a plurality of actors and interests which operate within an intersystem involving a number of subsystems (Callahan, "A Systems Approach to Long Term Care," 1981). Given the strength of provider interests, efforts to implement coordination mechanisms will require a process for gaining acceptance among these providers. Diamond and Berman (1981) have detailed major issues relating to the establishment of the S/HMO which are useful in anticipating obstacles that may arise given attempts to establish a new entity in the long term care system. In addition to political issues and concerns about provider incentives, they identify a number of organizational issues including establishment of referral agreements with local providers, financial management, and quality of care issues.

While plans to undertake this type of environmental analysis should be considered by the VA, development of specific procedures are beyond the scope of this chapter. They are mentioned to point out the complexities of organizational change within the community as well as within the VA when attempting collaboration to meet long term care needs. It is also important to note that the long term care environmental assessment should identify what services are already being provided in the community since the VA may not want to duplicate existing services for which an elderly veteran is eligible. This type of long term care system assessment will assist regional VAs in selecting among the options presented above.

ELIGIBILITY OPTIONS

An important determinant of how much use will be made of VA resources is that of eligibility. Although eligibility legislation has placed an umbrella over veterans aged 65+, most older veterans do not use VA benefits directly (VA, Health Care of the Aging Veteran: A Report of the Geriatrics and Gerontology Advisory Committee, 1983). Rather, VAMCs tend to be used by veterans without other insurance coverage and those with low incomes. In this way, the VA functions as "a safety net for veterans who are not full participants in the social system" (GGAC Report, p. 23). Age, in fact, shows the weakest effect on utilization. Because of the characteristics of the veterans who used the VA as reported in the GGAC report and considering findings of national demonstrations in coordination, the following options are outlined with respect to current eligibility requirements. These options would require major changes in the way eligibility is now handled by the VA. They include ways of controlling demand for long term care and targeting based on functional vulnerability.

145

<u>VA as secondary payor for veterans covered by other</u>
<u>programs</u>. Under the current system, the VA acts as the
primary payor if the veteran chooses to receive care from
the VA even if he/she may be eligible for coverage from
other programs such as Medicare. One option to prevent
cost shifting from community programs to the VA and to
prevent excessive demand for long term care from veterans
turning 65 would be for the VA to become the secondary
payor for long term care for veterans entitled to other
non-VA benefits such as Medicare, Medicaid, or private insurance. This would allow the VA to maximize other entitlements for aged veterans. This type of approach,
known as coordination of benefits, has been used successfully in the HMO Medicare demonstrations.

   <u>Develop and implement targeting strategies</u>. In order
to implement coordination projects with the community, the
VA may wish to take a more comprehensive look at eligibility requirements. Current eligibility for major VA medical benefits is determined by a complex set of categories
based on service-connected/non-service-connected characteristics, war served in, type of medical benefit needed,
and priorities for care in an inpatient and outpatient
setting. These eligibility regulations, while useful in
providing acute care to the total veteran population, seem
far less appropriate for use in deciding long term care
benefits for an elderly veteran. As most of the early
long term care demonstrations point out, community based
services are most cost effective and most likely substitutes for nursing home care when they are targeted to
those most in need based on functional capacity and unmet
need for assistance in daily activities. Since the VA is
currently the primary resource for veterans with limited
alternatives, eligibility criteria should also be developed with this kind of restriction on demand in mind.

   The VA must also examine eligibility to insure consistency between VA hospital care and VA long term care.

   The results of long term care experiments strongly
suggest that the VA provide services based on an assessment of need. "A major source of variation in the elderly's use of services can be attributed to functional disability and level of chronicity" (Randall, et al., 1981,
p. 3). Research also indicates that a person's ability to
handle every day activities is a much better indicator of
what a person needs than a medical diagnosis in long term
care settings. Researchers at Yale have developed cate-

gories based on functional disability called Resource Utilization Groups that are being tested for estimating nursing home costs, similar to the new Medicare DRG system for prospective hospital reimbursement.

While the VA may not be able or willing to change current entitlements, there may be other ways of addressing this problem. Specifically, the VA could set up criteria within current categories that will ensure that when services are limited, they be targeted to those veterans most in need of them based on functional impairment. Finally, consideration should be given to expanding written long term care eligibility guidelines to include not only services the VA pays for, but also services such as residential care which the VA administers but are paid for by the veteran. The success of the case management strategies previously described will require a clear-cut policy on targeting.

PAYMENT AND COMPENSATION OPTIONS

In addition to providing medical services, the VA administers a vast array of benefit programs including a large compensation program for veterans with service-connected disabilities and a pension program. There are several ways in which the VA could expand its income maintenance and compensation program to enable veterans to purchase services that are available in the community and not currently provided by the VA. Services such as home health aides and homemakers, essential to maintaining patients in their own homes, can presently be purchased only with the patient's funds. Some form of supplemental financial assistance should be available to home-bound veterans who are not financially eligible to receive those services through other programs and who need these services for successful home placement. A second consideration is review of the adequacy of the Aid and Attendance benefits, particularly as they affect the ability of an old, frail spouse to cope with an invalid husband. While the chapter in this book, "Serving the Family of the Elder Veteran," addresses serving the elder veteran's spouse, it is also important to view the older spouse who is caring for an elderly veteran as a critical determinant of the success of a home placement. While some supplemental financial assistance is available to home-bound veterans eligible for Aid and Attendance benefits, the adequacy of these benefits and the eligible population should be care-

147

fully reviewed (U.S. VAMC - Coatsville, 1981). Given an era of fiscal constraint, the actual cost of increases in certain financial benefits currently authorized, may be more feasible than new programs which require new funding authority.

It is important to note that these strategies imply a minimal amount of community interaction in that the individual veteran would simply purchase already existing community services. None require any capital expenditures or organizational changes by the VA and their impact on medical, social, and cost effectiveness variables could be measured.

Need for Incentives to Maintain Veterans in the Community

In addition to the various strategies identified for VA and community collaboration and for using the VA payment function and eligibility guidelines to support long term care planning, it is also important to point out the need to develop incentives for veterans and their families to choose care in the home rather than institutional care in a VA facility. Though not fully developed, the following strategies would provide the necessary incentives to offer veterans and families a real choice. They are to:

1) provide adequate reimbursement for spouses caring for a veteran at home;
2) provide transportation for access to VA facilities for outpatient care;
3) provide easy access for brief VA hospitalization when necessary;
4) promote tax credits to keep beneficiaries at home;
5) support adequate funding for non-VA non-institutional services at federal, state, and local levels.

IMPLICATIONS FOR THE VA

In addition to the specific options identified for community collaboration, the review of past demonstrations in long term care coordination suggests a number of other areas of importance to VA planning.

As the discussion of the channeling project and the S/HMO indicated, the Medicare program is moving closer to coverage for long term care services. Proposals have been put forth in Congress to set up a separate Medicare program, Part C, to pay for long term care for the aged and disabled. Given these directions along with the high percentage of veterans covered by Medicare (81%), particular attention should be paid to changes in the Medicare program as the VA moves forward with its long term care planning effort. While the VA should also work with the states in the Medicaid Community Care Waiver projects (2,176 waivers), a much smaller number of veterans are eligible for Medicaid (4.2%).

Second, the VA will need to develop decision making criteria for choosing when VA benefits versus non-VA benefits will be pursued.

Strengths of the VA system should also be remembered as planning goes forward. These include: 1) the VA's vast network of social workers capable of assisting veterans to access services for which they are eligible, 2) the large numbers of social workers with geriatric expertise, and 3) the VA's understanding of the importance of housing in the array of long term care services as evidenced by their past development of domiciliary care and residential care.

The review of available research findings from prior long term care demonstrations emphasizes the need for well designed and controlled studies. The VA has a number of advantages in launching its own research program in geriatric health services research since: 1) the VA can learn from mistakes of earlier studies and use the information from those studies to identify key issues for the VA; 2) the VA maintains control over its own facilities and it can exercise greater control over program and evaluation design; and 3) the VA can follow the lead of the channeling project by including a "process evaluation" to assess VA response to change. Also, critical to the VA is research which examines differences between the VA population and other, previously studied populations which have implications for long term care service delivery.

Given the strengths outlined above and elsewhere in this chapter, the VA is in a strong position to take a comprehensive organizational approach to long term care service delivery where deemed desirable. Because the VA has a greater degree of control over its own facilities, great potential is evident for working in a capitated model combined with specific targeting and case management approaches. Financial incentives for developing long term care programs at the local level must accompany national level decisions regarding long term care policy.

Conclusion

The VA now faces an opportunity comparable to that following World War II when it affiliated with medical schools across the country to provide high quality acute care to veterans while promoting medical research and education for health professionals. Now, nearly 40 years later, the VA faces the challenge of how to develop a long term care system for aging veterans that will maintain the high standards of excellence that have operated in the interim period. The VA must now examine how to best take advantage of the opportunity to work with the community to link acute and long term care in ways that will maximize resources.

As the VA becomes more involved with providing long term care to the aging veteran, coordination of services with community groups will become essential. The VA will need to study funding sources and eligibility criteria further in order to identify all community resources available and to provide direction for innovative collaborative arrangements with the community. As inter-organizational relations are developed with the community and as efforts by the VA to coordinate community services with its hospital and extended care facilities, the VA will begin to fill the gaps in services that still exist in the VA service system, enabling more rational and comprehensive plans of care to be provided to the aging veteran.

To the extent that this is recognized as a priority area by the VA, we can anticipate increasing VA and community support of a wider range of options so that broader issues related to the coordinating and integrating of services to "at risk" elderly can be addressed and resolved.

APPENDIX A

MEDICARE

Medicare is an entitlement program for persons eligible by virtue of having paid into the Social Security Trust Funds. Under Title XVIII of the Social Security Act, Medicare pays for much of the acute hospital inpatient and outpatient services and physician visits for individuals having coverage under Parts A and B. Eighty-one percent of veterans are covered by Medicare. Medicare coverage for skilled nursing and home health services is only for short term convalescent care, not for long term care. As of October 1, 1983, hospice care for the terminally ill will also be covered by Medicare.

MEDICAID

The Medicaid program is operated under Title XIX of the Social Security Act and provides acute and long term care services to individuals who qualify by virtue of having an income below predetermined eligibility levels. The program is funded by the federal government out of general revenues with a share paid by the states. Because of the means test, most Medicaid recipients are poor or have become poor by virtue of having a long term illness. Medicaid pays for most acute care and for long term skilled nursing care. Intermediate care facility coverage is optional for each state. Medicaid has become the primary funding source for publicly assisted long term nursing home services in the United States. However, because of many long term care demonstrations pointing out both the high and frequently inappropriate cost of institutional care, Congress passed Chapter 2176 in August of 1981 enabling state Medicaid programs to apply for federal waivers in order to provide more cost effective non-institutional services as a substitute for nursing home care.

TITLE XX/SOCIAL SERVICES BLOCK GRANTS

Until the passage of the Social Services Block Grants, most states funded social services under Title XX of the Social Security Act. Seventy-five percent of the cost of these services was paid for by the federal government with states picking up the remaining 25%. There is wide variation in the type and amount of service from state to state. Title XX frequently pays for a variety of community based and in-home social services used by elderly with chronic needs. These services include homemaker, chore, transportation, home health and personal care, etc.

OLDER AMERICANS ACT

Funds are received by all states under Title III of the Older Americans Act to provide social and nutritional services to the elderly in their homes and communities. These services have no income eligibility requirements. All Americans aged 60 or over can receive these services, although efforts are made to target to those in greatest social or economic need. Services provided under the Older Americans Act include homemaker, home health, chore, transportation, information and referral, legal services, congregate meals, home delivered meals and many more.

While many state and local governments fund programs for the elderly above and beyond those mentioned above, the Medicare, Medicaid, Social Services Block Grant, and Older Americans Act programs are the primary funders of long term care services in the community.

REFERENCES

Beatrice, D. "Case Management: A Policy Option for Long Term Care." In Reforming the Long Term Care System, pp. 121-163, Callahan, J.J. and Wallack, S.S. (Eds.). Lexington: D.C. Heath and Company, 1981.

Branch, L.G. "Understanding the Health and Social Service Needs of People Over 65." In Center for Survey Research Monograph, Center for Survey Research, University of Massachusetts and the Joint Center for Urban Studies of Massachusetts Institute of Technology and Harvard University, Boston, 1977.

Branch, L.G., Callahan, J.J. and Jette, A. "Targeting Home Care Services to Vulnerable Elders: Massachusetts Home Care Corporations." Home Health Care Services Quarterly, 2(2) p. 41, Summer, 1981.

Callahan, J.J. "Delivery of Services to Persons with Long Term Care Needs." Paper prepared for Administration on Aging Symposium, Levinson Policy Institute, Brandeis University, Waltham, Massachusetts, October 5, 1979.

Callahan, J.J. "Single Agency Option for Long Term Care." In Reforming the Long Term Care System, pp. 163-185, Callahan, J.J. and Wallack S.S. (Eds.). Lexington: D.C. Heath and Company, 1981.

Callahan, J.J. "A Systems Approach to Long Term Care." In Reforming the Long Term Care System, pp. 219-237, Callahan, J.J. and Wallack, S.S. (Eds.). Lexington: D.C. Heath and Company, 1981.

Callahan, J.J. The Channeling Demonstration: Summary Statement on Issues – Environment, Intervention and Outcomes (March, 1981). Handout presented at workshop "State Government and Aging Concerns," Annual Meetings of the Gerontological Society of America, Boston, November, 1982.

Callahan, J.J. and Wallack, S.S. Reforming the Long Term Care System. Lexington: D.C. Heath and Company, 1981.

Comptroller General. The Elderly Should Benefit from Expanded Home Health Care But Increasing these Services Will Not Insure Cost Reductions. G.A.O., Washington, D.C., December 7, 1982.

Diamond, L.M. and Berman, D.E. "The Social/Health Maintenance Organization: A Single Entry, Prepaid, Long-Term Care Delivery System." In Reforming the Long Term Care System, pp. 185-218, Callahan, J.J. and Wallack, S.S. (Eds.). Lexington: D.C. Heath and Company, 1981.

Diamond L., Gruenberg, L. and Morris, R. "Elder Care for the 80's: Health and Social Service in One Prepaid Health Maintenance System." The Gerontologist, 23(2), pp. 148-155, April, 1983.

Gottesman, L.E., Isizaki, B. and MacBride, S.M. "Service Management: Concepts and Models." The Gerontologist, 19(4), p. 378, August, 1979.

Jurgovan and Blair, Inc. Summary of Observations. Medicare/HMO Demonstration Project. HCFA Contract Number 500-81-0017, Washington, D.C., November, 1982.

Kane, R.L. and Kane R.A. "Care of the Aged: Old Problems in Need of New Solutions." Science, 200, pp. 913, 915-919, 1978.

Meltzer, J. and Farrow, F. "Federal Policy Directions in Long Term Care." Paper prepared for Symposium on Long Term Care Policy Options, Williamsburg, Virginia, June 11-13, 1980.

Morris, J. Massachusetts Elderly: Their Vulnerability and Need for Support Services and the Role of the Commonwealth's Home Care Corporation. Report prepared for the Massachusetts Department of Elder Affairs. Department of Social Gerontological Research, Hebrew Rehabilitation Center for the Aged, Boston, April 12, 1982.

Morris, J. Serving the Vulnerable Elderly in Massachusetts: The Role of the Commonwealth Home Care Corporation. Report prepared for the Massachusetts Department of Elder Affairs. Department of Social Gerontological Research, Hebrew Rehabilitation Center for the Aged, Boston, December, 1982.

National Academy of Sciences, Committee on Health Care
Resources in the VA. Health Care for American Veterans. Report submitted to the Assembly of Life Sciences, pp. 23-32, National Academy of Sciences, Washington, D.C., 1979.

Piktialis, D. and Callahan, J. "Organization of Long Term
Care: Should There Be Single or Multiple Focal Points
for Long Term Care Coordination?" Prepared for presentation at the conference "The Impact of Technology
on Long Term Care," sponsored by Project Hope Center
for Health Information. Office of Technology Assessment and the National Health Policy Forum, Milwood,
Virginia, February, 1982.

Randall, M., Lehrer, T., Abrahams, R. and Gruenberg, L.
"Utilization Profiles of the Elderly." Working Paper,
University Health Policy Consortium, Brandeis Univer-
sity, Waltham, Massachusetts, June, 1981.

Rucklin, H.S., Morris, J.N. and Eggert, G.M. "Management
and Financing of Long Term Care Services: A New Approach to a Chronic Problem." New England Journal of
Medicine, 306(2), p. 101, January 14, 1982.

Sager, A. "Learning the Home Care Needs of the Elderly:
Summary." Paper prepared for Levinson Policy Institute, The Florence Heller School for Advanced Studies
in Social Welfare, Brandeis University, Waltham, Massachusetts, March, 1980.

Sager, A., Pendelton, S., Lees-Low, C., et al. Living at
Home: The Roles of Public and Informal Supports in
Sustaining Older Adults. Levinson Policy Institute,
Brandeis University, Waltham, Massachusetts, March,
1982.

Sapolsky, H. and Wallack, S. "The Veterans' Health Care
System." In Federal Health Program, pp. 195-203, Altman, S. and Sapolsky, H. (Eds.). University Health
Policy Consortium, Lexington: D.C. Heath and Company,
1979.

Stasson, M. and Holakan, J. "Long Term Care Demonstration
Projects: A Review of Recent Evaluations." Working
Paper, 1227-2, The Urban Institute, Washington, D.C.,
February, 1981.

Trieger, S., Galblum, T. and Riley, G. HMOs: Issues and Alternatives for Medicare and Medicaid. Dept. of Health and Human Services, Health Care Financing Administration, Office of Research Demonstrations and Statistics, Baltimore, Maryland, 1981.

U.S. Congress, House Committee of Veteran Affairs, 1977. The Aging Veteran: Present and Future Medical Needs. Pub. #7. Washington, D.C.: USGPO, January 5, 1978.

U.S. Congress, Senate, Special Committee on Aging. "Adult Day Care Facilities for Treatment, Health Care and Related Facilities." A working paper prepared by Brahna Trager. Washington, D.C.: USGPO, 1976.

U.S. Department of Health and Human Services, Health Care Financing Administration, Office of Legislation and Policy. Long Term Care: Background and Future Directions. Baltimore, Maryland, January, 1981.

U.S. Department of Health and Human Services. A Comparative Study of Long Term Care Demonstrations. Human Services Monograph Series. Project Share, Washington, D.C., 1981.

U.S. Veterans Administration. Health Care of the Aging Veteran: A Report of the Geriatrics and Gerontology Advisory Committee. Washington, D.C., April, 1983.

U.S. Veterans Administration. Patient Treatment and Program Developments in the Care of the Aging Veteran. Geriatric Department of Medicine and Surgery Liaison Coordinating Committee, Washington, D.C., April, 1983 (Draft).

U.S. Veterans Administration Medical Center - Coatsville. The Aging Veteran Population: Interorganization Relations. Report of a Panel Presentation "The Old Veteran's Boom: Planning Services for Aging Veterans and Their Spouses." Seventh National Association of Social Workers Professional Symposium, Philadelphia, November 21, 1981.

Vladeck, B. "Understanding Long Term Care." New England Journal of Medicine, 307(1), p. 890, September 30, 1982.

Von Behren, R. *Adult Day Health Services*, Final Report, Department of Health Services, Sacramento, California, 1978.

Weil, P. "Comparative Costs to the Medicare Programs of Seven Prepaid Group Practice Plans." *Milbank Memorial Fund Quarterly*, pp. 339–365, Summer, 1976.

Weissert, W. "Costs of Adult Day Care: A Comparison to Nursing Homes." *Inquiry*, 15, pp. 10–19, March, 1978.

Weissert, W., Wan, T. and Liveratos, B. *Effects and Costs of Day Care and Homemaker Services for the Chronically Ill: A Randomized Experiment*. NCHSR Research Report Series. Department of Health Services Research, DHEW Publication No. (PHS) 79–3258, Washington, D.C., February, 1980.

Weissert, W., Wan, T., Liveratos, B. and Katz, S. "Effects and Costs of Day Care Services for the Chronically Ill." *Medical Care*, 18, pp. 567–584, June, 1980.

6. Mechanisms of Access and Coordination

Margaret A. Mac Adam, M.S.
Diane S. Piktialis, Ph.D.

Introduction

It was in 1866 that Congress established six national homes for disabled volunteer soldiers who had served in the Civil War. In 1930, the Veterans Administration was created "to administer veterans' laws effectively, expeditiously, and with sympathetic understanding, and to exercise constructive leadership in the field of veterans' affairs" (U.S. Congress, House Committee on Veterans Affairs, 1982b, p. 69). During the past one hundred years many changes have taken place in the age and composition of veteran cohorts, the delivery of services for those with chronic disease, and the development of publicly-supported non-VA health care systems. The current decade offers challenge and opportunity for the VA to assess its current programs in light of the needs of aged World War II veterans.

The purpose of this chapter is to examine the topics of access and coordination in long term care. While the issues are related, they are treated separately in order to identify the most salient features of each. The problems of access and coordination must be understood within the context of long term care. Therefore this chapter begins with a brief description of the VA and non-VA long term care service systems and identifies the major factors shaping current policy formulation. The approach is to move from consideration of each topic in the larger long term care arena to specific concerns within the VA program. The chapter concludes with a set of recommendations for improvements in access and coordination.

I. Problems of Access and Coordination in Long Term Care

Long term care refers to a set of personal support services provided over an extended period of time for those incapable of sustaining themselves without such care. Callahan has identified a minimum set of non-acute medical services that may be required by disabled individuals. In addition to institutional, home health, case management, and housing services, they include: adult day care, chore services, home-delivered meals, protective services, telephone reassurance/daily checking, transportation, information and referral services, and emergency mental health support (Callahan, 1981b). These services are available in varying quantities through thousands of local agencies of various types. The multiple needs of long term care clients are likely to require services from more than a single agency, which in turn necessitates coordination.

A. VA Extended Care Programs

The flow of patients within the VA extended care program warrants description in that it differs from the non-VA system; in order to be eligible for most extended care services, a veteran must have been hospitalized in a VA hospital first. Thus, there is the potential for close coordination and flexibility between the acute and extended care systems. Moreover, there is an ordering of services in terms of maximizing self-care and patient independence. Because the VA offers many levels of care [see below] the VA has the flexibility to transfer patients within its own system to more or less intensive levels of care as patient needs change.

The VA offers extended hospital, nursing home, and non-institutional services for veterans.

1. Extended Hospital Care

Within VA hospitals and in several state homes, the VA provides intermediate or extended hospital care when acute

160

care is no longer necessary. This program provides care to patients who need long term physician involvement and hospital based support services. Within VA hospitals, 10,557 beds are available for intermediate care while about 600 beds are available in state homes. This program has been growing because patients in unstable conditions are often referred to the VA when the private sector has not provided adequate care.

2. VA Geriatrics and Extended Care Programs

The VA Office of Geriatrics and Extended Care oversees a variety of long term care programs for veterans. They include nursing home care (VA, community, and state), domiciliary care, hospital based home care, adult day care, residential care, and the Geriatric Research, Education and Clinical Centers (GRECCs). There is also a hospice program in Los Angeles funded under this division. Each of these programs is described briefly below.

(a) Institutional Extended Care Programs

i. VA Nursing Home Care, authorized under Public Law 88-450, is provided in 9,239 beds at 99 VA medical centers across the country. In FY '82, the VA served 15,072 veterans in 9,239 beds (8,486 Average Daily Census) with skilled nursing home care. About 62% of the veterans receiving this care were aged 65 or older. In the next five years, the VA expects to add 3,000-4,000 additional beds to this program. This program provides a higher level of care than is usual in community nursing homes according to the National Academy of Science (1977).

ii. The Community Nursing Home Program provided skilled and intermediate care to approximately 31,658 patients (9,525 ADC) in FY '82. About 56% were 65 or older. The VA contracts with local nursing homes for this service and thus is able to provide care closer to the veteran's own home and community. This program is also expected to increase its census in the next five years. Length of stay is limited to six months for non-service-connected veterans (unless the VA medical center director extends the stay) and is indefinite for service-connected veterans.

iii. State Nursing Home Care is a unique program of the VA which assists state governments to build and operate nursing homes. In FY '82 the VA assisted 27 states to provide care in 41 state homes to about 11,934 veterans (6,428 ADC). Seventy-five percent were expected to be aged 65 or older. During the next five years, the VA expects to increase patients treated in this program by 15%.

The VA is experiencing a decline in the ratio of new nursing home beds to growth in the elderly veteran population (U.S. Congress, House Committee on Veterans Affairs, 1982b). The VA's goal is to provide for 20% of the veterans' needs for nursing care but is actually providing for 14-15% of the need. The Medical District Initiated Program Planning (MEDIPP) system will provide new information about needs and resources for institutional care [see below] on a district level.

iv. Domiciliary Care in VA facilities provides medical and other professional care for ambulatory veterans who are disabled but do not require the skilled services of a nursing home or hospital. In FY '82, about 14,535 veterans were treated in 16 VA domiciliaries which had an average daily census of 7,087. Since 1972, the supply of domiciliary beds in VA facilities has been declining in part because many of such facilities are over 50 years old and no longer meet fire, safety, and privacy standards. About 30% of VA domiciliary patients are 65 or older. The VA expects that there will be 5,851 new or remodeled beds available in the next five years.

In addition to VA domiciliaries, 32 states provided domiciliary care in 43 state homes to about 9,550 veterans (4,493 ADC) in FY '82. In the state domiciliary care program approximately 51% of patients are 65 or older.

(b) Non-Institutional Extended Care Programs

i. Hospital Based Home Care. Thirty VA medical centers (VAMCs) provide medical, nursing, social, rehabilitation, and dietetic services to disabled homebound veterans. In FY '82 over 6,500 patients were treated in this program through 144,100 home visits made by health professionals.

ii. Adult Day Health Care. Recently the VA has started several models of adult day care programs in an effort to facilitate the return of disabled veterans to their own homes. Both a medical model which stresses rehabilitation and a social model which emphasizes respite

162

care for family members and maintenance of functioning are in operation now [see below].

      iii. <u>Residential Care</u>. The residential care program provides room, board, personal care and general health supervision to veterans who cannot live independently. In 1982 an approximate average daily census in the program was 12,800 in 3,124 approved homes across the country. Ten to fourteen percent of the patients placed in residential care are general medical/surgical patients.

The residential care program is paid for by the veteran himself from his pension or service-connected disability check. The VA does not provide direct financial support but does locate and inspect homes and monitor the veteran after placement. Most of the patients currently in residential care have psychiatric disorders. The program offers an inexpensive "foster care" model for veterans who have types of ailments which do not require ongoing medical supervision.

(c) Geriatric Research, Education and Clinical Centers (GRECCs)

The GRECC program, established under Section 302 of Public Law 96-330, consists of eight centers funded to attract and develop professional staff in the field of gerontology and geriatrics, and to integrate research and educational achievement in geriatrics into the VA clinical system. The GRECC program is not a line program of the VA but is a special effort to improve clinical, research and training capabilities in the area of geriatric care. Geriatric evaluation units (GEUs) have been established at most of the GRECCs for diagnosis, research, and therapy. Six GRECCs have implemented GEUs with a broad base in internal medicine and in psychiatry including one with an emphasis on Alzheimer's disease. The concept of special geriatric evaluation units is beginning to be implemented by some VAMCs which do not have a GRECC.

(d) Hospice

The VA is operating one hospice program for the care of the terminally ill at the Los Angeles Wadsworth VA Medical Center.

3. Eligibility for VA Extended Care Services

Eligibility for all VA health services is based on three broad criteria: (1) veteran status, (2) degree of disability, and (3) service-connection of disability. (Note: Eligibility for services within the VA is a complex subject beyond the scope of this chapter. A few comments on eligibility are provided which indicate general principles of eligibility.)

In 1970, Public Law 91-500 amended eligibility criteria for VA services by permitting veterans with non-service-connected disabilities aged 65 years or over to be eligible for hospital, nursing home, and domiciliary care regardless of their ability to pay on a space available basis. Currently 12-16% of elder veterans avail themselves of this entitlement depending on the type of care and age of the veteran (VA, 1983b). However, this provision does not override other higher priority criteria such as need for care for a service-connected disability.

The next section of this chapter describes the non-VA long term care service system.

B. Non-VA Geriatric and Extended Care Programs

The focus of delivery of the non-VA long term care system rests at the state level. The availability of Medicaid funds to meet the needs of the disabled has forced states to develop planning and service delivery systems in response to the growing pressure for care of the elderly. In general, the non-VA long term care system is comprised of two main sectors: institutional and non-institutional.

1. Institutional Care

The institutional sector is made up of chronic disease hospitals and nursing homes. Nationally there are two million long term care beds of all types: 1,406,000 nursing home beds (comprised of 83% nursing care beds and 17% personal care and domiciliary care beds); and 302,100 long-stay hospital beds (76% psychiatric beds, 7% chronic disease and 17% "miscellaneous" including rehabilitation, tuberculosis and other). There are an additional 320,000 residential care beds (57% for the mentally retarded, 20% for the emotionally disturbed, 9% for drug abusers or alcoholics, and 14% other)(U.S. DHHS, 1981a). In 1978 there were 18,000-20,000 nursing homes and 614 long term hospitals in the country (Callahan, 1981b).

The construction of new beds has not kept pace with the nation's increasing elderly population. The shortage of nursing home beds, which is marked in some regions of the nation, has led to pressure to keep some elders in acute care hospitals until a suitable placement can be made. Pressure also is being felt by families and the community sector to care for certain frail elders who are waiting for an institutional placement.

2. Community Service System

The non-institutional long term care sector is composed of four major subsections: the certified home health agencies which provide nursing, home health aide, speech, physical and/or occupational therapy to clients who need these services; home care agencies which provide case management and certain purchased social services to eligible elders; the Area Agencies on Aging which are federally mandated to plan and coordinate services for elders; and a large number of supportive services including housing programs which offer subsidized and, in some cases, supportive living arrangements to elders. At the local level, these four groups of providers should work closely together to offer community based, long term care services. Each of them is described below in more detail.

(a) Home Health

Home health agencies are organizations which provide health-related services to patients in their homes with the goal of promoting, maintaining, or restoring health. The states are authorized by Medicare to certify agencies who wish to collect Medicare reimbursement for home health services. In Massachusetts, for example, Medicare was the source of payment for 62% of home health cases, Medicaid reimbursed 12% of all cases, and private funds accounted for the remainder (Commonwealth of Massachusetts, 1981). Services provided by home health agencies include skilled nursing, home health aide, physical, occupational, and speech therapy. Nationally, 2,100 home health agencies are serving more than 700,000 individuals per year (Callahan, 1981b).

165

(b) Home Care

Many states are now offering to provide care management and coordination of non-institutional and social support services for the frail elderly (Massachusetts, New York, Georgia, Maine, Pennsylvania, Connecticut, Wisconsin and California, for example). Additionally, some programs can directly authorize the provision of certain social services (homemaker, chore, transportation, laundry, home delivered meals, for example) for eligible clients. Most of these services are targeted to those who are vulnerable -- that is, clients who have functional deficits which place them in an at-risk category. The goal of these programs is to allocate local service resources to prevent unnecessary nursing home placements.

(c) Area Agencies on Aging

Created under the Older Americans Act, Area Agencies on Aging (AAAs) are federally designated organizations which are mandated by law to coordinate and develop comprehensive service delivery systems to serve elderly persons in greatest social or economic need. There are more than 600 AAAs across the country. The activities of AAAs include planning, grants management, and monitoring of locally funded service programs, local service system development, coordination and advocacy. As more emphasis is placed on community based and in-house service delivery, the mandate of AAA's to develop coordinated systems is becoming increasingly important. Over 11 million elders receive services funded through AAAs (Callahan, 1981b).

(d) Supportive Services

i. Housing. The literature describes a range of various types of housing or residential environments that would meet the needs of people who are becoming increasingly frail. In general, supportive housing should provide at least one meal per day, opportunities for companionship, and some limited supervision. Home health and other services such as homemaker/home health aides may be delivered in these residential environments as well. Included within this broad description are rest homes and congregate housing sites.

ii. Adult Foster Care is similar in concept to the VA's Residential Care Program. Individuals receive money for providing room, board, companionship and unskilled personal care in a family-like setting to frail elderly and disabled persons who are at imminent risk of institutionalization. Provider organizations can include hospitals, home care agencies and family service associations. Adult Foster Care clients usually have medical conditions which require assistance with activities of daily living (ADLs) and the supervision of medications.

iii. Other Services. As mentioned above, the potential range of services which long term care clients may need is extensive. In addition to the major service sectors described here, most communities offer important services such as day care, homemaker, chore, meal, telephone reassurance and hospice programs.

3. Eligibility for Community Care Services

Eligibility for major long term care services is determined by the funding source and may include age, income, condition -- singly or in combination. Standards used by each state to determine eligibility vary widely. Table 1 lists the eligibility standards for specific target groups for major federal programs.

In summary, Table 2 lists the extended care services offered by the VA and non-VA service systems. As can be seen there is considerable overlap in services with the notable exception of in-home supportive services not provided by the VA.

Clearly, the VA and the non-VA systems are moving in parallel directions as the impact of aging clients is felt in both systems. In the area of planning, the VA has initiated MEDIPP which resembles the comprehensive coordinated health planning goals of the Health Systems Agencies (HSAs) set up in 1975 [see below]. In the area of geriatric research education and clinical services, the VA has established the GRECCs while the AOA has funded the Long Term Care Gerontology Centers in nine medical schools across the country. In the area of service delivery, the VA has promoted multidisciplinary case management and the development of non-institutional alternatives such as residential care, hospital based home care, and day care. In the non-VA sector, case management, financial management caps and community service alternatives are also being developed.

167

Table 1

E L I G I B I L I T Y   S T A N D A R D S
FOR SPECIFIC TARGET GROUPS
FOR TITLES III, XVIII, XIX, XX, AND SSI, CMHC PROGRAMS

	TITLE III, OR OLDER AMERICANS ACT	SSI, TITLE XVI OF SOCIAL SECURITY ACT	MEDICARE, TITLE XVIII OF SS ACT	MEDICAID, TITLE XIX OF SS ACT	TITLE XX OF SS ACT	CMHC
Aged	60+ Individuals in greatest economic and social need.[1]	65+	65+	Same criteria as for SSI in 35 states.	Each state defines target populations in its own way.[2]	No specific emphasis or exclusion. Programs establish their own fee schedules.
Blind	Emphasis on vulnerable elderly.[1]	Eligible if meet specific visual acuity standards.	Eligible if entitled to certain social security disability or railroad retirement benefits.	Same as above	Same as above	Same as above
Disabled	Same as above	Eligible if unable to work for specified time as result of disability.	Same as above	Same as above	Same as above	Same as above

Mentally Disabled	Same as above	Eligible if meet speci-fied IQ standard for levels of functioning.	Same as above	Same as above Special provi-sion low-income mentally retarded.	Same as above Focus is on young adults.
Special Groups	None	Children with impairments comparable to these speci-fied for adults.	People requir-ing dialysis or kidney transplants, & in social se-curity or rail-road retirement programs.	Same as above	Same as above None

1 Programs may establish fee schedules but no individual may be denied service because of unwillingness to pay.

2 States choose the various levels and services for which fees are charged.

From: DHHS, Office of the Assistant Secretary for Planning and Evaluation; Working Papers on Long-Term Care; October, 1981.

169

Table 2

COMPARISON OF LONG TERM CARE SERVICES
OFFERED BY THE VA
AND NON-VA SERVICE SYSTEMS

VA	Non-VA
• Extended Hospital Care	• Chronic Disease and
• Nursing Home	Rehabilitation Hospitals
• Residential Care	• Nursing Home
• Domiciliary	• Foster Care, Board and Care
• Adult Day Health Care	• Congregate Housing
• Hospital Based Home Care	• Day Care
	• Home Health Agencies
	• Home Care Programs
	• Social Support

C. **Fragmentation of the Existing System and Factors for Change**

Identification of problems in the delivery of long term care services is not a new phenomenon, nor are the problems themselves different. In particular, the problem of fragmentation had been identified as early as 1956 by the Commission on Chronic Illness. Callahan (1981b) has highlighted one concise description of the problem in the work of the Commission:

> No single agency in any community can meet all the complex needs of the long term patient; without some central organization concerned with those needs, gaps and overlaps in long term care are almost inevitable. The task of such a central agency is formidable because of the wide range in needs of the long term patient, the multiplicity of ways through which care is financed, conflicting interests and pressures, the existence of outmoded facilities, and other factors... Chronic illness is everyone's problem and, by the same token, no one's clear responsibility...for the long term patient, the absence of a single responsible agency is a major lack... the individual does not know where to turn (p. 148).

170

Both the VA and non-VA systems are working to meet the needs of aged clients within similar constraints: limited resources, complex priorities for care, and existing incentives to institutionalize. However, there are three characteristics of the present delivery system which underlie the need to address problems of access and coordination:

- Disabled people participate in different subsystems (health, housing, income maintenance) and therefore there is a need for coordination among the subsystems.

- The personal care subsystem is particularly poorly organized and yet is the system of most importance to a disabled person.

- In many instances the long term care individual is a marginal client to the service providers upon whom he depends because most providers are not established, with a major goal, to meet the needs of the chronically impaired (Callahan, 1981b).

The dynamics of the long term care service system are changing rapidly. Three factors which shape current thinking in the area are financing, utilization, and targeting.

Somers (1982) identified three major demographic factors which underlie the growing focus on long term care: increasing life expectancy for the elderly, the dominance of chronic disease as the major cause of morbidity in the United States, and the "shrinking" of the American family. These factors are affecting the financing, utilization, and targeting of services which all long term care providers offer.

1. Financing

During the 1970s, the VA as well as the non-VA health delivery systems were affected by several phenomena in patient management which enabled them to improve efficiency: increased patient turnover, reduced lengths of stay, optional modalities for care, more ambulatory care, and more outpatient surgery. Many of these changes have been prompted by rapidly rising medical care expenditures. In particular, the share of the federal budget being expended on health care is now a source of great concern. The federal share of public funds grew from 51% in 1965 to 67% in 1973 due to a combination of program growth, financing changes, inflation, and new entitlements (Freeland and Schendler, 1981). The Congressional Budget Office recently calculated that the Medicare budget will rise to $112 billion by 1988, an increase of almost 100% from the current level of $57 billion. More importantly, the Social Security Trust Fund for health insurance is expected to be depleted by 1989 (Rivlin, 1983). In 1977, 94.4% of veterans over 65 years of age had health insurance, 81.1% were covered by Medicare (VA, 1979). Therefore, the anticipated financing problems in the Medicare program are likely to motivate many elderly veterans to seek care from the VA.

2. Utilization

A second area of change is in utilization of long term care services by the elderly. In the population as a whole, assuming current use rates, the projected growth of nursing home utilization by age will increase 54% over the next 20 years and 132% by 2030 (U.S. DHHS, 1981b). Historically, the VA has attempted to care for approximately 20% of the veterans' need for nursing home care. It is estimated that by 1990, in order to meet 20% of the need the VA will require from 20,000 to 22,000 beds, almost double the supply of beds in 1982 (U.S. Congress, House Committee on Veterans Affairs, 1982b).

3. Targeting

A third trend is the need to target resources to those most in need. Targeting methodologies will become more effective as consensus is developed about the most appropriate clients for publicly funded long term care services. Currently every financing program has its own eligibility criteria which reflect the political strength of various constituents. If public resources are not able to accommodate the demand for service, it is likely that resource allocation will become a major public policy debate. For the VA, this question is taking shape around the appropriate priority level for services to the non-service-connected veterans.

Explicit in resource allocation discussions is an understanding of the vital role that family members and informal support systems play in the provision of long term care services. Shanas (1982) has put to rest the myth that old people are alienated from their families and children. She found that for every individual living in a nursing home, there are two living in the community who are being taken care of by their families and friends. The Cleveland GAO study concluded that the importance of family and friends is evidenced by the fact that greatly or extremely impaired elderly who live with their spouses and children generally are not institutionalized, whereas those who live alone usually are (Comptroller General, 1977a). As the role of the family becomes clearer, it is evident that public programs must support rather than supplant family care.

In response to these trends the VA has moved in two directions which anticipate the shape of long term care service delivery in the future. First, the VA has recognized the need to maintain a continuum of care from both the acute and long term care sectors. An integrated system, which can be managed and controlled, requires access to a full array of services when needed. A second development in the VA's long term care system has been early recognition of the social dimension of long term care. In particular, the VA has developed an array of treatment modalities which in and of themselves provide a primary answer to the needs of many long term care patients. During the 1980s, non-VA long term care service providers are moving into both of these areas to gain control over a full range of services and to develop noninstitutional alternatives.

Critics of today's long term care system identify two major problems which plague the existing system: fragmentation of service delivery across a variety of services, providers, financing mechanisms, funding sources, and eligibility requirements, and, secondly, financial incentives which favor medical over social services, and institutional over non-institutional care. Careful attention to these issues is imperative for both VA and non-VA long term care service providers.

II. Coordination Issues

A. General Review of Coordination

A major barrier to change in access and coordination of health care services for the elderly is organizational complexity. The previous discussion of range of services,

173

eligibility criteria and mechanisms for delivery highlight several factors which contribute to the problem.

Resistance to coordination among agencies is rooted in the political-economic context of agency survival. Benson, et al., (1973), studied the relationships among social welfare agencies in Missouri and found "the agencies are enmeshed in a complex system of relations in which they pursue a supply of resources" (pp. 121-122). Aiken, et al., went on to develop two suggestions for successful coordination: development of a coalition which brings in new money and leaves previous funding undisturbed, and/or the creation of domain consensus about the interdependence of services. In other words, successful coordination takes place when the strategy either incorporates all interests or accommodates them. Their research also concluded that

> the most basic lesson regarding service delivery which can be learned from the experiences of these five projects is that particular structures are appropriate for coordinating some elements in a service delivery system (information, clients, programs and services, or resources), but inappropriate for coordinating other elements. When the service delivery structure does not match the element to be coordinated, it is highly unlikely to be successful (Aiken, et al., 1975, p. 147).

Wilson (1981) has identified two approaches to coordination of various aspects of the health care system: case coordination and structural coordination. At the micro level, case coordination enables individual patients to obtain multiple services of numerous organizations. The community long term care system can be so disorganized, that the case coordination function can serve as the focal point of a mix of medical, rehabilitation, and social services provided at the patient level. At the case coordination level, social welfare literature has described many reasons for interorganizational failure to achieve the goal of integrated services. Callahan highlighted the following thirteen points from the literature as "lessons" which are pertinent to today's problems of service delivery:

"1. No one program model suits all communities.

2. The majority of users of innovative multipurpose or case coordination projects are <u>not</u> the at-risk population for which that particular program was designed.

3. The agency which coordinates other agencies should not operate direct services.

4. Coordination is very expensive, as well as difficult. Don't try to coordinate too many agencies at once.

5. Public/voluntary funding contracts can work, but successful coordination requires moderate stress.

6. Consumer and community involvement is difficult, takes time, and is a two-edged sword. Different degrees of community control are indicated for different kinds of objectives.

7. Co-location does not equal coordination. Unification of different services under one administration does not guarantee coordination.

8. Authority helps but does not guarantee coordination. Cooperative models rarely succeed.

9. Accountability mechanisms are difficult to install and maintain, but can be productive in time.

10. A coordination system should be evolutionary and cumulative.

11. The potential efficiency and effectiveness of a coordination program cannot be evaluated during the first and second years.

12. The leader of a coordination project must be a super being with optimum political skills, administrative competence, missionary fervor, and familiarity with the entire range of professional interventions and management techniques. In addition, the leader must, during the early phases of the new project, be primarily process-oriented and, in later phases, be primarily task-oriented.

13. At all levels of coordination, it is crucial that there be frequent and genuine interpersonal con-

tact between representatives of agencies who are essential to the program's success" (Callahan, 1981b, pp. 161-162).

Wilson (1981) concludes that "coordination must be seen as a political process by which health care professionals and organizations mobilize and form linkages in response to health problems and issues" (p. 61). These writers agree that the actual mechanics of coordination and access will depend on the political-economic context of the problem.

In his testimony before the House Committee on Veterans Affairs, Dr. Donald Custis, at the time Chief Medical Director, succinctly summarized the major political-economic reasons for the VA's concern about the needs of aging veterans. The first reason is demographic. The projected increase in the number of veterans over age 65 is from 3.3 million in 1981 to 7.7 million in 1990 and about 9 million in 2000. In 1981, almost 25%, or 798,000 of all veterans received care from the VA. By 1990, about 1.8 million veterans could be seeking help from the VA if the pattern of utilization remains the same. Dr. Custis concluded his demographic analysis with the statement that "it is evident that even if we leave the matter there, our system would be experiencing overall demands for care that would exceed our current ideas about adequate resources" (U.S. Congress, House Committee on Veterans Affairs, 1982b, p. 7). A second factor which will affect the pool of potential users of VA services is the availability of alternative health services, particularly Medicare and Medicaid. Eighty-one percent of elderly veterans are covered by Medicare and 4.2% by Medicaid. As these major financing programs experience funding constraints, it is probable that increasing numbers of eligible veterans will turn to the VA for services. Storey (1983) described the results of cutbacks in Medicare and Medicaid programs on elderly beneficiaries: (1) cuts may increase a beneficiary's out-of-pocket costs for services and/or private insurance, (2) beneficiaries may receive less service, and (3) they may have to rely more on family support to meet health care expenses or to avoid institutionalization. A fourth effect, recognized by Dr. Custis, is to tilt veterans toward the VA for services.

At the macro level, structural coordination establishes a set of organizational relationships characterized by cooperation, joint programs, mutual referrals and joint planning and policy making. Wilson identified the most pervasive examples of structural coordination efforts as the HSAs established by the National Health Planning and Resources Development Act of 1974 (Public Law 93-641). Within the VA, the MEDIPP process is an example of structural coordination. The flexibility of all coordination efforts is constricted by limitations imposed by local, state, and federal forces. Eleven factors limiting local coordination efforts were developed by Gardner and reported by Callahan:

"1. The workings of the national economy as it affects the resources available to policy makers;

2. The deliberate results of national policy, such as a support for categorical grants or regulatory policies requiring environmental impact statements;

3. The inadvertent effects of national policy, such as a support for suburbanization which resulted from the Highway Act in the tax structure;

4. The role of state government;

5. The role of public opinion and constraining local actors;

6. The views of outside political actors themselves, unions, interest groups and individual citizens;

7. Geography of the city and region (e.g., the degree to which the city's boundaries incorporate or are separate from the metropolitan economy, allowing linkage of local dollars outside the locality itself and in the region);

8. Demography, since the make-up of a population constrains its policy;

9. The city's own resources in light of both actual fiscal strength and its taxpayers' perceptions of their tax burdens;

10. Time as a constraint on short-range policy making;

11. Judicial decisions as they set the legal boundaries of local policy" (Callahan, 1981b, pp. 163-164).

177

The interaction of horizontal and vertical constraints on coordination efforts highlights the need to take action at all levels if effective change is to take place.

B. Coordination in Long Term Care

The institutional long term care system is relatively well organized because it is so heavily dominated by public payments through the Medicaid programs. The single largest problem for consumers and professionals is the lack of a central clearing house on nursing home bed availability at the local level.

Non-institutional programs on the other hand are not dominated by any particular funding source; Medicare, Medicaid, Social Service Block Grants, Title III of the Older Americans Act, federal and state housing and transportation programs, and state-funded social service programs all participate in providing extended care services to the elderly. At the local level, with the exception of demonstration programs, no single agency coordinates the entire array of community based, long term care services. In fact, each major program has its own legislatively mandated eligibility requirements, benefit package, provider participation restrictions, administrative structures, and service delivery mechanism.

At the local level, the array and fragmented nature of health and social service delivery can be both confusing and frustrating. Assemblyman Art Torres of California observes that in the community care system "when a problem arises, the average person is faced with an array of fragmented services offered by a large number of providers in a totally disjointed, disorganized, inefficient non-system" (Torres, 1982). A typical description of the problems arising between two of the local service systems can be described as follows:

A patient needing skilled nursing care or home health aide service is likely to be referred by a doctor or hospital discharge planner to a certified home health agency. That agency is under no obligation to provide or even arrange for any service other than home health care. Although the home health agency can and may refer the patient to a social service agency if social services are required, the burden of coordinating those services is usually on the patient or his family. Agencies sometimes do not make such referrals until home health benefits have been exhausted. In these circumstances, patients may do without needed services. If the home health agency does make the referral, the social service agency might send its own provider(s). So an individual might receive health aide services from the home health agency and home-maker services from another social service agency. The confusion is compounded if the patient requires nutrition services (yet another agency) or dental care.

Because this problem is so pervasive in the current community care system, and appears to result in ineffi-cient use of scarce resources, several states have initi-ated comprehensive case management programs (California, New York, Georgia) while the Health Care Financing Admin-istration (HCFA) and the AOA are funding the National Long Term Care Channeling Demonstration Program, a major re-search project in coordinated case management. These and many earlier demonstrations to address this issue are dis-cussed in depth in another chapter in this book, "Experi-ments and Demonstrations of Sharing and Coordination."

Veterans and VA staff face the same problems as other consumers and advocates as they attempt to penetrate the community care system. The VA has responded by assigning Social Work Community Coordinators to identify community resources for aged veterans, by developing directories of community resources for use by social workers, and by par-ticipating with AAAs and HSAs in efforts to improve coor-dinated planning and development.

C. VA Models of Coordination

The VA has developed many coordinated programs. This chapter will discuss those which particularly emphasize coordination with non-VA resources: (1) Medical District Initiated Program Planning process (MEDIPP), (2) Geriatric Research, Education and Clinical Centers (GRECCs), (3) Sharing of Specialized Medical Resources, (4) State Nurs-ing Home Program, (5) Spinal Cord Injury Units, (6) Social Work, (7) Community Based Care Programs, and (8) Voluntary Services.

1. Medical District Initiated Program Planning Process (MEDIPP)

In 1981, the VA Department of Medicine and Surgery im-plemented a five-year district planning process designed to formulate plans at the district level for the provision

179

of health care. The VA has established six goals of the MEDIPP process:

- To be responsive to the health care needs of veterans;

- To be reflective of resource needs, as determined at the medical district level;

- To be based on local and national demographic analyses;

- To be supportive of the approved mission of each VA health care facility in a district;

- To be built upon specific professional and supportive programs and activities; and

- To be reflective of current directives and policies, as set forth in the Chief Medical Director's Guidance.

Within the VA, the MEDIPP process has been designed to promote coordination, collaboration and cooperation at all levels of the Department. At the local and district levels, it can be expected that the MEDIPP process will encourage close scrutiny of local resources both within and without the VA. The third cycle of MEDIPP is currently underway and will impact the VA budget request in 1985. The MEDIPP process provides the VA for the first time, with an internal structure for interacting with other community health planners, particularly those in the AAAs and the HSAs.

Additionally, the VA continues to participate as a non-voting member in the community and national planning efforts of HSAs and the State Health Planning and Development Agencies. Although the VA is exempt from the Certificate of Need program, it has been the policy of the VA to notify local HSAs of its construction plans.

2. Geriatric Research, Education and Clinical Centers (GRECCs)

Beginning in 1974, the Geriatric Research, Education and Clinical Center program attracted professionals to teach and conduct basic and clinical research on aging. Each center provides education in geriatrics and may experiment with alternative means for providing care to the aged. Eight GRECCs were funded from the original authorization. Seven more were authorized by the VA Health Care Amendments of 1980, although funding constraints have slowed the development of new GRECCs. The VA has focused on strengthening the current GRECCs with available resources.

In some ways, the GRECCs are similar to the Long Term Care Gerontology Centers which are funded by the AOA of the U.S. Department of Health and Human Services. These centers are located in nine medical schools across the country to provide research and education services. The research projects of the Long Term Care Gerontology Centers typically are in the area of service delivery rather than clinical care. The AOA has recently announced that the Long Term Care Gerontology Centers will be asked to develop new models for long term care service delivery systems for the non-VA service system.

3. Sharing of Specialized Medical Resources

In 1966, the VA was granted authority to share underutilized, specialized, scarce and costly resources in VAMCs with community hospitals, federal and state hospitals, clinics, and blood and organ banks. In return the VA was permitted to purchase similar community resources for the care of veterans. Public Law 98-785 required no reduction in service to the veteran and that provision be made for reciprocal reimbursement. By the end of FY '81, 109 VAMCs had entered into 368 sharing agreements with community health care facilities with an annual cost amounting to $30,257,000. Sharing agreements have resulted in better cooperation between VA hospitals and community health providers and in improved utilization of scarce medical specialists and facilities. Up to this time, the VA has purchased more community services, primarily hospital services, than it has provided to community hospitals.

4. State Home Program

The VA helps states to defray the costs of building and operating homes through construction grants and per diem payments. State homes include state-operated hospitals, nursing homes and domiciliaries providing care primarily to disabled veterans incapable of earning a living. In FY '82, there were 41 homes in 27 states and the District of Columbia. Of the 41 homes, all provided dom-

iciliary care, 38 provided nursing home care and seven
provided hospital care. Many of the homes accept veteran-
related dependents which helps to avoid separation of a
family unit and provides a more normal atmosphere in the
home. Veterans in state homes usually contribute toward
the cost of their maintenance in the home. The state home
program has provided $81 million for construction of 6,041
nursing home beds and $11 million for 833 domiciliary beds
from the beginning of the program up to July 1, 1981. An
additional $16 million has been obligated for renovations,
including life safety projects. In FY '82, the state home
program had an average daily veteran census of 4,493 for
domiciliary care, 6,428 for nursing home care, and 580 for
hospital care. In each of the participating state homes,
up to 25% of the bed occupancy may be used to care for non-
veterans.

Because the VA pays only part of the cost of care provided to veterans in state homes, this form of care costs
the VA less than to provide the care directly or to contract with community nursing homes. A recent evaluation
of this program by the Comptroller General (1981) found
that the VA could reduce per diem payments by verifying
the level of care needed by veterans admitted to state
homes and could develop other funding mechanisms for some
of the cost of care of veterans. However, the report did
find that, even with current use patterns, state homes are
a cost effective alternative to providing care in VA facilities.

5. Social Work

The social work function in the VA is extensive. During FY '82, 1,595,720 cases were treated by VA social
workers. Basic patient care services include patient
screening, social assessments, and treatment of psychosocial problems. Additionally, social workers provide
discharge and after-care planning, education, research and
community resource development and coordination.

Social work services in the VA have been well developed. For example, in 1983, the VA clarified the role of
the social worker in discharge planning and emphasized
procedures which included:

- Multidisciplinary planning,
- Quality of life concerns for the veterans,
- Patient/family involvement,

182

- Referrals to community agencies and resources, and
- Referrals to VA community care programs (VA, 1983a).

The social work service at each VAMC carries a primary responsibility for accessing, integrating, and coordinating VA and community resources for the ill and disabled. The social work case management program is particularly focused on the aged in addition to prisoners of war, spinal-cord injured, blind, and dialysis patients. The objectives of the case management program are:

- Provision of individualized appropriate range of health services,
- Improved utilization of acute care beds,
- Increased turnover rates,
- Reduced lengths of stay, and
- Reduced dependency of veterans on VA with concomitant improved quality of life (VA, 1983c).

In 1983, each medical district assigned a social worker to function as a community service coordinator to help to develop new programs and cooperative community arrangements. In Region 3, for example, the Medical District Community Coordinators have assisted in developing workshops related to the needs of the elderly, participated in developing state standards for residential care homes and have begun to develop a computerized community resources directory. As the role of the community service coordinators becomes established in the MEDIPP process within each VAMC, these staff can be expected to play an important role as change agents in VA relations with community programs.

6. Spinal Cord Injury (SCI)

The VA has pioneered the field of spinal cord injury medicine in the United States. Currently, the VA operates 19 SCI units which employ a multidisciplinary mode in the management of SCI patients. The VA SCI system treats approximately 85% of all SCI service- and non-service-connected veterans. Interagency agreements with the Armed Forces, civilian hospitals and non-SCI VA hospitals have been signed which permit admissions from those sources to VA SCI units. The SCI program exemplifies the role of the VA as a clinical leader in a specialized branch of medicine with coordinated follow-up for life-long monitoring.

183

7. Community Care Programs

At the local level, the VA is encouraging the development of community based care programs for older veterans:

(a) Adult Day Health Care

Adult Day Health Care is a new development within the VA. The VAMC in North Chicago, Illinois, has a comprehensive program located on the medical center grounds, while a day care program of the Loma Linda, California Medical Center is provided in the Ucaipa American Legion Post. The Loma Linda Day Care Program is particularly noteworthy because it began as a VA operated program and was successfully transferred to the community as a state-certified day care program, open to veterans, non-veterans and American Legion members. This project was a joint undertaking of a VAMC, a veterans service organization and the community at large. Other program models are operating at VAMCs in American Lake, Washington, Palo Alto, (Menlo Park Division), California, and Butler, Pennsylvania. The Menlo Park "Elder Veterans Day Center Day Respite Program" accepts elderly people who need intensive nursing care. A primary goal of the program is to provide respite care for family members and to delay institutionalization. The program operates three days a week serving about 20 men a day.

(b) Case Management

In the California Palm Springs area, the VA is cooperating with the Palm Springs Senior Center to develop a new program to serve the needs of the frail, chronically ill, at-risk and elderly person. The goal of the DAWN (Desert Area Wellness Network) program will be to provide the client group with case management services designed to postpone or avoid premature institutionalization. The program intends to develop an organized and cooperative network of providers using available community agencies and resources. The Veterans Hospital at Loma Linda has offered to contribute the time of a professional social worker to serve as DAWN's program director. This project may demonstrate the assistance a local VAMC can offer to community based programs designed to serve frail elders.

(c) Respite Care and Family Support Programs

At the Brentwood Division of the West Los Angeles Medical Center, VA staff are working with Alzheimer's patients and their families to assist them in four areas: help in achieving an accurate diagnosis, treatment of concurrent medical problems, assistance in managing the dementing illness, and referrals to needed community services. This program is typical of the kind of activity which can be developed to support families caring for disabled veterans. At the Marion VAMC in Indiana, there is a support group for the wives of Alzheimer's patients. This program is geared to help family members understand the disease process and to learn coping mechanisms for adjusting to the change in family life experienced by those with a relative with the disease. Some VAMCs offer respite care for family members who are the primary caretakers of aged veterans. For example, in Gainesville, Florida, medical and social work staff have a multidisciplinary model in a nursing home unit which includes family support groups, respite care, and a community health resources guide for family members. The respite and family support programs are designed to support and assist family caregivers in day to day delivery of care by providing information, emotional support, and relief from the full burden of care.

8. Voluntary Service

The VA has a special Voluntary Service which is 35 years old. More than 77,500 volunteers contributed 10.9 million hours of service in FY '82, many of them devoted to caring for the aged, long term patients, and the terminally ill. Volunteers participate in a wide variety of activities including intergenerational programs, telephone reassurance for homebound veterans, and letter writing for impaired patients.

In summary, it can be seen that the VA has embarked on various approaches to develop coordinated service delivery. The programs described above illustrate approaches to coordinated planning within the VA (MEDIPP); involvement of non-VA geriatric professionals in VA clinical care and research (GRECCs); sharing of hospital resources; funding of states to provide long term care; development of case management services; development and provision of clinical care in an area which has led to national leadership (SCI); development of non-institutional alternatives in long term care; and use of volunteers.

D. Recommendations to Improve Coordination

The literature has identified two major barriers to increased coordination of health services for the elderly:

- The large number of organizations to be coordinated, and
- The competitive political-economic environment.

These two factors operate within the VA system as well as within the larger health care system of this nation. The challenge for the VA is to develop specific strategies to increase internal VA capacity for coordination activities as well as to bridge organizational domains. Steps the VA could take to address access and coordination issues therefore can be grouped into two categories: inter-VA and intra-VA recommendations. Within each of these categories are short- and long-range efforts. Short-range recommendations address themselves to an incremental approach to be implemented while the necessary steps are being taken to develop the support needed for more fundamental change in the long run.

1. Intra-VA Coordination Recommendations

(a) Planning

i. Short-Range. Recognizing the cross-cutting nature of provision of care to those who are chronically impaired, hence the need to address the simultaneous delivery of income maintenance, health, and social services, the VA should initiate an internal study of barriers to intra-agency long term care planning.

ii. Long-Range. The ultimate focus of such a study should be implementation of coordinated policy directions in compensation and pensions, housing assistance, and health care for the aged veteran. These three areas, in particular, offer the VA an excellent opportunity to build on one of its most significant strengths -- the control over eligibility for and level of benefits that veterans receive from the VA.

(b) Service Delivery

i. Short-Range. At national, regional, and district levels, the VA should continue to encourage the development of non-institutional alternatives such as day care, residential care, and respite care. The Hospital Based Home Care Program should be expanded to include more VAMCs.

ii. Long-Range. The VA should work with its constituent groups and the Congress for permission to offer non-medical personal care services (homemaker, meals, transportation, etc.) to veterans able to live in the community. These services should be either provided directly by the VA or contracted with existing community providers.

(c) Case Management

i. Short-Range. VA social work should promote the use of case managers to assess client needs and to be responsible for coordinated service delivery. Recently, new assessment and care planning instruments have been developed which could prove to be useful models for VA social work. A client tracking system should be initiated within the VA through the social work department. The VA should also initiate new demonstration programs in case management which use models similar to the DAWN project in California.

ii. Long-Range. VA social workers should become the focus for case management services which are designed to provide coordinated efficient long term care for aged veterans. The functions of a strong case management service should include preplacement screening, assessment, care planning, and monitoring. Serving as the focus for case management services, the social worker would work with other health professionals to develop care plans based on the requirements of the individual case.

(d) Research, Education, and Clinical Care

i. Short-Range. The potential impact of the GRECCs has been validated in the report of the Geriatrics and Gerontology Advisory Committee which found that, despite limitations to funding "...they seem to be operating reasonably effectively" (VA, 1983b, p. 71). It is important then, given the small number of GRECCs, that the VA publicize the work of the GRECCs and support implementation of GRECC findings in the larger VA system.

ii. Long-Range. The GRECCs, when fully funded, can become models for geriatric evaluation, clinical research and education within the VA and the most effective aspects of the model can be adopted throughout the system.

The extent to which these suggestions for greater coordination are successful will depend upon the ability of VA staff to generate support for change among the affected units of the VA. To this end, techniques of information sharing, consensus building, and resource negotiation can be used.

2. Inter-VA Coordination Recommendations

(a) Planning

i. Short-Range. At the national level, the VA should continue and increase its participation in aging and health planning and coordinating groups. In particular, the VA should consider developing interagency working agreements with the HCFA and the AOA of the Department of Health and Human Services. These agreements could provide a focus for expanded dissemination of research, clinical and service delivery models. Ultimately, the VA, HCFA and AOA could combine resources to demonstrate new cost effective models of long term care. The National Long Term Care Channeling Demonstration Project is an example of a coordinated, jointly-funded project between AOA and HCFA.

At the local level, the VA should actively participate in the work of local HSAs, State Health Coordinating Councils and AAA Advisory Councils. These groups, located in each community and state, attempt to establish goals for institutional bed supply and encourage the establishment of community based and in-home services. From the VA perspective, familiarity with existing community resources which can supplement or replace the need for VA services will further enable the VA to respond to the needs of veterans with VA and non-VA services. From the community perspective, the VA can be a provider of services, information, and training in geriatrics and gerontology. Moreover, the VA can "loan" staff to work on community projects such as health fairs, conferences, and new programs as appropriate.

ii. Long-Range. The chapter entitled, "Experiments and Demonstrations in Sharing and Coordination," makes two recommendations for planning: (1) that the VA take the lead in coordination of community services, and (2) that the VA participate as an equal partner in community planning for long term care services with non-VA providers at the state and local levels. Planning would encompass both resource allocation and service coordination.

(b) Service Delivery

i. Short-Range. The VAMC Loma Linda, California, social work staff have developed the concept of "coalitional networking" to describe one approach to large community resource innovation. This process brings together existing and potential service providers under the leadership of the VA to develop community resources for the elderly. The steps involved in coalitional networking are all established community organizing techniques:

1. Identify need and feasibility;
2. Establish a transition to community based service delivery; and
3. Identify common goal-sharing opportunities in the community.

The VA can encourage staff at VAMCs to use the Loma Linda model to develop new community resources for veterans. However, the VA should allow local VAMCs to respond flexibly to the particular needs and resources of their communities. This may include the development of new models.

ii. Long-Range. The long-range recommendations in coordinated service delivery are (1) that the VA take the lead as the focal point for community care of veterans, and (2) that VA and non-VA providers share in the provision of care where appropriate.

(c) Case Management

i. Short-Range. Many community programs are being established in the states which emphasize the role of case managers to assess needs, plan and implement services, monitor quality of care, and reassess continued need for service. New screening instruments have been developed to identify at-risk elders as well as to assess and provide case planning services. Automated client

189

tracking systems are also being implemented in many areas. The VA social work service which participates in social work education and training opportunities could take the lead to share information on case management and client monitoring systems. Currently, there is no organized vehicle for the timely dissemination of improvements in case management practice at the regional level.

ii. Long-Range. The VA eventually could participate in multidisciplinary screening and/or assessment with non-VA providers. Additionally, it has been recommended in the "Experiments and Demonstrations in Sharing and Coordination" chapter that the VA develop collaboration between VA home services and community care providers for both resource allocation and case management.

(d) Research, Education, and Clinical Care

i. Short-Range. The VA's internal research and education projects, extensive data base, and the activities of the GRECCs, offer many opportunities for the VA to develop a leadership role in geriatrics and gerontology. In particular, the VA could work with the National Institutes of Health (especially the National Institute on Aging) and the AOA to share research findings.

ii. Long-Range. A longer-range recommendation in this area is that, where appropriate, the GRECCs could form local sharing arrangements with the Long Term Care Gerontology Centers funded by the AOA.

III. Access Issues

In a report entitled Long Term Care: Background and Future Directions, the Office of Policy Analysis at HCFA prepared an excellent overview of barriers to access in long term care (U.S. DHHS, 1981b). According to HCFA, the present long term care system suffers from problems of cost, accessibility, and quality of services. In the area of accessibility, there are four constraints on equal access to the full range of long term care services by those in need:

1. Bias toward institutional and medical care;
2. Discrimination against Medicaid and heavy care patients;
3. Geographic variability in access to service; and
4. Unmet needs.

Additionally, this report identifies competition among public payors and access issues specific to the VA service system.

A. Bias toward Institutional and Skilled Medical Care

In the past ten years, numerous studies have indicated that a substantial proportion of nursing home patients could be maintained at home or in non-institutional settings if support services were available. Within the VA, it has been estimated that up to 28% of nursing home residents could be served in the community if appropriate supportive programs were available (VA, 1983d).

In the community long term care system, Medicaid eligibility criteria favor provision of benefits in a nursing home for two reasons. First, in 16 states, only those receiving public assistance (SSI) can become eligible for Medicaid while living in the community, no matter how great their medical or long term care needs are. In almost all these states, however, persons can become eligible for Medicaid if they are in a nursing home. In the other 34 states, there is a spend-down provision which enables those not on cash assistance to qualify for Medicaid but only if their medical expenses are large enough to reduce their remaining income below the Medicaid eligibility standard. A common problem in most states is that the Medicaid eligibility standard is so low that people who become eligible for Medicaid support in the community may not have enough income remaining to meet day-to-day living expenses.

Until recently, spouses and parents were financially responsible for Medicaid patients only when they lived in the same household. If the Medicaid applicant lived in an institution, family members were not responsible for care. In 1982, the federal government changed the Medicaid regulations to allow the states to impose financial liability on certain family members.

Within the VA, some of these same incentives apply. For a service-connected veteran who meets the medical need criteria, the VA covers nursing home care of indefinite duration. For a veteran without a service-connected disability, the VA covers a six-month stay in a community nursing home and under extenuating circumstances, the length of stay can be extended beyond the six months. While living in the community the veteran supports himself

191

using his own resources, although some financial support may be provided through the Aid and Attendance or Special Monthly Pension for Spanish-American and WWI veterans.

A second major bias toward institutionalization is the predominance of medical care financing programs. Medicaid, like the VA health care system for the aged veteran, is an open-ended entitlement program for a select population. Funding for social services or non-medical housing alternatives on the other hand is very limited and not as open-ended as medical care financing. Within the VA, budget allocations made to the medical centers are based on average daily census of occupied beds which creates incentives to favor institutional over non-institutional service delivery. Additionally, Section 4101 of Title 38, U.S.C. states that "the primary functions of the Department of Medicine and Surgery shall be to provide a complete medical and hospital service...for the medical care and treatment of veterans." The medical orientation of the VA is evident in the options available to older veterans' health needs. The six programs offered to aid veterans with extended care needs are: Hospital Extended Care, Nursing Home Care, VA Domiciliary Care, Residential Care Homes, Hospital Based Home Care, and Adult Day Health Care. Not every VAMC has all six extended care programs available. For example, VA nursing home care units were available at 92 of the 172 medical centers in 1980, and hospital based home care was available in only 30 centers (Haber, 1981). While the VA intends to expand its census in these six programs by 16.8% by 1988, growth is planned in the VA nursing home, state nursing home and state home domiciliary care programs (VA, 1983b). The availability of non-institutional alternatives such as geriatric day care is limited to a few demonstration programs.

B. Discrimination against Medicaid and Heavy Care Patients

Ironically, it is those most in need of institutional care who may experience the most difficulty in obtaining it. Public pay patients who require heavy care compete for beds at a disadvantage to private pay or public "light" care patients. As a result, many community hospitals are facing a back-up of heavy care public pay patients who are awaiting nursing home placement.

The VA extended care programs offer a wide array of services for heavy care patients and so have fewer incentives to discriminate in favor of less disabled veterans.

192

However, the VA has stated that case mix considerations require a balance of light and heavy care patients for two reasons: 1) work load and staffing patterns would have to be changed if more frail patients are admitted, and 2) it is depressing for morale if a facility becomes over-loaded with heavy care patients. Therefore, the VA has attempted to maintain a balance of patients in its facilities.

C. Geographic Variability in Access to Service

Access to services is also limited by the unequal distribution of long term care resources across the country. A DHHS report states that the nursing home bed supply varied from 23.9 beds per thousand elderly in Florida to 118.5 beds per thousand elderly in Nebraska in 1980 (U.S. DHHS, 1981b). A study by Scanlon in 1980 found that most variations in resources do not appear to be related to need (U.S. DHHS, 1981b).

The availability of non-institutional services also varies across the states. Massachusetts, New York, and several other states have actively encouraged the development of community care programs in the past five years. New York, for example, accounts for over 75% of all Medicaid home health expenditures in the nation (U.S. DHHS, 1981b).

The VA is faced with similar geographic variation in both bed supply and availability of non-institutional alternatives. In the 1979 Survey of Veterans, 13.1% of veterans using non-VA medical services said they did so because the VAMC was too far away. As described earlier, only 43 VAMCs have hospital based home care programs, adult day health care programs are still isolated demonstration programs, and other noninstitutional alternatives are variably distributed across the country. The full range of both institutional and non-institutional long term care services is not equally available to veterans.

D. Unmet Needs

Many people who need services do not receive them. The availability of family and friends to provide services hampers measurement of the need for formal, government-approved services. The National Health Interview Survey of 1977 of the non-institutional population found that 5% of those surveyed who were aged 65+ reported a need in at least one activity of daily living (bathing, eating, dressing, toileting). For most of these people (88%) family and friends provide the necessary help. However, between 4% and 12% (depending on the service) report that they do not receive the needed assistance most of the time (U.S. DHHS, 1981b).

E. Competition among Public Payors

Problems in access to long term care can be exacerbated when public programs compete among themselves for resources. In the area of institutional long term care, the VA currently reimburses community nursing homes at a higher rate than the Medicaid program. All other things being equal then, the VA client will be more welcome by nursing home administrators than the Medicaid recipient. In the next five years, the VA plans to expand its census in community nursing homes by 32.2% (VA, 1983b). Because the supply of nursing home beds is not expected to rise as quickly as the elderly population, there may be competition among payment sources for access to beds. Another aspect of this issue is competition among health providers to maintain their share of the market. If, as some anticipate, cutbacks in Medicare and Medicaid coverage encourage a higher proportion of veterans to use VA resources, there will be a concomitant loss of patients in the non-VA system. The effect of a patient shift on provider behavior may reveal itself in several ways:

- Increased numbers of physicians may wish to be affiliated with the VA as staff.

- Non-VA hospitals may wish to participate in the VA sharing program and/or may be encouraged to provide services for HMOs.

- Increased numbers of community nursing homes may wish to contract with the VA for nursing home care.

F. VA Access Issues

Some veterans who may be eligible for veterans health benefits may not be referred to VA centers by private physicians who do not receive payments for attending inpatients in VAMCs. "Thus, there is an incentive not to refer a patient to the VA as long as the patient's resources cover non-VA medical center costs and physicians fees" (Broberg, 1981, p. 5).

194

A second access issue which affects the choice of VA or non-VA care is the extent and choice of health care required by a veteran's spouse. Because the VA does not provide care to non-veteran spouses, some married veterans may choose to use the same medical providers as their spouse and to forego their VA benefits because of convenience.

Some veterans have more incentives to use VA resources than non-VA resources. These may include financial incentives and quality of care. Broberg (1981) made rough extrapolations from the 1979 Survey of Veterans data regarding World War II veterans and found "that nearly one-half of black veterans, one-half of women veterans and from one-fifth to one-third of white male veterans will need to give serious consideration on economic grounds alone to availing themselves of VA services" (pp. 4-5). An earlier study by Epstein (1980) concluded that "the VA serves numerous veterans who are not served by other programs — for whatever reason — and provides a superior benefit" (p. 28).

Access to VA facilities by veterans is controlled by complex eligibility rules which emphasize three criteria: 1) veteran status, 2) degree of disability, and 3) service connection of disability. Users who emerge from the eligibility criteria include three groups: 1) veterans receiving compensation for service-connected disabilities, 2) those who are receiving VA pensions for non-service-connected disabilities, most of whom are 65 or over, and 3) all other eligible veterans without service-connected disabilities.

G. Recommendations for Access

A literature review has identified five major access issues in long term care services for the elderly:

1. Bias toward institutional and skilled medical care,
2. Discrimination against Medicaid and heavy-care patients,
3. Geographic variability in access to services,
4. Competition among public payors, and
5. Specific VA access issues.

Using the conceptual framework previously developed for the discussion of recommendations for improved coor-

195

dination, suggestions for decreasing barriers to equal access have been divided into intra- and inter-VA categories.

1. Intra-VA Efforts to Improve Access

(a) Bias toward Institutionalization

The VA represents the largest care system under unified management in the nation. It has the advantage over the non-VA system of being able to implement policy more directly. If the VA decides to address the needs of aging veterans from a comprehensive perspective, it follows that each Medical District should have a full range of VA/community programs available. Funding at the district level should be awarded on the basis of total program census rather than inpatient occupancy rate.

(b) Discrimination against Medicaid and Heavy Care Users

The VA does not discriminate on the basis of Medicaid or other public funding. Rather, VA eligibility criteria reflect space available priority to service the non-service-connected 65+ veteran. Thus, there is some evidence of unequal access to service due to demographic and resource variables (VA, 1983c). The VA should monitor client utilization patterns in an effort to maintain equal access to services for veterans with similar needs and conditions.

(c) Geographic Variability

The VA should not establish an isolated program of geriatric care but should continue to utilize and encourage the development of community programs. Each Medical District should have access to a full range of services, institutional and non-institutional. Flexibility should be granted at the district level to develop these programs directly or by contract. Thus, in a service-rich environment, the VA may wish to purchase existing community services; while in a service-poor environment, the VA may wish to develop new programs itself, or encourage other community agencies to do so as appropriate.

As a first step, however, the VA should clearly establish a set of core services to which every veteran should have equal access. These service requirements should then be flexibly provided depending on local community needs and resources.

(d) Competition among Public Payors

The VA can view itself either as the provider of the last resort or as a primary option to the eligible veteran. Under the first view, the VA should establish the entitlement of veterans to services funded and provided by non-VA programs and should encourage veterans to use those resources. The VA would view its own resources as a safety net for veterans, when specific needed services are not available from other sources. Currently, there is no clear policy on this issue. Those veterans who for a variety of reasons seek care from the VA and qualify for service may view the VA as their primary provider. Certainly, even they should be urged toward non-VA services when it is in their own best interest. This issue is likely to become more thorny as Medicare and Medicaid tighten eligibility and reimbursement.

(e) Specific VA Access Issues

i. Private Physician Control over Referrals. The VA should inform both consumers and providers of care available from the VA to encourage appropriate referrals.

ii. Care for Non-Veteran Spouses. The VA should consider utilization of VA facilities by spouses. This may involve implementation of third-party billing or special trade or sharing arrangements in that it does not appear to be financially feasible for the VA to add care for spouses without considering new financial arrangements.

iii. High Users of VA Services. Veterans who are particularly economically disadvantaged have higher participation rates in the VA system. As mentioned above, the VA should re-examine its service priorities to ensure the use of the VA by those in greatest economic need.

iv. Eligibility. VA eligibility criteria which reflect a space available priority to serve the non-service-connected 65+ veteran may result in unequal access to one or more long term care services. The chapter "Experiments and Demonstrations in Sharing and Coordination" includes a number of options for modifying current eligibility guidelines for the population needing long term care.

2. Inter–VA Efforts to Improve Access

(a) Bias toward Institutionalization

The VA should actively encourage other service systems to offer non-institutional alternatives to the aged. In particular the VA should participate financially in the development of new community based programs.

(b) Discrimination against Medicaid and Heavy–Care Users

The VA offers model programs through its GRECC GEU, Extended Hospital Care, and VA Nursing Home programs. The VA has extensive experience in meeting the needs of heavy-care patients and should publicize the impact of these programs on quality of care, patient outcome, and satisfaction measures.

(c) Geographic Variability

The VA should work with state governments to assure equitable distribution of services across the nation.

(d) Multiplicity of Programs

The VA should become involved in planning and legislative efforts to streamline long term care service delivery by actively participating in federal and state planning and policy formulation.

(e) Competition among Payors

[See above: Intra–VA Efforts to Improve Access] Especially in the community nursing home programs, the VA should examine its payment structure for economy.

(f) Specific VA Access Issues

[See above: Intra–VA Efforts to Improve Access]

198

REFERENCES

Aiken, M., et al. Coordinating Human Services. San Francisco: Jossey-Bass, 1975.

Altman, S. and Sapolsky, H. (Eds.). Federal Health Programs. Lexington, Massachusetts: D.C. Heath and Co., 1975.

Benson, K., et al. Coordinating Human Services: A Sociological Study of an Interorganizational Network. Research Series No. 6. University of Missouri, June, 1973.

Broberg, M. "Some Factors to Be Considered in Meeting the Needs of World War II Veterans." Professional Social Workers Symposium: The Aging Veteran Population; Inter-Organizational Relations. Philadelphia, November, 1981.

Callahan, J. "A Systems Approach to Long-Term Care." In Reforming the Long-Term Care System, Callahan, J.J. and Wallack, S.S. (Eds.), pp. 219-237. Lexington, Massachusetts: D.C. Heath and Co., 1981a.

Callahan, J. "Delivery of Services to Persons with Long-Term Care Needs." In Policy Options in Long Term Care, Meltzer, Farrow, and Richman (Eds.), pp. 148-181. Chicago: University of Chicago Press, 1981b.

Commonwealth of Massachusetts, Department of Public Health, Office of State Health Planning. State Health Plan for Massachusetts, Policy Summary. April, 1981.

Comptroller General, Conditions of Older People: National Information System Needed. GAO, Washington, D.C., 1977a.

Comptroller General. The Well-Being of Older People in Cleveland, Ohio. HCD-77-70, GAO, Washington, D.C., 1977b.

Comptroller General. State Veterans Homes: Opportunities to Reduce VA and State Costs and Improve Program Management. HRD-82-7, GAO, Washington, D.C., October 22, 1981.

199

Comptroller General. The Elderly Should Benefit from Expanded Home Health Care But Increasing These Services Will Not Insure Cost Reductions. GAO, Washington, D.C., December 7, 1982a.

Comptroller General. Preliminary Findings on Patient Characteristics and State Medicaid Expenditures for Nursing Home Care. 82-4, GAO/IPE, Washington, D.C., July 15, 1982b.

Epstein, W. "The Social Work Planner in Long-Term Health Care: A Case Study of Institutional Geriatric Care in the Veterans Administration." Social Work in Health Care, 6(1), pp. 23-35, Fall, 1980.

Freeland, M. and Schendler, C. "National Health Expenditures." Health Care Financing Review, Winter, 1981.

Fries, J. "Aging, Natural Death and the Comprehension of Morbidity." New England Journal of Medicine, 303(3), July 17, 1980.

Galblume, T.W. and Trieger, S. "Demonstrations of Alternative Delivery Systems under Medicare and Medicaid." Health Care Financing Review, 3(3), March, 1982.

Gruenberg, L. and Stuart, N. "Medicare Expenditures for the Chronically Impaired Elderly: Implications for National Long-Term Care Policy." Presentation at the 35th Annual Meeting of the Gerontological Society of America, Boston, Massachusetts, November, 1982.

Haber, P. "Geriatrics and Extended Care in the VA." Professional Social Workers' Symposium: The Aging Veteran Population: Inter-Organizational Relations. Philadelphia, November, 1981.

Jones, W. "The Aging Veterans." In Aging and Retirement: Prospects, Planning and Policy, McCheskey and Borgatta (Eds.), pp. 47-59. Beverly Hills, California: Sage Publications, 1981.

Kane, R. and Kane, R. "The Extent and Nature of Public Responsibility." In Policy Options in Long-Term Care, Meltzer, Farrow and Richman (Eds.), pp. 78-118. Chicago: University of Chicago Press, 1981a.

Kane, R. and Kane, R. "Long-Term Care: Can Our Society Meet the Needs of Its Elderly?" Annual Review of Public Health, 1, pp. 227-53, 1981b.

Mac Adam, M. "Background Paper: Non-Institutional Long-Term Care in Massachusetts." Massachusetts Association of Home Care Programs/Area Agencies on Aging, Somerville, Massachusetts, March, 1983.

Morgan, D.M. "Community Outreach in Long-Term Care." Dimensions in Health Service, 59(5), pp. 21-25, May, 1982.

National Academy of Science. Health Planning in the U.S.: Issues in Guideline Developments. Washington, D.C., March, 1980.

National Academy of Science, National Research Council. Study of Health Care of American Veterans. Washington, D.C., July 8, 1977.

Rivlin, A. "CBO Director: Health Budget Future Is Grim." The Nation's Health, July, 1983.

Sayles, L.R. and Chandler, M.K. Managing Large Systems: Organizations for the Future. New York: Harper and Row, 1971.

Shanas, E. "The Family Relations of Old People." National Forum, Fall, 1982.

Somers, A. "Long-Term Care for the Elderly and Disabled: A New Health Priority." New England Journal of Medicine, 307, July 22, 1982.

Storey, J. Older Americans in the Reagan Era: Impacts of Federal Policy Changes. The Urban Institute Press, 1983.

Torres, A. Press Release on Torres-Felando Long-Term Care Reform Act, California, September 27, 1982.

U.S. Congress, House Committee on Veterans Affairs. VA Sharing Program. Washington, D.C.: U.S. Government Printing Office, 1980.

U.S. Congress, House Committee on Veterans Affairs. VA Medical Program. Washington, D.C.: U.S. Government Printing Office, June 9, 1981.

U.S. Congress, House Committee on Veterans Affairs. Budget Proposed for Fiscal Year 1983. Washington, D.C.: U.S. Government Printing Office, 1982a.

U.S. Congress, House Committee on Veterans Affairs. Oversight of the VA's Extended Care and Geriatric Programs. Washington, D.C.: U.S. Government Printing Office, July 14, 1982b.

U.S. DHHS, Administration on Aging. Policies and Program Directions for 1982-84. AOA-IM-82-36, Washington, D.C., August 26, 1982.

U.S. DHHS, Assistant Secretary for Planning and Evaluation. Working Papers on Long-Term Care. Washington, D.C., October, 1981a.

U.S. DHHS, Health Care Finance Agency. Long-Term Care: Background and Future Directions. 81-20047, Baltimore, Maryland, January, 1981b.

U.S. Veterans Administration. The Aging Veteran: Present and Future Medical Needs. Washington, D.C., October, 1977.

U.S. Veterans Administration. 1979 Survey of Veterans. Washington, D.C., 1979.

U.S. Veterans Administration. Annual Report, 1982. Washington, D.C., June, 1983.

U.S. Veterans Administration. Department of Medicine and Surgery. Circular 10-82-133, Washington, D.C., 1983a.

U.S. Veterans Administration. Health Care of the Aging Veteran: A Report of the Geriatrics and Gerontology Advisory Committee. Washington, D.C., April, 1983b.

U.S. Veterans Administration. Program Evaluations: Social Work Response. Washington, D.C., 1983c.

U.S. Veterans Administration. Summary: Health Care for the Aging Veteran. Integrating VA and Community Resources. Suncoast Gerontology Center, Tampa, Florida, May 4-6, 1983d.

Wegmiller, D. "Shared Service Programs Are on the Rise." Hospitals, pp. 147-49, April 1, 1980.

Weissert, W. "Toward a Continuum of Care for the Elderly: A Note of Caution." Public Policy, pp. 331-340, Summer, 1981.

Wilson, P. "Expanding the Role of Social Workers in Coordination of Health Services." Health and Social Work, 6(1), pp. 57-64, February, 1981.

Wolf, R. "Appropriate Placement and Long-Term Care Health Planning." American Journal of Public Health, 70(11), November, 1980.

7. Attitudes and Behaviors of Service Providers Toward Elder Patients in the VA System

Terrie Wetle, Ph.D.
Sue E. Levkoff, Sc.D.

Introduction

Practitioners in the Veterans Administration system are increasingly becoming the caretakers of older veterans. The overall veteran population is aging dramatically; the number of veterans 65 years and older will have tripled from 1981 to the year 2000. And, those veterans over age 85, who make the most dramatic demands on the health care system, will increase sixfold by the year 2000 (VA, Annual Report 1982). Health care providers within the VA medical setting face complex challenges in their future activities as the caretakers of this aging patient population. The provision of comprehensive and coordinated health care services to geriatric patients is dependent not only on system level characteristics, but also on characteristics at the individual provider level. Some of the most influential of such characteristics are the attitudes and skills of service providers.

This chapter reports on survey research undertaken to examine how attitudes held by health care providers within the VA medical care setting influence their behaviors with older patients. Specifically, we will examine the attitudes that physicians, nurses, and social workers hold toward their geriatric patients and explore if, and how,

such attitudes relate to decisions made in the clinical
setting. First, a brief overview of the relevant literature on attitudes toward older people is provided. Second,
the methodology for this research is presented, including
an overview of the theoretical framework, sampling design,
and survey findings. Finally, the implications of the
study findings are discussed, with special focus on options for VA service organization, in-service training for
VA health care providers and VA geriatric policy.

Past Research

A comprehensive review of the literature on attitudes
of health care providers toward older people is not within
the scope of this chapter. Three such reviews have been
published over the last fifteen years (McTavish, 1971;
Bennett and Eckman, 1973; Lutsky, 1980), and another unpublished review has been made available (Adelson and
Kraus, 1983). The overall conclusions of these reviews
are highlighted below.

The two early reviews (McTavish, 1971; Bennett and
Eckman, 1973) focus on traditional attitude research as
initiated more than 25 years ago and provide interesting
examples of the widely divergent interpretations and dis-
tinctive views exemplified in such research. In McTavish's review, studies are presented according to type of
measurement used. McTavish's general assessment of the
research findings is that the emphasis tends to be on aspects of studies which suggest a higher level of negative
attitudes about old people. Stereotypes uncovered included views that old people are generally ill, tired, not
sexually interested, mentally slower, forgetful, less able
to learn new things, withdrawn, grouchy, and isolated.
However, he also suggests that views of the elderly are
not uniformly negative, but of a multidimensional nature.
While the attitudes held about the elderly were typically
found to be multidimensional, there was no consistency in
the nature or content of provider orientations. Correlates of attitudes were also examined but associations
were weak and inconsistent.

Bennett and Eckman (1973), reviewing many of the same
early attitude studies, come to a far stronger conclusion
about the prevalence of negative attitudes toward the elderly. They state unambiguously that negative views of
aging are shared by young and old alike and that attitudes
toward aging may be critical for adjustment and survival.

They further suggest that the net result of these processes may be the observed responses in the United States today of neglect and rejection of the aged.

In the third review, Lutsky (1980) concentrates on
more recently published literature than the earlier reviews, covering the years from 1976 to 1979. His review
of attitudes toward old people is quite extensive. Across
all the research domains he surveys, including beliefs,
perceptions, and evaluations, he notes that a number of
misconceptions and negative beliefs are held, but that the
aged are infrequently viewed in a strongly negative fashion. Attitudinal evaluations of the aged were found to be
consistently more positive or neutral than negative. His
overall assessment of attitudinal research is closer to
that of McTavish's, whose conclusion suggests that some
attitudinal rejection exists, than to Bennett and Eckman's
strongly pronounced and unequivocal negative statement.
Lutsky further concludes that the substantial diversity
and complexity in attitudes toward the elderly is a function of both object and perceiver characteristics as well
as the method used.

Two sets of findings reviewed by Lutsky are worth noting for the purposes of this research: those related to
beliefs about old people and those related to attitudinal
evaluations of old people. Much of the early attitude research has been criticized (Kogan, 1979) because of the
confounding of attitudes as beliefs about old people (that
is, misinformation), with attitudes as evaluations of old
people (that is, stereotypic views which reflect rejecting
judgments). The Facts on Aging Quiz developed by Palmore
(1977) was an attempt to respond to this possible confusion in attitude research. This quiz tests an individual's knowledge of 25 facts about aging. Application of
this quiz in a variety of populations suggests that certain misconceptions about aging are indeed widespread. It
is again worth noting, however, that some of the misconceptions found in the earlier review by McTavish (1971)
(e.g., most old people are senile, have no interest or capacity for sexual relations, cannot learn new things) were
not generally supported in these later studies.

Perhaps the most widely recognized source of information on the public's beliefs about old people is the national study conducted by Louis Harris and Associates for
the National Council on Aging (1975). This survey demonstrated that old and young hold beliefs regarding older

207

people in general that are <u>not</u> reported by the old in referring to themselves. Thus, individual elderly reported fewer social and economic problems for themselves than they reported for elderly people in general.

Lutsky's review of the attitudinal evaluations of older people allows specific focus on the attitudes of health care professionals. Professionals with prior experience in working with older people were found to be neutral or positive in their attitudes toward elders. In contrast, those professionals uninvolved with geriatric patients were found to have more negative attitudes; even those with relatively neutral attitudes were unwilling to consider making a career change to work in geriatrics or with patients over 65.

The review compiled by Adelson and Kraus (1983) focuses exclusively on the attitudes of health care providers toward geriatric patients. In contrast to the reviews cited previously, they conclude that health care professionals in all disciplines (medicine, nursing, social work, etc.) often hold negative attitudes and stereotypes of the geriatric patient. They stress those studies of professional attitudes that follow in the tradition of Butler's theory of ageism (Butler, 1975). They suggest that while negative attitudes seem to be pervasive across health professions, the content of these attitudes differs due to variations in training and the social learning process that accompanies professional education. Studies cited indicate that doctors and psychiatrists tend to emphasize physiological deterioration, while social workers and nurses stress the social isolation and dependency which accompany aging. The review also found that health care providers' negative attitudes and stereotypes of aging were reflected in their career choices. Numerous studies cited demonstrate the reluctance of various occupational groups including nurses, physicians, social workers, and psychologists to work with geriatric patients.

Adelson and Kraus also examine the existing literature to determine the effects of health care providers' age, education and experience on their subsequent attitudes toward the older patient. They conclude that there are weak, but positive correlations between provider age and positive attitudes as well as between education or training and positive attitudes, and a significant association between past experience working with the elderly and positive attitudes.

Adelson and Kraus stress the importance of research focused on understanding the relationship between practitioner attitudes and their behavior toward geriatric patients. They state that negative attitudes have significant implications for the quality of care resulting in negativism, defeatism, and professional antipathy, the withholding of services, the provision of unnecessary services and the lack of recognition of individual needs. The need for research that examines the relationship of other factors in the treatment environment that may influence practitioner behaviors, such as the number of staff or the socioeconomic status of the patients, is stressed.

Several studies not described in these literature reviews have addressed the relationship between the attitudes and behavioral intentions of health care providers (Robb, 1979; Crane, 1975). Crane (1975) examined how physicians perceive patients and how their perceptions influence their treatment decisions. Her findings suggest that physicians do not rely solely on physiological aspects of illness, but also consider social and psychological considerations, such as the patient's capacity to resume former roles and interact with others. Crane's findings also reflect the influence of the patient's age on the physician's willingness to resuscitate patients as well as to use major diagnostic and treatment procedures. She found that patients under age 40 were most likely to be treated aggressively while those over 79 were the least likely to receive such treatment.

Theoretical Framework and Objectives

The framework for this research is based on two different perspectives from cognitive psychology -- attitude theory and social judgment theory. An underlying assumption of most attitude research is that self-reported attitudes can be used to predict behavior. Thus, cognitive theory suggests that attitudes affect the behaviors of health care providers toward their older patients in the clinical setting. According to McDavid and Harari (1974), an attitude has three components: a basic cognitive component (an idea or belief), an affective component (a value), and a behavioral component (a predisposition or inclination in a behavioral direction). It is the intent of this research to examine the relationships among these components.

209

The second perspective upon which this research is based is that of social judgment theory. The social judgment paradigm is particularly useful for the purposes of our research because it is concerned with how clinicians reason about the problems with which they deal and how this reasoning process might be improved. Within this paradigm, attitudes represent one of many different possible determinants of clinical decision making.

We have set the following four objectives for this research project. Each objective is based directly on the theoretical constructs described above:

1. To describe how health care providers within the VA medical setting perceive their older patients. According to attitude theory as defined by McDavid and Harari (1974), this information provides the cognitive base on which affect and behavioral predispositions rest. Information illustrative of this conceptual perception of older patients includes: the physical and behavioral characteristics of older patients, the particular age marking the onset of old age, and the characteristics describing the onset of old age.

2. To describe those aspects of working with older patients that health care providers within the VA medical system find especially rewarding and/or frustrating. Once the conceptual category of older patients has been defined, we will then determine how providers feel about different aspects of working with such patients. According to McDavid and Harari (1974), this information fits into the affective dimension of attitude. Information is collected on how rewarding and/or frustrating providers find, among other factors: the close relationship with the older patient, handling their multiple problems, the chronic nature of their problems, and working with the cognitively impaired.

3. To identify the behavioral intentions of health care providers within the VA medical setting toward their older patients. Following the McDavid and Harari framework, once we know how providers perceive their older patients and what they find rewarding or frustrating about working with them, we can attempt to identify how they might tend to act toward them, or what their behavioral predispositions would suggest. We rely on social judgment theory to examine the behavioral predispositions of health care providers toward their older patients. Specifically,

210

we use several case vignettes to illustrate the hypothetical outcomes of decisions made in the clinical setting.
We also ask providers to indicate how comfortable they are
with a number of non-intervention decisions, such as do
not resuscitate orders, withholding of life supports, the
termination of life supports, and the withholding of IVs
for hydration.

4. To identify the determinants of a range of clinical decisions involving older patients. The social judgment approach allows us to describe how health care providers use and weight different factors which influence
their decision making processes. A variety of factors are
hypothesized to interact and influence the decision making
of providers with their older patients, such as institutional constraints, eligibility for services, staff cooperation, family considerations, etc. (Table 1). We will
also attempt to determine whether the attitudes health
care providers hold toward their older patients are important determinants in their decision making.

Research Design

The research design for this study consists of a survey of physicians, nurses and social workers at VA facilities. To achieve an optimum response rate, health care
providers were mailed copies of the survey instrument and
data were collected through pre-arranged telephone interviews. Of the 294 individuals selected to participate in
the survey, 251 were successfully interviewed, giving an
85.4% response rate. The mean time taken to complete the
telephone interview was 15 minutes; most respondents read
through the questionnaire and determined the responses before the scheduled interview. Forty-seven individuals
chose to mail in their questionnaires instead of answering
the survey by telephone interview. The next two sections
describe the development of the survey instrument and the
sampling methodology.

1. Instrumentation

The research instrument, a survey questionnaire, was
initially developed and pretested in a pilot study supported by Harvard University's Division of Health Policy
Research and Education. Further refinements have since
been made in the questionnaire to address the unique concerns of the VA. The survey instrument is composed of two
major components: 1) items addressing the attitudes of

211

Table 1
VARIABLES WHICH INFLUENCE HEALTH CARE PROVIDER DECISIONS

I. Medical Considerations

    A. Medical risk to the patient
    B. Expected quality of life after treatment
    C. Degree of pain and suffering

II. Institutional and Societal Constraints

    A. Potential legal liability
    B. Formal rules of the institution
    C. Informal rules of the institution
    D. Eligibility for service

III. Patient Factors

    A. Prior wishes of the patient
    B. Patient characteristics
        1. Current cognitive function
        2. Pre-existing dementia
        3. Age of patient
        4. Societal worth of patient
    C. Family considerations

IV. Health Provider Factors

    A. Professional discipline
    B. Prior training in geriatrics
    C. Age of provider

health professionals toward both older patients and toward providing health care services within the VA, and 2) clinical vignettes which measure the behavioral intentions of these same providers.

Questionnaire items addressing the attitudes of health care providers were developed using a phenomonological approach. Based on findings from the literature and on experience in clinical practice, the research staff developed an open ended instrument and interviewed a small but diverse group of health care providers (15 interviews). From the responses to these open ended questions, closed ended items addressing provider attitudes were designed. These attitudinal variables were then pretested in interviews with 50 health care providers, including physicians, nurses, and social workers. Descriptive analyses were performed, and only those variables which had variation of response were maintained.

To measure the behavioral intentions of health care providers, we have relied on the use of standardized, structured cases, which we have called clinical vignettes. The use of clinical vignettes, a standard practice in social judgment theory, allows the researcher to describe how a clinician uses and weights information to make a judgment about some criterion event, for example, a diagnosis or treatment. The vignettes for this study were developed through clinical observations made in a variety of decision making episodes involving older patients. They simulate the actual decisions facing health care providers in their day-to-day practice with older patients. In these clinical vignettes, providers are asked to make hypothetical, specific treatment decisions. Providers are further asked to indicate the relative importance of a number of factors influencing their decision making.

The use of vignettes has several advantages for researchers interested in examining the factors influencing judgments in a variety of clinical situations. First, the structured nature of the case allows the researcher to maintain a degree of control not available in the actual clinical setting, permitting the disentanglement of the effects of provider and patient variables. Second, the use of hypothetical vignettes allows the researcher to obtain a broad sampling of clinical cases in a limited time frame. Third, the data collected from the structured vignettes lend themselves well to statistical analyses and to comparisons among health care providers. Fourth, the costs incurred are much less than costs associated with participant observation methods. Fifth, due to the staged process of the vignettes, in which additional pieces of information are added under the researcher's control, analyses can distinguish the effects of individual variables on clinical decisions (Elstein and Bordage, 1980). And finally, it is believed that the identification of information relied on in making decisions will enable practitioners to better understand how they select and combine information to reach decisions, improving their decision making and ultimately improving the quality of health care geriatric patients receive.

213

2. Sampling Framework

The sample of physicians, nurses, and social workers chosen for this study was selected from two VA medical center (VAMC) acute care hospitals and a combined VA acute care and long term care facility, using a multistage cluster sampling approach. The VAMCs, the primary sampling units, were chosen purposively on several criteria. The VA acute care facilities were chosen because they are large medical centers with close contact with major medical schools. The combined VA acute/long term care facility was chosen because of the presence of the long term care program. These facilities were selected from diverse geographic locations to improve the generalizability of the research findings.

In the final stage of the multistage sampling framework, the secondary sampling units, the health care providers were randomly selected from each facility's staff roster for inclusion in the study. Lists of all physicians, nurses, and social workers were obtained from each of the facilities. The total population of physicians from specific services which were known to provide the bulk of health care to geriatric patients was chosen. Due to the small numbers of social workers at the facilities, the entire population of social workers was surveyed. Due to the large number of nurses, a random sample (approximately two-thirds) of all nurses was selected. The resulting sample included 96 physicians, 121 nurses, 31 social workers, and 3 Ph.D. psychologists.

Research Findings

In this section, we provide descriptive statistics on the attitudes of service providers toward their older patients and toward working within the VA system, as well as on the relationship between attitudes and behavior. Descriptive analyses will either combine all the professional disciplines together, or will examine questions separately for physicians, nurses, and social workers.

Patients Most Preferred

As the review of the literature suggests, when asked with which age group of patients health care professionals most prefer to work, the majority of providers chose those under the age of 65 (Table 2). When all professional disciplines are combined, the middle aged are ranked as the

Table 2
AGE GROUP OF PATIENTS MOST PREFERRED

Age Group	N	%
18–44	56	22.3
45–64	103	41.0
65+	45	17.9
No Preference	47	18.7
TOTAL	251	100.0

Question: Please indicate the age group of patients with whom you prefer to work.

most desirable patients, with the fewest number of respondents ranking the aged as their most desirable patient group. An interesting comparison can be made by examining these responses by specific disciplines (Table 3). While the majority of individuals from each of the separate professions indicated that the middle aged group was considered most preferable to work with, differences did emerge regarding the age group which was considered next most desirable. The second largest response category among physicians was the young adult group, whereas for social workers and nurses, those over age 65 were the group next most preferred. Interpreting the data slightly differently, by adding together those physicians who indicated a preference for old with those who reported "no preference," 43% would "not mind" working with older patients.

Table 3
PATIENT GROUP MOST PREFERRED

Physicians	%	Nurses	%	Social Workers	%
18–44	26.0	18–44	17.4	18–44	25.8
45–64	30.2	45–64	52.1	45–64	35.5
65+	10.4	65+	21.5	65+	29.0
No Pref	33.3	No Pref	9.1	No Pref	9.7
TOTAL	100.0	TOTAL	100.0	TOTAL	100.0

Question: Please indicate the age group of patients with whom you prefer to work.

A preference for working with younger rather than older elders is also evidenced in data which examine with
which category of older adults professionals most prefer
to work (Table 4). A consistent pattern emerged, with the
largest percentage of each discipline professing they most
preferred working with the young-old, followed by the old-
old, and finally by the very-old.

Table 4
OLD AGE GROUP MOST PREFERRED

Age Group	N	%
65-74	144	57.4
75-84	38	15.1
85+	24	9.6
No Preference at all	45	17.9
TOTAL	251	100.0

Question: Among patients over age 65, with whom do you
prefer to work?

Rewarding and Frustrating Aspects of Older Patients

In spite of the fact that old patients were not deemed
by a majority as the most desirable patient population
with which to work, several general characteristics of
working with older patients were found to be very rewarding (Table 5). Well over 75% of all those interviewed
found patient appreciation of their services to be very
rewarding. Other characteristics of working with the
elderly that were found to be very rewarding included:
having a close personal relationship, coordinating care
with other staff, working with family members, and handling their complex problems, each mentioned by at least
half the sample. Other characteristics were mentioned as
being very rewarding by many fewer respondents. For example, providing services to the cognitively impaired,
managing their diminished response to treatment and the
chronic nature of their problems were each mentioned as
being very rewarding by less than one-third of the study
sample. It is interesting to speculate on the characteristics reported most often as being rewarding compared to
those mentioned least often. None of those characteristics mentioned most often as being very rewarding are spe-

Table 5
CHARACTERISTICS OF OLDER PATIENTS VIEWED AS REWARDING

Characteristics	%
Patient appreciation	83.3
A close personal relationship	71.3
Working with their family members	62.9
Coordinating care with other staff	54.2
Handling their multiple and complex problems	50.2
Providing services to the cognitively impaired	29.1
Managing their diminished response to treatment	15.6
The chronic nature of their problems	13.6
Their own negative feelings toward old age	6.4
The limited availability of resources	3.2

Question: Working with older patients may be both rewarding and frustrating. When experienced with older patients, how rewarding do you find...

cific to working with older patients, and could in fact be regarded as positive aspects of working with any patient group. On the other hand, those characteristics mentioned least often as being very rewarding are indeed integral characteristics of geriatric care.

Several aspects of working with older patients were also found to be very frustrating (Table 6). The limited availability of resources was most often indicated as being very frustrating (mentioned by over two-thirds of all respondents). Other characteristics mentioned as being very frustrating, and cited by at least one-third of the sample included: the aged's negative feelings toward old age, providing services to the cognitively impaired, managing their diminished response to treatment and the chronic nature of their problems. Approximately one-quarter of respondents indicated that handling their multiple and complex problems was very frustrating. These characteristics, most often mentioned as being very frustrating, seem to be common aspects of geriatric care.

In addition to asking respondents generally which characteristics of working with older patients they found most rewarding and/or frustrating, we also asked them to consider their experience in working specifically within the VA medical care system (Table 7). Of all the aspects

217

Table 6
CHARACTERISTICS OF OLDER PATIENTS VIEWED AS FRUSTRATING

Characteristics	%
The limited availability of resources	71.0
Their own negative feelings toward old age	40.3
Providing services to the cognitively impaired	36.3
Managing their diminished response to treatment	34.3
The chronic nature of their problems	33.9
Handling their multiple and complex problems	23.9
Coordinating care with other staff	16.3
Working with their family members	9.6
Patient appreciation	2.8
A close personal relationship	2.0

Question: Working with older patients may be both rewarding and frustrating. When experienced with older patients, how frustrating do you find...

of working within the VA, the coordination of long term care for older patients without service-connected disabilities was mentioned most frequently by the respondents as being difficult. Close to one-half of respondents indicated that the spouses of patients need services. Approximately one-third of respondents indicated that problems with staff influenced the quality of care they provided to their older patients. Equal numbers indicated that paperwork interferes with serving older patients, and that training was almost never available to improve their skills in working with older patients. Fewer than 20% of respondents indicated that complex eligibility requirements made it difficult for them to deliver services to older patients or that the coordination of long term care for persons with service-connected disabilities was difficult.

Again, it is interesting to compare responses across professional disciplines (Table 7). Among physicians, the coordination of long term care for the non-service-connected disabled is most often reported as a problem (mentioned by almost 60%). Several physicians indicated that coordination of long term care is difficult for all patients, regardless of disability status. It was noted that additional support systems for non-institutional placement of elderly are needed. Over 40% of all physi-

Table 7
CHARACTERISTICS OF WORKING WITHIN THE VA SYSTEM

Characteristics	All %	MDs %	RNs %	SWs %
Coordination of long term care is difficult for older patients without service-connected disabilities.	50.3	58.9	11.2	58.1
Spouses of your older patients need services.	47.7	41.6	46.6	71.0
Problems with staff influence the quality of care provided to older patients.	36.0	25.3	45.5	29.0
Paperwork interferes with serving older patients.	35.2	26.4	42.9	35.5
Training is not available to improve your skills in working with older patients.	32.7	39.6	28.3	9.7
Complex eligibility requirements make it difficult for you to provide services to your older patients.	18.9	26.4	15.3	12.9
Coordination of long term care is difficult for older patients with service-connected disabilities.	13.8	18.9	11.2	3.2

Question: "Considering your experience working in the VA System..." – Percent indicating usually or always.

cians reported that spouses of their patients need services and close to 40% indicated that training is almost
never available to improve their skills in working with
the elderly. Some physicians were not aware if training
was available. Problems with staff and paperwork were
mentioned by less than 25% of physicians as interfering

219

with their ability to provide services to older patients. Physicians who did mention problems with staff and paperwork suggested that increased use of paramedical services might alleviate some of these stresses.

For nurses, problems are seen from a very different perspective. Problems with staff, the fact that families of patients need services, and problems with paperwork were all reported as problems more frequently than the coordination of long term care for the non-service-connected disabled. Although the lack of adequate training was mentioned by more than 25% of nurses as being a problem, it was not as important as other perceived difficulties. At each institution, understaffing was cited by nurses as a major problem. Several nurses commented that lack of adequate nursing staff hampers the provision of quality care to older patients. Nurses seemed to feel that they spend too much time on paperwork and not enough time on patient care activities. From the nursing perspective, lack of adequate nursing staff not only affects the quality of patient care, but also limits training opportunities, since additional staff are required for coverage when seminars are offered. Nurses voiced their desire for in-service training sessions covering care of the elderly, psychology of aging and quality of care. Several nurses indicated that the lack of adequate long term care options for placement was the major obstacle in providing care to older patients.

The one characteristic mentioned by most social workers was that spouses of their older patients needed services. This might be expected, given their training focus on seeing the patient in a family context. As with physicians and nurses, social workers reported difficulty in coordinating care for those with non-service-connected disabilities. A relatively large percentage of social workers, like nurses, also reported that problems with paperwork interfered with their ability to provide services to elderly patients.

On first review of the data, we were surprised to discover that eligibility requirements did not emerge as an important factor in respondents' decision making nor as a problem in delivering services to older patients. However, probes revealed that respondents were referring to those patients already admitted into the hospital, and who thus had already met mandatory eligibility requirements. The fact that complex eligibility requirements were not seen as a major impediment in the provision of care to older patients by over 80% of respondents can be elucidated by respondents' comments. It appears that nurses as well as physicians assume that if patients are admitted, they are eligible for care. Physicians indicated that doctors do not know if patients have service-connected or non-service-connected disabilities, although they acknowledged that the hospital administration might worry about such issues. Nurses, on the other hand, seemed to be aware of patients' disability status, but insisted that there was no difference in the quality of care provided.

To test whether physicians, nurses, and social workers differed significantly in their experience working in the VA system, chi-square tests of significance were performed. There were significant differences across disciplines in the following four characteristics: problems with staff (X^{2*} = 11.69; p = .02), the coordination of services for patients with non-service-connected disabilities (X^2 = 11.0; p = .02), the availability of training (X^2 = 9.56; p = .048), and the fact that spouses of patients need services (X^2 = 9.18; p = .056).

Clinical Decisions

Another major focus of this research was to examine how respondents felt about certain clinical aspects of working with older patients. Specifically, we were interested in ascertaining how comfortable respondents were with difficult treatment decisions. In the care of seriously impaired older patients, a point is often reached when one is no longer comfortable with further medical intervention. Respondents were asked to rank a number of non-intervention decisions according to their degree of comfort. The ranking of non-intervention treatment decisions varied little across professions (Table 8). Examining the modal response category for each decision, there was consistency across professions with regard to the following: do not resuscitate orders (most often given a one, or "most comfortable"), withholding of surgical procedures (most often given either a two or one), withholding of IVs for hydration (most often given a four or five), withholding of antibiotics (most often given a three), and termination of life supports (most often given a seven, or "least comfortable"). The withholding of life

---

* X^2 calculated for 4 degrees of freedom throughout the chapter.

221

Table 8
DEGREE OF COMFORT WITH NON-INTERVENTION PROCEDURES

	Physicians			Nurses			Social Workers		
	Median	Mode	Mean	Median	Mode	Mean	Median	Mode	Mean
Withholding surgical procedures	2.2	1	2.9	2.5	2	3.3	2.5	2	3.2
Do Not Resuscitate orders	1.9	1	3.0	1.7	1	2.6	1.7	1	2.5
Withholding life supports	4.2	6	4.4	4.7	4	4.6	4.7	4	4.6
Withholding antibiotics	4.1	3	4.3	3.5	3	3.7	3.5	3	3.7
Withholding of tube feeding	4.6	5	4.5	5.2	6	5.0	5.2	6	5.0
Termination of life supports	6.6	7	5.7	6.6	7	5.5	6.6	7	5.5
Withholding of IVs for hydration	5.8	4	5.7	5.2	5	5.2	5.1	5	5.2

Question: In the care of seriously impaired older patients, a point may sometimes be reached at which further medical intervention is thought to be inappropriate. Non-intervention may take a variety of forms, some of which professionals may be less comfortable with and feel to be less appropriate than others. Please rank the following seven non-intervention decisions according to how comfortable you would feel with each.

supports was ranked as equally uncomfortable for nurses and social workers (given a four), but ranked as much less comfortable for physicians (given a six). The withholding of tube feeding, on the other hand, was somewhat more uncomfortable for both nurses and social workers than for physicians.

As stated earlier in this chapter, the ultimate purpose of this study of attitudes is to further clarify the way in which cognitions, values and feelings influence the way health care providers interact with their older patients, and influence the decision making process. To address this question, providers were asked to respond to two different case vignettes, and on each to indicate both their treatment decision and how each of thirteen factors influenced their decision making process. In the first vignette, individuals are asked to make an intergenerational choice between two patients, a 35 year old and a 75 year old, both in need of the one remaining bed in the Intensive Care Unit. While close to 40% of the respondents refused to make a choice (often indicating that they would somehow find a way to treat both), of the remaining respondents, approximately 70% recommended the 35 year old man, and 33% recommended the older man. Interestingly, when asked directly how important age was as a factor in their actual choice of patients, it did not rank as a critical force either among physicians who ranked it sixth, nor for nurses who ranked it tenth in importance, nor for social workers who ranked it eleventh.

In order to gain an understanding of the factors which influenced this intergenerational choice, respondents were asked to indicate the relative degree to which they were influenced by a variety of factors believed to be important in decision making. A disparity did appear in the ranking of the factors by physicians, nurses and social workers (Table 9). Physicians, as might be expected, placed the greatest importance on technical medical criteria, with over 80% naming the medical risk to the patient as very important in their decision making. Other factors mentioned as being very important by over two-thirds of all physicians included: expected quality of life following treatment, prior wishes of the patient, degree of pain and suffering and pre-existing dementia. Physicians placed least importance on factors such as the formal rules or informal practices of their institution, eligibility requirements, and potential legal liability. When nurses and social workers were queried about these

223

Table 9
FACTORS VERY IMPORTANT IN DECISION MAKING – ICU

Factors	MDs %*	RNs %*	SWs %*
Medical risk to patient	84.6	90.7	87.6
Expected quality of life following treatment	71.6	89.9	73.4
Prior wishes of patient	71.1	88.2	76.7
Degree of pain and suffering	67.4	85.7	83.3
Pre-existing dementia	67.1	60.2	56.7
Age of patient	56.6	49.6	43.3
Family considerations	52.3	68.9	53.4
Current cognitive function	50.0	58.9	46.6
Formal rules of your institution	37.5	58.5	73.3
Societal worth	31.1	23.9	30.0
Potential legal liability	28.9	59.6	40.0
Informal practices of your institution	19.3	46.6	53.3
Eligibility for service	18.6	22.9	46.6

*Percent indicating that the factor was "important" or "very important" on a 5 point scale (1 = "not at all important" and 5 = "very important").

Case Vignette:

Two patients have just been admitted to your hospital, a 75 year old man and a 35 year old man. Both require treatment in the Intensive Care Unit (ICU).

Both have clear cognitive function. Neither is married. The prognosis for each is equivalent.

Question:

In making this difficult decision, how important is each of the following to you?

same factors, they placed a similar emphasis on the medical risk to the patient, degree of pain and suffering, prior wishes of the patient and expected quality of life. However, a higher percentage of nurses and social workers indicated that other factors such as family considerations, potential legal liability, and the formal and informal rules of their institution were important considerations in their decision making.

In another treatment decision, we asked respondents how strongly they would support intubation for an 85 year old man whose chronic obstructive pulmonary disease had taken a terminal course. Although few respondents supported life saving treatment in this case, differences did emerge by profession, with over 27% of social workers indicating they would very strongly support such life saving treatment, and less than 10% of physicians and less than 15% of nurses indicating the same. Respondents were again asked to indicate the relative influence of a number of factors in their decision making (Table 10). In this vignette, physicians, nurses and social workers all seemed to be very influenced by expected quality of life after treatment, degree of pain and suffering, and prior wishes of the patient. As in the other vignette, nurses and social workers continued to place more emphasis on the formal and informal practices of the institution and potential legal liabilities than did physicians.

Finally, we were interested in discovering whether there were any differences between what individuals said was important in their general decision making with older patients, and their behavior when faced with a specific treatment decision. We were particularly interested in discovering whether any differences existed in the stated importance of the age of the patient depending on whether the respondent is presented with a general situation or a specific treatment decision. When all disciplines are combined, 36% of respondents indicated that age was a very important factor in making difficult treatment decisions with older patients. This is in contrast to the specific clinical vignettes. In the ICU example, age was mentioned as being most important by over a half of the sample (52%), and in the vignette regarding a demented patient needing life saving intubation treatment, age was mentioned by just under one-half of the sample (48%). This pattern differs by disciplines. For physicians, the pattern is consistent, with age being mentioned as important in the general case by approximately one-third of respondents

225

Table 10
FACTORS VERY IMPORTANT IN DECISION MAKING
(Dementia Patient)

Factors	MDs %*	RNs %*	SWs %*
Expected quality of life following treatment	87.2	90.9	76.6
Degree of pain and suffering	80.9	92.5	93.3
Prior wishes of patient	80.7	85.1	83.9
Pre-existing dementia	78.8	69.7	46.7
Family considerations	70.2	71.9	76.7
Current cognitive function	64.2	72.0	60.0
Medical risk to patient	59.1	75.2	70.0
Age of patient	44.2	53.7	36.7
Formal rules of your institution	43.6	61.6	73.4
Societal worth	38.3	34.4	23.3
Potential legal liability	34.1	56.2	60.0
Informal practices of your institution	26.9	47.1	63.4
Eligibility for service	18.9	20.0	37.9

*Percent indicating that the factor was "important" or
 "very important" on a 5 point scale (1 = "not at all
 important" and 5 = "very important").

Case Vignette:

Mr. L. is an 85 year old widower. He is disoriented,
bedridden, and incontinent as a result of severe senile
dementia.

He develops acute respiratory failure associated with
chronic obstructive pulmonary disease, which has taken a
progressive and probably terminal course.

Question:

In your decision concerning Mr. L., how important is
each of the following to you?

(31%), and by 57% and 44% for the ICU and dementia cases, respectively. This same pattern emerged far less strongly among nurses and social workers: among nurses, age was mentioned by 40% in the general case, and by 50% and 54%, respectively, for the ICU and the dementia cases; among social workers, age was mentioned by 37% in the general case, and by 43% and 37%, respectively, for the ICU and the dementia cases.

There were several significant differences in the importance of certain factors across all the decision making situations. Chi-square tests of significance revealed that physicians, nurses and social workers consistently differed in the importance they ascribed to potential legal liabilities, formal rules of their institution, and the informal practices of their institution. Clearly, nurses, and to a lesser degree social workers, feel more constrained by these factors than do physicians.

While physicians, nurses, and social workers differed across all decision making situations with respect to these three factors, there was more variability with respect to certain additional characteristics. In the ICU case, additional significant differences were found in the importance ascribed to: expected quality of life ($X^2 = 13.9$; $p = .009$), prior wishes of the patient ($X^2 = 12.16$; $p = .016$), family considerations ($X^2 = 10.08$; $p = .039$), patient's pain and suffering ($X^2 = 13.2$; $p = .01$), and eligibility requirements ($X^2 = 10.5$; $p = .03$).

In the case involving the demented patient, physicians, nurses, and social workers differed in the importance ascribed to the medical risk to the patient ($X^2 = 13.14$; $p = .01$) and to pre-existing dementia ($X^2 = 14.17$; $p = .007$). Finally, in the general decision making situation the disciplines only differed with respect to the importance of pre-existing dementia ($X^2 = 11.49$; $p = .02$).

Thus, it appears that while providers may be consistent in the importance they ascribe to certain factors, such as legal liability and the formal rules of their institution, they may be less consistent in the importance they ascribe to other characteristics. The relative importance of these other characteristics seem to be dependent on the specific type of decision being made.

Conclusion

These preliminary findings indicate opportunities for the VA to improve service to elder veterans by increasing the knowledge, resources and skills of the staff who provide care to them. An examination of characteristics of working within the VA system revealed that a large percentage of individuals perceive their ability to provide services to older patients constrained by the amount of paperwork required and by staffing problems. Nurses seemed particularly overburdened by these factors. A large number of physicians indicated that adequate training was not available within the VA to improve their skills in working with older patients. Moreover, efforts to change the VA system should take into account current values and attitudes of care providers. The majority of providers indicated that of all age groups, they least preferred working with older patients. Some efforts should be made to make the experience of working with older patients more rewarding, perhaps by removing perceived constraints in providing geriatric care within VA facilities.

REFERENCES

Adelson, R. and Kraus, C. "Attitudes of Health Professionals toward the Geriatric Patient: A Literature Review."
Unpublished working paper, 1983.

Bennett, R. and Eckman, J. "Attitudes toward Aging: A
Critical Examination of Recent Literature and Implica-
tions for Future Research." In The Psychology of Adult
Development and Aging, Eisdorfer, C. and Lawton, M.P.
(Eds.), pp. 575-597. Washington, D.C.: American Psy-
chological Association, 1973.

Butler, R.N. Why Survive? Being Old in America. New York:
Harper, 1975.

Crane, D. "Decisions to Treat Critically Ill Patients: A
Comparison of Social versus Medical Considerations."
Milbank Memorial Fund Quarterly/Health and Society, pp.
1-33, Winter, 1975.

Elstein, A.F. and Bordage, G. "Psychology of Clinical
Reasoning." In Health Psychology - A Handbook, Stone,
G.C., Cohen, F., and Adler, N.E. and Associates (Eds.),
pp. 333-367. San Francisco: Jossey-Bass, Inc., 1980.

Harris, L., et al. The Myth and Reality of Aging in America. Washington, D.C.: National Council on Aging, 1975.

Kogan, N. "Beliefs, Attitudes and Stereotypes about Old
People: A New Look at Some Old Issues." Research on
Aging, 1, pp. 11-36, 1979.

Lutsky, N. "Attitudes toward Old Age and Elderly Persons."
Annual Review of Geriatrics, pp. 287-336, 1980.

McDavid, J.W. and Harari, H. Psychology and Social Behavior.
New York: Harper Row, 1974.

McTavish, D.G. "Perceptions of Old People: A Review of
Research Methodologies and Findings." The Gerontologist,
pp. 90-101, Winter, 1971.

Palmore, E. "Facts on Aging: A Short Quiz." The Gerontologist, pp. 315-320, Summer, 1977.

229

Robb, S.S. "Attitudes and Intentions of Baccalaureate Nursing Students toward the Elderly." Nursing Research, 28, pp. 43-50, 1979.

U.S. Veterans Administration, Administrator of Veterans Affairs. Annual Report 1982. Washington, D.C.

8. Serving the Family of the Elder Veteran

Terrie Wetle, Ph.D.
Linda Evans, Ph.D.

Introduction

The purpose of this chapter is to explore how the Veterans Administration might assist families of elderly veterans. Specifically, two basic questions are addressed: (1) what programs or services might the VA implement for supporting family caregivers, and (2) how might the VA provide care to the spouses of elderly veterans?

Currently, families provide substantial caregiving assistance to elders residing in the community. Interest in providing formal support for family caregivers is premised on three assumptions: (1) living in the community is preferred to institutional life, (2) many elderly persons can be maintained in the home for less cost than in an institution, and (3) the quality of care and willingness of caregivers to provide services in the home can be enhanced through such support.

Provision of care by the VA to needy spouses of elder veterans will also be explored in this chapter. The rationale is that provision of such care is more humane and efficient than the dual health care systems used by many elderly couples -- one VA and one non-VA.

231

In efforts to plan for health care needs of the increasing numbers of elders and to improve the health care
system, the VA and other care providers are confronted
with several major questions. How can care to elders with
multiple conditions be most efficiently coordinated? Is
it desirable to shift from institutional care to in-home
care? How can the VA and community share resources?

Modifications in the present health care system must
take into account the family circumstances of those requiring care. Possible options for family support are
presented in this chapter, preceded by a discussion of the
context within which such programs would be developed including what is known about family caregiving patterns,
the types of family support programs already tried in the
United States and abroad, and VA efforts on behalf of elderly veterans and their families to date.

I. Caregiving Patterns -- An Overview

A. Family Caregiving

Adult children are providing assistance to elders in
functional decline both within their own and the elders'
homes (Dono, et al., 1979). GAO (1977) studies, indicate
that 90% of older persons' personal care needs are being
met by family and friends. As might be expected, older
persons who live with adult children tend to be in poorer
functional condition than those residing in their own
homes (Fendetti and Gelfond, 1976; Gelfond, et al.,
1978). The amount of care that the family provides ranges
from periodic checking in to extensive full-time care.
One study (Newman, et al., 1976) estimates that caregiving
time among adult children ranges from one to five hours
per week to more than 40 hours per week.

Sex roles and female longevity converge so that women
are more likely to be both care receivers and caregivers.
Women typically provide more direct care for chronically
ill parents and parents-in-law than men (Shanas, 1979;
Brody, 1978). However, changing social patterns (e.g.,
entry of increasing numbers of women into the labor force,
increased rates of divorce which may weaken family ties)
lead to decreased availability of these traditional caretakers. There is already some evidence that incentives
may be necessary in the future to encourage family care of
elders. For example, one recent study did not find widespread support for filial responsibility norms, particu-

larly among middle-aged and black Americans (Hanson, et al., 1983). Job obligations exert pressure on these two groups as well as on persons whose marriages have been disrupted by divorce, widowhood, or remarriage. Cicirelli (1983), for example, compared adult children in these categories with those with intact marriages and found children with disrupted marriages to perceive lower parental needs, feel less filial obligation, and feel more restrained in helping - primarily because of job responsibilities.

In addition to limited availability of family to provide care, care providers experience substantial stress related to their caretaking efforts. Stresses and costs of family care are related in part to unpreparedness for burden, dependency issues, communication problems and conflict of multiple demands (Cohen, 1983). Female caregivers often have children to care for and work responsibilities outside of the home (Robinson, 1983; Soldo and Sharma, 1980). Other stress points are excessive demands on time and energy and resultant feelings of lowered life satisfaction, isolation, and restricted mobility (Fengler and Goodrich, 1979; Isaacs, et al., 1976). Additionally, some caregivers have to manage their feelings toward other family members who do not give regular help (Clark and Rakowski, 1983). Despite these stresses, a large proportion of community based care continues to be provided by families to their elder members.

B. Spouse Caregiving

Institutionalization of an elderly person depends more upon the absence of a spouse than on the absence of a child (Palmore, 1976). Adult children frequently provide care to mildly or moderately impaired elders while severely disabled elders are more likely cared for by a spouse (Getzel, 1981). With respect to commitment and tolerance, a marriage is the most viable, comprehensive, and long term support available in old age (Johnson and Catalano, 1982). As a group, "caretaking" couples are disproportionately below or near the poverty level and have a proportion of caregivers in poor health that exceeds that of all other categories of caregivers. In some instances support arrangements are mutual. Independent households are often sustained even when the health and functional capacities of both husband and wife have seriously deteriorated. Again, women typically provide more direct care

233

for a chronically ill spouse, acting as caregivers more often than as care receivers (Fengler and Goodrich, 1979).

As with adult children, the spouse caregivers experience considerable stress. One longitudinal study of spouses providing care revealed that the caregiving spouse's health deteriorated in 50% of the cases examined (Johnson and Catalano, 1982). Another study of wives caring for disabled husbands identified the wives as "generally worried, frustrated, sad, resigned, and impatient" (Fengler and Goodrich, 1979). Working wives experienced "role overload" and most wives had low morale. Caretakers are also more likely to suffer from stress-related diseases, including ulcers and alcohol abuse.

Efforts to provide support to family caregivers including counseling, skills development, respite and backup services have increased both the capacity and willingness of family members to continue to provide in-home care.

C. Policy Implications

To date, most discussions regarding the targeting of social services have focused upon elders without families, and some policy makers have gone so far as to suggest that in the future, the majority of formal social services should be confined to this group (Nelson, 1982). This approach has reflected both scarcity of available resources and services, as well as concern over greatly increased demand as formal services are substituted for those provided by family members. A somewhat less extreme argument is that services should be targeted to those at highest risk of institutionalization, and designed in such a way as to supplement and enhance, rather than replace, family care.

Targeting of services raises two difficult questions: to whom, and how? If services are to be targeted only to those with no kin available to provide care, the opportunity to enhance family care and perhaps delay or even avoid institutionalization is lost. Such a policy could also lead to circumstances of abandonment in which family members including spouses would reluctantly withdraw all support and caregiving in order for their loved one to qualify for the targeted "kinless" group. Such a policy raises difficult ethical and political issues as has been demonstrated by negative response to repeated efforts to hold family members responsible for the costs of nursing home care. The difficulties in implementing such regulations are many and have met with major resistance from family members and the elderly themselves. Efforts to target services to those most at risk for institutionalization have met with only partial success, due mainly to limited capacity to accurately identify those most likely to be institutionalized in a given period. Recent studies, for example, indicate different high risk categories for targeting. Cantor (1983) found spouses to be the highest risk group; Soldo and Myllyluoma (1983) located families providing care to an unmarried relative as the most vulnerable to dissolution. Yet development of effective assessment tools for this type of targeting continues, particularly as preliminary data indicate that family supports may indeed be effective in delaying institutionalization and reducing formal service utilization.

II. Support Programs for Family and Spouse

As a result of recent emphasis upon an investigation of community alternatives to institutional care, a number of innovative family support programs have been initiated around the country. There are several premises underlying this approach. One is that elders should be maintained within their homes in a known community for as long as possible. Certainly elders prefer this arrangement and it is argued that overall costs of care are substantially reduced. Although evidence exists that elders do indeed prefer to avoid nursing homes, assumptions about cost reduction remain unproven. Simple cost comparisons between different placements at one point in time are impressive. For example, State of Michigan personnel estimate that their Adult Home Health program costs $2,500 per client per year in comparison with $6,000 for adult foster care and $12,000 for nursing home placement (Haas, 1982, p. 2). However, these simple cost comparisons have a number of weaknesses. First, they assume that only those persons who would otherwise be institutionalized are receiving the community service. Second, they do not add in other costs of remaining at home (rent, food, etc.) that are covered by the institutional bill. However, if indeed much of the community support and care is provided through individual or family resources, community based services may prove to be cost effective in terms of "public" spending.

235

A. Tax Incentives and Family Reimbursement

Support to families may take many forms which cover a wide spectrum, from the least to the most restrictive (and most intrusive). At the less restrictive end of the spectrum is providing elders or caregiving families with cash grants or tax breaks, allowing them to choose and pay for services and providers (assuming multiple options exist in their geographic area). However, tax strategies presume baseline financial solvency, and many needy persons have little or no income to be taxed and are frequently not tax payers (Maryland Office on Aging, the Comptroller's Office, 1977)(for this same reason, recent promotion of IRAs as protection for old age will bypass America's less affluent). Thus, tax advantage programs may be targeted toward middle income persons who may not be able to afford to purchase services but do not qualify for Medicaid. At the national level, several such tax bills have periodically been introduced. One bill proposed a tax credit to the elderly for 50% of the average daily benefit paid for nursing home care under Medicare and Medicaid -- if they were eligible for nursing home care, but remained in the community; another bill would have provided a standard deduction of $250 (in 1977) for anyone caring for an old person in the home (Maryland Office on Aging, 1977). On the state level, Arizona and Maryland have explored tax benefits such as financial aid, and Oregon initiated a tax credit for caregivers in 1979 (Whitfield, 1981).

Unlike tax proposals which remain untried for the most part, direct cash grants have been made available to caregivers in several states, including Florida, California, Colorado, Washington, Nebraska, and Utah. Some are targeted toward any family member, some toward spouses, and some toward any caregiver. They also differ with respect to requiring co-residence for eligibility. The California In-Home Supportive Service program provides enough money to purchase services while the Washington state program provides only a small supplement to the caregiver providing direct care (Whitfield, 1981). The VA has played a leadership role in providing supplemental financing to veterans who are disabled and qualify for the Aid and Attendance Program. More than 170,000 individuals receive this benefit, allowing them to purchase additional services or supplement family income.

B. Hospital Based Programs

Probably the greatest potential for minimizing inappropriate nursing home placements lies in linking hospital discharge planning with community services or agencies responsible for authorizing home care (Crystal, 1982). Unfortunately, such coordination is rare. Caro (1982), for example, reports that services were arranged for only 40% of seriously disabled elders released from six New York City hospitals in his study of post-release care. If there were family members readily available, hospital personnel assumed family members would accommodate elder care needs themselves or arrange for help. Since none of the hospitals recorded functional level, it is not clear how well hospital personnel could have advised family members about follow-up arrangements had they been asked. Hospital personnel are most likely to address the home service needs of those older patients whose relatives insist that it is a precondition for the patient leaving the hospital (Armitage, 1981). Administrators justify this inattention to impaired elders with families on two grounds. First, they have limited staff available for such work, and second, existing personnel concentrate their efforts on the difficult-to-place institution-bound patient, thus assuring release of their beds to others. From a cost perspective, hospital administrators do not see a comparable pay-off for home-service liaison work (Caro, 1982).

More encouraging than hospital-release procedures is the hospital based home assessment approach. Home assessments have been part of the United Kingdom's geriatric clinics for a number of years, but have only recently been tried in the United States. The Family Practice Program of the Bowman Gray School of Medicine in Winston Heights in Salem, North Carolina, has undertaken home visits with geriatric patients (Aaron and Elliott, 1982). The purpose of the program is to develop a bio-psycho-social model of health and illness; toward this end all house calls have been made with a physician/family therapist team. Results indicate that meaningful information was obtained on traditional geriatric issues (functional status, medications, and quality of support) and more subjective data were gleaned (personality, beliefs, life styles, and relationships) that affected subsequent medical care. Also, problems such as depression and dementia were easier to explore in the home. Family based care is enhanced in such a program through better understanding of treatment and care and through relieving the strain of frequent visits to physician offices and hospital clinics.

C. Agency Based Programs

Agency based services fall into two major types -- those directed at the elderly client such as escort service, household maintenance, and personal care, and those directed at the caregiver which include group work with kin and friends, respite care, and technical assistance. Obviously, any formal service provided to the elder constitutes an area of potential relief to a caregiving relative or friend. While a variety of home care and caregiver assistance programs are being tried around the country, a program that offers an unusual array of services ranging from the task-oriented to training in advocacy is presented for illustration. That program is the Natural Supports Program under the auspices of the Community Service Society of New York (Mellor, 1982; Mellor and Getzel, 1980; Mellor, et al., 1981; Gross-Andrew and Zimmer, 1977; Zimmer and Sainer, 1978; Horowitz, 1978; Getzel, 1982).

The Community Service Society, a nonprofit, nonsectarian social agency, is operating the Natural Supports Program as a time limited demonstration and research project. The intention is to investigate the implications for family life of the care of a disabled older member as well as the effect of supplementary organized services. Families are eligible to participate when there is a functionally disabled member over 60 years of age, at least one family member identified as the primary support, and the income of the elder and spouse is not more than $8,000, including interest income. An initial meeting takes place in a family member's home and includes the elder and all interested family. At this time, self-care and family-provided care are assessed as well as family members' articulation of needed supplementary benefits and services. A contract letter is developed to confirm agreements reached and to outline the roles to be played by the informal and formal sectors. The most frequently identified service need of families is a form of home care -- that is, some combination of personal care and chore help. When provided, such care allows the caregiver periodic respite from the ongoing demands of caregiving. House modifications are made in some instances to facilitate client mobility. These services are theoretically targeted for the client and are provided within a family

238

case work model with some individual and family counseling. Because elders are not inclined toward seeking counseling, other family members are used as the vehicle for getting the older member involved in such activities.

Counseling and group work are also made available for caregivers with the intention of improving elder care, preventing breakdown of caregivers and facilitating caregiver advocacy in the long run. These meetings are open and findings from this project as well as other community outreach or group work approaches indicate that caregivers often attend such gatherings for information -- at least initially (Steuer and Clark, 1982). They seek information on how to handle disabilities, what the likely course of disease is, and general knowledge about aging-related problems. Programs designed to empower the caregiver usually offer this information as well as skill-building related to crisis management and seeking community services. Even though caregivers tend to join groups only to gather information, if they stay engaged, emotional support is often cited as the single most important benefit of the group. Within the Natural Supports Program, some participants have gone on to form peer groups with little formal oversight and eventually have become involved in advocacy activities within the political arena. Thus, caregivers may not recognize emotional support as a need, but over time, such support appears to decrease depression, isolation, and guilt and can lead to efforts to change the social, economic, and political context of their caregiving. Both the case and the group work methods used within this program are helpful in reducing caregiver stresses. Formal provision of personal care, for example, decreases adult children's tensions associated with parent-directed physical contact and permits greater caregiver mobility. Similarly, group meetings for community caregivers diminish their isolation and enhance skills for dealing with everyday caregiving problems and obstacles. In these various ways, perceptions of burden can be lessened and willingness to continue care, extended.

The United States has been slow to undertake the continuum of care issue in comparison with other countries such as Japan, England, and Sweden. Japan pursues an explicit public policy of financial, psychological, and practical support to the caregivers of elderly parents. These include:

1) Tax deductions or exemptions for caregiving as well as additional tax credits when the elder is impaired;

2) Loans to caregivers needing to build or remodel their homes to accommodate the elder;

3) Special equipment, such as special beds or bathtubs, telephones, or water heaters required by families caring for elders;

4) Short-term nursing home stays; and

5) Day care services for the impaired (Little, 1982; Japanese Government, 1982; Maeda, 1983).

England provides a system of geriatric medical centers for needs assessment and has many personal social services available to elders, such as domestic help, shopping assistance, meal service, laundry service, recreation centers, and transportation. The use of these services eases the burden of care for family members. Volunteer services are also widespread in England. For years, Sweden has provided payments to family caregivers and employed over 80,000 home helpers for elderly and caregiver assistance (Kane and Kane, 1976).

D. The Veterans Administration's Programs

Coordinating care within or across the local, state, and national levels of government is problematic. However, the VA is in a position to both build upon its institutional and medical expertise and better coordinate its medical center services with those available at the local level. The VA, in other words, has the potential for integrating medical and social care and for establishing a nationally coherent, yet locally-sensitive and flexible long term care strategy. The VA has already taken some steps in these directions.

Through a number of program innovations and selected evaluations, VA personnel have learned three very important facts. First, a patient's socioeconomic status and a social worker's involvement, rather than medical condition, are the best predictors of successful post-hospital placement (Rodell, 1979). Second, gaps in care continuity, which lead to insufficient or incorrect placement choices, are costly in that they often result in an unnecessary return to hospitals (Geriatric Liaison Coordinating Committee, 1983). Third, through the careful interdisciplinary diagnostic functional assessment and placement efforts of the geriatric evaluation units, the well-being of elderly veterans can be enhanced. Thus, acute care and chronic care are closely intertwined and, within the VA, successful placement begins with admission to a hospital (VA, 1982f; Rubenstein, et al., 1981).

In addition to the institutional care provided in VA hospitals, nursing homes, domiciliaries, and state veterans homes, the VA authorizes Residential Care Homes and provides Hospital Based Home Care within the community. More recently the VA has implemented programs for Adult Day Health Care, Respite Care, Palliative Care, and expanded education and support groups for caretakers (Neher, 1983; VA, 1976; Steuer and Clark, 1982). These services provide a continuum for patients requiring constant surveillance through those unable to perform daily maintenance to those living at home whose health must be monitored only periodically.

The weakest link in the VA system is in the area of home care supports -- primarily because the VA is legislatively prohibited from providing "non-medical" services. For this reason, only one existing VA benefit, the Aid and Attendance Program, touches on non-medical services; recipients may purchase non-medical services with the Aid and Attendance benefit if they so choose. Both the Day Ambulatory Service for Health (DASH) and the Desert Area Wellness Network (DAWN) represent demonstrations of the coordinated and collective efforts of the VA and community resources. Thus far, however, VA input to these types of programs has necessarily been limited to organizational and technical assistance.

III. Policy Options Available to the VA

In this section two questions are addressed: (1) how might the VA support family caregivers, and (2) in what ways might the VA provide care for needy spouses? While some possible services for spouses are described in the discussion of caregiver supports, the issue of whether spouses could receive more direct care is addressed in a later section. Practical and ethical considerations surround both of these questions.

A. Options for Supporting Family Caregivers

Supports for family caregivers take three basic
forms. The first is the provision of financial support to
families or elders living with family members. The second
category involves services provided to caregivers to enhance their caretaking skills and tolerance to stress.
These would include counseling, support groups, skills
development, respite care and advocacy training. The
third category of supports involves the provision of services to the dependent elder which supplements care provided by family members. These include personal care services, home health, homemaker and chore services, friendly
visitors, therapies, etc. Each category of service is
discussed below.

1. Financial Supports to Family Caregivers

There is renewed interest in providing financial supports to family care providers. Current federal proposals
and state level programs of this sort were discussed earlier in this chapter. The major VA mechanism for
providing such financial supports is the Aid and
Attendance Benefit which provides financial supplements to
qualified veterans receiving:

- Veterans compensation for service-connected disabilities,
- Disability pension for non-service-connected disabilities, or
- Certain qualified family members receiving sur-
  vivor benefits.

While the eligibility requirements for this benefit
are complicated and confusing, the supplemental financial
assistance may, in many cases, provide incentives to families to continue to provide in-home care. Expansion of
eligibility for this benefit, along with coordination or
provision of service supports to caregivers, are likely to
enhance home based family care. Aid and Attendance also
provides an example of VA support for veterans' family
members, in that dependents and spouses are taken into
consideration in the calculation of benefits and surviving
spouses also may qualify for benefits.

A somewhat different way in which the VA might use
financial supports to help delay or prevent nursing home
care would be to share domiciliary costs with the veteran.

242

More veterans might avail themselves of this type of care if they received some financial assistance. With respect to any type of financial support, the Department of Veterans Benefits might be a potential vehicle for implementing the program, perhaps on a demonstration basis, and for assuring program evaluation.

2. Service Supports to Family Caregivers

While major purposes of family caregiver service support programs are to improve the quality of life for care providers and the quality of care for the elder, they are also viewed as having the potential to expand the family's willingness to continue to provide care at home, thereby reducing expenditures for formal services and avoiding or delaying high institutional expenditures. These supports include technical assistance in learning new skills, counseling, family mental health services or personal supports, and a variety of respite or emergency caretaking services. For the most part, these services are provided directly to the care provider, though some (e.g., respite care) may involve the elder as well. Services of this sort recognize the substantial efforts made by family caregivers and the potential stresses of caretaking. Current demonstrations of family caretaker support programs lean heavily on volunteer services and "self-help" groups which bring together caregivers for mutual support, information sharing and other activities. Current examples of such programs within the VA are programs at the Brentwood Division of the West Los Angeles Medical Center and the Marion VA Medical Center which offers support to spouses and families of patients with Alzheimer's disease.

The VA has two options for providing service supports to family care providers. One option is to develop VA programs which use VA staff and volunteers to provide counseling and skills development. These programs would most likely emanate from VA medical centers (VAMCs) and outpatient clinics but would be most effective if offered in the client's home and in geographic locations close to home. A continuing difficulty for caregivers is to leave the house for any purpose because of the ongoing care requirements of their dependent family member. The availability of telephone reassurance and contact has been noted as being very supportive by many family members, particularly those who are housebound by their caretaking responsibility. Use of telephone contacts certainly would expand the impact of a VA support program and reduce fiscal and personal costs (e.g., travel, inconvenience) and is likely to be quite effective if supplemented by home or clinic visits. Such services would represent an extension of the life-line concept already in use with some veterans and of the contact person approach offered to patients and family members at some VA medical facilities. VA experience suggests that future volunteer-based services will be enhanced when Volunteer Resource Needs Assessments are performed early and when planned medical facility support underpins volunteer training, supervision, and morale maintenance. The potential value of the VA's impressive pool of volunteers cannot be over emphasized.

Another approach for the VA in developing supports for caretakers is to develop sharing arrangements with community agencies. This strategy would require legislative changes. The exact "format" (e.g., contracts, pooling of resources, "trading of services") of such sharing arrangements is discussed in other chapters in this book. It should be recognized, however, that programs to support family caregivers are not common in community service systems across the country and, in fact, will be a novel idea in many communities. This provides the VA with a good opportunity for early involvement in the planning and implementation of such programs, serving as a full partner, and perhaps innovator, in the community development process. Further, a project such as this lends itself well to sharing arrangements in which a VAMC may provide family support services to a combination of veterans and non-veterans in its immediate geographic area in exchange for similar services provided to veterans by community agencies in areas which are not geographically convenient to the VA facility.

The VA might approach sharing arrangements through coordination with the Administration on Aging (AOA) at the national level and through experimental programs on the local level where VA social workers could serve as case managers, guiding clients through the labyrinth of non-VA and VA services.

3. Services Which Supplement Family Care

The VA has before it a rich array of options for supplementing family care. Strictly speaking, any service which eases the burden of caregivers falls into this category, including: home health care, chore services, day hospitals, friendly visitors, and even temporary institutional care. The delivery of this broad array of services in the continuum of long term care is discussed in other chapters, but a few issues are particularly relevant to this discussion.

First, for supports to care providers to be most cost effective, they should supplement, not supplant, family services. Unfortunately, because family capabilities and the elders' needs for assistance vary so widely, it is not possible to identify specific services which substitute rather than supplement. In some families, personal care services such as bathing, toileting and dressing are considered to be a natural and comfortable part of family life, but these same family members may feel overwhelmed by technical tasks such as dressing changes for wounds, colostomy care, injections, or suction of secretions. Another family may become proficient in these technical skills, but feel uncomfortable with personal care that violates family taboos of privacy and modesty. A case-by-case assessment of needs, capacities, and family expectations is required.

In addition to the usual array of home health and social services that may be used to supplement and enhance family care, respite care services are particularly important in family care situations. Respite care provides a "time-out" for family care providers. The duration of the respite may be for a few hours to a month or more. It may be a regularly scheduled event or available on an "emergency" basis only, and it may be provided in the home of the elder or in other settings, including nursing homes and acute care hospitals. The care itself may require highly trained professionals for elders with complex medical or behavioral problems; on the other hand, many elders have respite care requirements which could easily be met by non-professional staff and volunteers with minimal training.

The VA has a number of options before it for providing respite care, some requiring legislative changes. VAMCs already provide "unintentional" respite care for families in crisis who bring in an elder for admission to the acute hospital for more or less "real" medical problems. A careful analysis of many of these cases will indicate that, although a medical problem may exist, the major factor in the hospitalization is the need for a "time-out" for family members. This occurrence is not unique to the VA; the Friday night drop-off of an elder family member to

245

the emergency room is not an uncommon experience for hospitals across the country. Unfortunately, this unplanned, "back door" respite may have a number of negative consequences. First, it is in the business of acute care hospitals to "work up" patients who are admitted to their care. The diagnostic procedures involved in such work-ups may have negative health consequences for the frail elder with a somewhat precariously balanced set of health problems. Secondly, acute hospitals are dangerous places for elders who are at increased risk for iatrogenic disease, nosocomial infection, accidents, and the development of confusion. This is not to say that acute hospitals should not be used for respite care. Rather, it stresses the importance of respite services which encourage families to plan ahead and allow care providers to appropriately define the purpose and nature of care in order to reduce these problems.

Further, "deliberate" respite care allows for the provision of needed services with appropriate levels of staffing and intervention. The VA already offers some deliberate respite care and has the potential to offer such care in a variety of its institutional and residential settings, including acute care, extended care, nursing homes, and perhaps even domiciliary care.

Respite care provided in the community whether in the home of the elder, in a group home, or in the home of a volunteer, may be preferable in many cases. It allows the elder to stay in familiar or home-like settings, and may cost less to provide. The use of elders for this purpose, either as volunteers or with moderate pay, has been effective in some communities.

Day hospitals and adult day care are other forms of support which supplement family caretaking. These services may be particularly useful in circumstances in which the family care providers are working during the day or when the daytime care requirements are too burdensome. Day care programs require careful planning and "marketing," and yet have proven effective in many communities. Current VA programs in adult day care include those located at Loma Linda, American Lake, Palo Alto, North Chicago, Butler, and the VA Outpatient Clinic in Boston. Still others are being planned.

Again, the VA may choose to initiate day care and day hospital programs at VAMCs or may choose to enter into

246

sharing arrangements with community agencies in order to access elder veterans to these services. If sharing arrangements are selected, coordination with the AOA at the national level and with the Department of Veterans Benefits for implementation purposes is likely to be beneficial.

B. Options for Caring for the Spouses of Elder Veterans

A continuing dilemma in caring for the older veteran is concern for the veteran's spouse. As was noted earlier, the married couple is the most enduring and committed of caretaking arrangements. Unfortunately, caretaking may continue long after personal and financial resources have been drained, at great cost to each spouse. The dilemma is further complicated by multiple entitlements and eligibilities which bring a number of providers and agencies into the caretaking environment. Sadly, there are also circumstances in which only one spouse may qualify for a range of care needed by both. Community based care providers report the moral difficulty of coming into a home to serve one elder and being unable to assist his or her spouse, even though care is clearly needed.

The VA is providing services to the family members of veterans in some circumstances. The Civilian Health and Medical Program (CHAMPVA) allows provision of medical care to the spouse or child of a veteran who is totally disabled or who has died as a result of a service-connected event (VA, 1982b). CHAMPVA is organized as an insurance program with the VA reimbursing outside providers. Recently, however, a sharing agreement between the VA and the Department of Defense has resulted in provision of direct care to spouses within Medical District 23. Family members are only eligible for CHAMPVA when they are not eligible for Medicare or Civilian Health and Medical Program of the Uniformed Services (CHAMPUS), and when the care is available in a VA facility.

Should the recent sharing agreement prove cost effective, the VA could consider a similar arrangement in other medical districts, as well as attaining eligibility for spouses of other elder veterans. Legislation would be required to allow such eligibility. As is discussed in the chapter, "Utilization of the VA by Elder Veterans: An Empirical Analysis," veterans who use the VA health system are less likely to be married than those veterans who do not (61% vs. 87%), but a majority of veterans who use VA health care are married. It is difficult to estimate potential demand; however, access to such a program could be needs-based, income-based, or a combination of factors.

Another option is for the VA to offer selected services only to those spouses whose veteran spouse (usually husband) qualifies for and needs the service. In this manner, home health services would only be provided to a wife whose husband is also receiving home health care. This option would also require legislation.

Nursing homes or residential care arrangements are other arenas in which spouses might be offered care. Cohabitation in VA care facilities could not only improve quality of life for couples, but might also result in some continued care provided by spouses to one another. Provision of services to non-veterans within VA facilities would involve legislative changes. VA personnel in Cleveland are currently investigating placement of couples in residential home care dwellings (Neher, 1983).

Expansion of VA health services to include spouses involves potential problems in addition to increased demand. The experience of female veterans in the VA health care system has been problematic. Because the vast majority of veterans are male, the physical plant and staffing patterns of VA hospitals are not geared toward female patients. Lack of female-oriented specialties (such as gynecology) as well as lack of privacy and restroom facilities for women have been noted. Structural and staff changes would be required to accommodate inpatient and outpatient care of female spouses. Some of these issues are currently being addressed by the VA Administrator's Special Advisory Group.

Certainly, as with other service modalities, the VA faces the option of providing care directly or entering into sharing relationships on a contract or fee-basis. The Department of Veterans Benefits might be viewed as a potential vehicle for implementing and evaluating any revised eligibility criteria. As with all suggested changes, a research design would need to be developed that could accurately identify cause-effect phenomena.

248

Conclusion

VA provision of medical care to needy spouses is an unconventional idea at this point and, along with caregiver support programs, necessarily entails major legislative changes. Such changes are required to permit the VA increased flexibility in coordinating care and support to veterans' family members both within VA facilities and the community. The payoffs of increased VA flexibility for veterans, their spouses, and the VA could be considerable. The family unit would be maintained longer than it otherwise might be, and the VA, in building upon its geriatric expertise, would be assuring quality medical care to older veterans and their spouses. With legislative authorization, the VA might also find it advantageous to explore exchange relationships with government agencies whereby the VA exchanges its medical knowledge and/or care for state reimbursement or coordinates and controls the allocation of state medical funds on behalf of veterans and their spouses. (Possible VA/community coordination patterns are addressed in other chapters within this book, as are the attendant legislative options and obstacles.) VA oversight of veterans' family needs on a case management basis, for example, could enhance medical assessment, curtail instances of redundant or parallel health delivery, and improve overall family health care. No matter what specific care delivery or reimbursement pattern may be eventually selected, increased VA familiarity with elder veterans' family needs holds great promise for improved medical care for these families. Ultimately, the major purpose and payoff of caregiver support programs and provision of care to needy spouses is improved quality of life for the elder veteran.

REFERENCES

Aaron, M.M. and Elliott, S.S. "The Home Assessment House Call for Elderly Patients." Paper presented at the 1982 Gerontological Society Meetings, Boston. Winston Salem, N.C.: Bowman Grey School of Medicine.

Administration on Aging. Facts and Figures on Older Americans, No. 5. DHEW Publication No. (OHD) 74-200005, pp. 4-6, Washington, D.C., 1974.

Armitage, S.K. "Negotiating the Discharge of Medical Patients." Journal of Advanced Nursing, 6, pp. 385-389, 1981.

Atchley, R.C. "Dimensions of Widowhood in Later Life." Gerontologist, 15(2), pp. 176-178, 1975.

Bell, W.G. "Policy and Practice in Long Term Care of Elderly: A Proposal for Change." Paper presented at the 1974 Annual Meetings of the Gerontological Society of America, Portland, Oregon.

Brody, E.M. Long Term Care of Older People: A Practical Guide. New York Human Services Press, 1977.

Brody, E.M. "The Aging Family." Annals of the AAPSS 438, pp. 13-27, 1978.

Brody, S., et al. "The Family Caring Unit: A Major Consideration in the Long Term Support System." Gerontologist, 18, Issue 6, pp. 556-561, 1978.

Brubaker, T., et al. "Forum on Aging and the Family: Discussion with F. Ivan Nye, Bernice L. Neugarten, and David and Vera Mase." Family Coordinator, 27, pp. 437-444, 1978.

Callahan, J., et al. "Responsibility of Family for Their Severely Disabled Elderly." Health Care Financing Review, Winter, 1980.

Campbell, R. and Chenoweth, B. "Health Education as a Basis for Social Support." Gerontologist, 21, Issue 6, pp. 619-627, 1981.

Cantor, M. "Caring for the Elderly: Impact on Family, Friends and Neighbors." Paper presented at the 1980 Annual Meetings of the Gerontological Society, San Diego.

Cantor, M. "Strain among Caregivers: A Study of Experience in the United States." Gerontologist, 23, pp. 597-604, 1983.

Caro, F.G. "Post-Hospital Care Arrangements for the Functionally Disabled Elderly." Paper presented at the 1982 Meetings of the Gerontological Society of America, Boston. (Available through the Community Service Society, New York).

Chevan, A. and Korson, J.H. "The Widowed Who Live Alone: An Examination of Social and Demographic Factors." Social Forces, 51, Issue 1, pp. 45-53, 1972.

Cicirelli, V.G. "Kin Relationships of Children and One Child Elderly in Relation to Social Services." Paper presented at the 1979 Meetings of the Gerontological Society, Washington, D.C.

Cicirelli, V.G. "A Comparison of Helping Behavior to Elderly Parents of Adult Children with Intact and Disrupted Marriages." Gerontologist, 23, pp. 619-624, 1983.

Clark, N.M. and Rakowski, W. "Family Caregivers of Older Adults: Improving Helping Skills." Gerontologist, 23, pp. 637-642, 1983.

Cohen, P.M. "A Group Approach to Working with Families of the Elderly." Gerontologist, 23, Issue 3, pp. 249-250, 1983.

Comptroller General. Report to the Congress of the United States: Entering a Nursing Home: Costly Implications for Medicaid and the Elderly. Report No. PAD-80-12. Washington, D.C.: General Accounting Office, November 26, 1979.

Congressional Budget Office. Long-Term Care: Actuarial Cost Estimate: CBO Technical Analysis. Washington, D.C.: U.S. Government Printing Office, 1977.

251

Crystal, S. America's Old Age Crisis: Public Policy and the Two Worlds of Aging. New York: Basic Books, 1982.

Davis, K. "Equal Treatment and Unequal Benefits. The Medicare Program." Milbank Memorial Fund Quarterly, 53, pp. 449-488, 1975.

Dono, J.E., et al. "Primary Groups in Old Age." Research on Aging, 1(14), pp. 403-433, 1979.

Emling, D.C. Adult Chore Services. Lancing, Michigan: Michigan Department of Social Services, November, 1976.

Fendetti, D.V. and Gelfond, D.E. "Care of the Aged: Attitudes of White Ethnic Families." Gerontologist, 16, pp. 545-549, 1976.

Fengler, A. and Goodrich, N. "Wives of Elderly Disabled Men: The Hidden Patients." Gerontologist, 19, pp. 175-185, 1979.

Gelfond, D.E., et al. "Two Generations of Elderly in the Changing American Family: Implications for Family Services." Family Coordination, 27, pp. 395-403, 1978.

General Accounting Office. Home Health -- the Need for a National Policy to Better Provide for the Elderly, Washington, D.C.: USGPO, 1977.

General Accounting Office. The Well-Being of Older People in Cleveland, Ohio. Washington, D.C.: USGPO, 1977.

Geriatric Liaison Coordinating Committee. Department of Medicine and Surgery. "Patient Treatment and Program Developments in the Care of the Aging Veteran." (Draft) Washington, D.C.: Veterans Administration, May, 1983.

Getzel, G.S. "Helping Elderly Couples in Crisis." Paper presented at the 1981 Meetings of the Gerontological Society, Toronto.

Getzel, G.S. "Group Work with Kin and Friends Caring for the Elderly." Paper presented at the 1982 Annual Meetings of the Gerontological Society, Boston. (Also available from the National Supports Program, Community Service Society, New York).

Golden, G. "Coping with Aging: Denial and Avoidance in Middle-Age Caregivers." Unpublished doctoral dissertation. Berkeley: University of California, 1982.

Gonyea, J., et al. "The Impact of Chore Services Termination on Family Caregivers." Paper presented at the 1982 Annual Meetings of the Gerontological Society of America, Boston.

Gross-Andrew, S. and Zimmer, A.E. "Incentives to Families Caring for Disabled Elderly: Research and Demonstration Project to Strengthen the Natural Supports System." Paper presented at the 1977 Annual Meetings of the Gerontological Society of America, San Francisco.

Haas, C.D. The Adult Home Health Services Module. Lancing, Michigan: Department of Social Services, 1982.

Hanson, S.L., et al. "Racial and Cohort Variations in Filial Responsibility Norms." Gerontologist, 23, pp. 426-631, 1983.

Hayes, W.C. and Mindel, C.H. "Extended Kinship Relations in Black and White Families." Journal of Marriage and the Family, 35, Issue 1, pp. 51-57, 1973.

Health Care Finance Administration. Long Term Care: Background and Future Directions. Washington, D.C.: U.S. Department of Health and Human Services, HCFA-81-20047, 1981.

Henderson, M. Outpatient of the Geriatric Kind, Final Report. Washington, D.C.: VA Health Services Research and Development, 1981.

Horowitz, A. "Families Who Care: A Study of Natural Support System of the Elderly." Paper presented at the 1978 Annual Meetings of the Gerontological Society of America, Dallas.

Horowitz, A. "Sons and Daughters as Caregivers to Older Parents: Differences in Performance and Consequences." Paper presented at the 1981 Annual Meetings of the Gerontological Society of America, Toronto.

Isaacs, B. and Neville, Y.   "Measuring Need in Old People."   Paper read at the Tenth International Congress of Gerontology, Jerusalem, 1975.

Isaacs, B., et al.   "The Stricken: The Social Consequences of Stroke."   Age and Aging, 5, pp. 188-192, 1976.

Japanese Government.   The National Report for the United Nations World Assembly on Aging.   Tokyo: Government of Japan, May, 1982.

Johnson, C. and Catalano, D.   "A Longitudinal Study of Family Supports to Peer Elderly."   Paper presented at the 1982 Annual Meetings of the Gerontological Society of America, Boston.

Kane, R.L. and Kane, R.A.   Long-Term Care in Six Countries: Implications for the U.S.   Washington, D.C.:   U.S. Department of Health and Human Services, NIA Publication No. 80-1207, 1976.

Kivett, B.R. and Learner, R.M.   "Perspectives on the Childless Rural Elderly: A Comparative Analysis."   Gerontologist, 20, pp. 708-716, 1980.

Kuypers, J.A. and Trute, B.   "The Older Family as the Locus of Crisis Intervention."   Family Coordination, 27, pp. 405-412, 1978.

Leurie, W.F.   Employing the DUKE OARS.   Methodology in Cost Comparisons: Home Services and Industrialization.   Durham, North Carolina: Duke University Center for the Study of Aging and Human Development, 2,2, 1978.

Little, V.C.   "The Family as a Source of Support for the Elderly."   Unpublished chapter.   West Hartford, Connecticut: University of Connecticut School of Social Work, 1982.

Litwak, E.   "Extended Kin Relations in an Industrialized Society."   In Social Structure and the Family, Shanas, E. and Streib, G. (Eds.).   Englewood Cliffs, New Jersey: Prentice Hall, 1965.

Maddox, G.L. "Families as Context and Resources in Chronic Illness." In Long-Term Care: A Handbook for Researchers, Planners and Providers, Sherwood, S. (Ed.). New York: Spectrum, 1975.

Maeda, D. "Family Care in Japan." Gerontologist, 23, pp. 579-583, 1983.

Maryland Office on Aging. Caring for Elderly Relatives, Tax Credits: Current Practice and Fiscal Impact. A working chapter. Baltimore, 1977.

Maryland Office on Aging, The Comptroller's Office. Report to the General Assembly: Tax Credits for Those Who Care for Elderly Relatives. Baltimore: Office on Aging, 1977.

Mellor, J. "Towards Self-Help Empowerment of the Caregiver." Position chapter, Natural Supports Program, Community Service Society of New York, October, 1982.

Mellor, J. and Getzel, G.S. "Stress and Service Needs of Those Who Care for the Aged." Paper presented at the 1980 Annual Meetings of the Gerontological Society of America, San Diego.

Mellor, J., et al. "A Partnership of Caring: A Blueprint for Social Action." Paper presented at the 1981 Annual Meetings of the Gerontological Society of America, Ontario.

Moran, A.E. and Soumerai, S.B. Care of the Aging Veteran: Development of the HSRD Research Agenda. Boston: VA GRECC, 1982.

Moroney, R.M. The Family and the State: Considerations for Social Policy. New York: Longlan, 1976.

Neher, J. (Ed.) Geriatric Planning: A Shared Approach. Topeka, KS: VA Medical District 22, Community Services, April, 1983.

Nelson, G. "Support for the Aged: Public-Private Responsibility." Social Work, 27, Issue 2, pp. 137-146, 1982.

Newman, S., et al. Housing Adjustments of Older People: A Report of Findings from the Second Phase. Ann Arbor, Michigan: Institute of Social Research, 1976.

Palmore, E. "Total Chance of Institutionalization among the Aged." Gerontologist, 16, pp. 504-507, 1976.

Patten, S. "Assessment of Client Functioning. (Draft No. 1)." University of Minnesota, Center for Health Services Research, 1979.

Robinson, B.C. "Validation of a Caregiver's Strain Index." Journal of Gerontology, 38, Issue 3, pp. 344-348, 1983.

Rodell, D.E. "Discharge Planning for Hospitalized Older Veterans." Evaluation Health Professional, 2, Issue 1, pp. 71-86, 1979.

Rubenstein, L.Z., et al. "Improved Care for Patients on a New Geriatric Unit." Journal of American Geriatric Society, 29, pp. 531-536, 1981.

Schorr, A. Filial Responsibility in the Modern American Family. Washington, D.C.: Department of Health Education and Welfare, Social Security Administration, Division of Program Research, 1960.

Schorr, A. Exploration in Social Policy. New York: Basic Books, 1968.

Schuckit, M., et al. "Unrecognized Psychiatric Illnesses in Elderly Medical and Surgery Patients." International Journal of Gerontology, 30, Issue 6, pp. 566-600, 1975.

Seelbach, W.C. "Correlates of Aged Parent's Filial Responsibility. Expectations and Realizations." Family Coordinator, 27, pp. 341-350, 1978.

Seiling, V. and Page, W.F. Health Characteristics of Veterans and Nonveterans: Health Interview Surveys, 1971-1974. Washington, D.C.: VA Comptroller Monograph No. 11, 1980.

Shanas, E. "Social Myth and Hypothesis: The Case of Family Relations of Old People." Gerontologist, 19, pp. 3-9, 1979.

Shanas, E. and Hauser, P. "Zero Population Growth and Family Life for Old People." Journal of Social Issues, 30, Issue 4, pp. 79-92, 1974.

Soldo, B. and Mossey, J. Validity of Derived Measures in a Study of Caregiving Using Secondary Data. Working Paper No. 5, Series CPR, MD-80/1. Washington, D.C.: Georgetown University Center for Population Research, Kennedy Institute of Ethics, January, 1980.

Soldo, B. and Myllyluoma, J. "Caregivers Who Live with Dependent Elderly." Gerontologist, 23, pp. 605-611, 1983.

Soldo, B. and Sharma, M. "Families Who Purchase vs Families Who Provide Care Services to Elderly Relatives." Paper presented at the 1980 Annual Meeting of the Gerontological Society Meeting, San Diego.

Special Committee on Aging, United States Senate. Nursing Home Care in the United States: Failure in Public Policy. Washington, D.C.: U.S. Government Printing Office, 1974.

Steuer, J.L. and Clark, E.O. "Family Support Groups within a Research Project on Dementia." Clinical Gerontologist, 1, Issue 1, pp. 87-95, 1982.

Streib, G. "An Alternative Family Form for Older Persons: Need and Social Context." Family Coordinator, 27, pp. 413-420, 1978.

U.S. Veterans Administration. "More than a Thousand Receive VA Hospital-Based Home Care." In Vanguard, Washington, D.C., September 21, 1976.

U.S. Veterans Administration. Office of Reports and Statistics. Veteran Population, March 31, 1982a, Washington, D.C.

U.S. Veterans Administration. Project Profiles: The Older Volunteer: Report Prepared for the National Council on Aging. Washington, D.C., May, 1982b.

U.S. Veterans Administration. Office of Reports and Statistics. Veteran Population, September 30, 1982c, Washington, D.C.

U.S. Veterans Administration. Office of Reports and Statistics. *Statistical Brief: A Comparison of Selected Characteristics of VA Nursing Home Patients and National Nursing Home Residents.* Washington, D.C., October, 1982d.

U.S. Veterans Administration. Department of Medicine and Surgery. Chief medical director's letters. IL-10-82-10. Washington, D.C., 1982e.

U.S. Veterans Administration. Department of Medicine and Surgery. *Social Work Service Responsibility in Discharge Planning.* Circular 10-82-133, Washington, D.C., 1982f.

U.S. Veterans Administration. Voluntary Services. *Volunteer Activities of the Older Veteran.* (In-house report), Washington, D.C., 1982g.

U.S. Veterans Administration. Voluntary Services (135). *Volunteer Services for the Older Veteran.* (In-house report), Washington, D.C., 1982h.

U.S. Veterans Administration. Office of Reports and Statistics. *VA Trend Data 1958-1982.* Washington, D.C., February, 1983a.

U.S. Veterans Administration. *Vanguard.* Washington, D.C., May, 1983b.

U.S. Veterans Administration. "Demographics of the Aging Veteran." Draft of Geriatrics and Gerontology Advisory Committee Report, Washington, D.C., 1983c.

Vinick, B. "Remarriage in Old Age." *Family Coordination,* 27, pp. 359-364, 1978.

Ward, R.A. "Limitations of the Family as a Supportive Institution in the Lives of the Aged." *Family Coordinator,* 27, pp. 365-374, 1978.

Whitfield, S. *Report to the General Assembly on the Family Support Demonstration Project.* Baltimore: Maryland Office on Aging, 1981.

Woehrer, C.E. "Cultural Pluralism in American Families: The Influence of Ethnicity on Social Aspect of Aging." *Family Coordinator,* 27, pp. 329-340, 1978.

Zimmer, A.H. and Sainer, J.S. "Strengthening the Family as an Informal Support for Their Aged: Implications for Social Policy and Planning." Paper presented at the 1978 Annual Meetings of the Gerontological Society of America, Dallas.

9. Functional Status and Service Use Among a Community Sample of Elderly Veterans

Laurance G. Branch, Ph.D.
Paul A. Scherr, Ph.D.
Nancy R. Cook, D.Sc.
James O. Taylor, M.D.

Introduction

The increasing numbers of older people present complex challenges to health system architects. The innovative programs and policies developed for aging veterans, indeed, might be the harbingers of national responses to the geriatric imperative. In this context health policy planners in the Veterans Administration have had a long-standing need for appropriate planning data. Over the years four vexing problems have re-emerged regularly.

Problem 1. Do elderly veterans differ from elderly non-veterans in their need and use of health care services and in the characteristics associated with utilization? If they do not significantly differ, existing data sources, most notably the annual Health Interview Survey (HIS) conducted by the National Center for Health Statistics, would be valuable sources of data for VA health planners. If elderly veterans and non-veterans are significantly different, special (and costly) data collection efforts are required.

Some older published works compared the health care utilization profiles of elderly Spanish-American War veterans with the general utilization rates reported from the

U.S. National Health Survey (a forerunner of the Health
Interview Survey) and the 1962 Survey of the Aged, while
controlling for the age of the respondents (Freeman, et
al., 1966; Richardson, et al., 1967). The findings that
aged Spanish-American War veterans used more services than
comparably-aged non-veterans are difficult to generalize
because the Spanish-American War veterans did not have the
same barriers to access that the pre-Medicare non-veterans
had.

More recently, the VA has continued this tradition of
analyzing the "Health Characteristics of Veterans and Non-
Veterans" by aggregating data from the 1971-1974 Health
Interview Surveys (Seiling and Page, 1980), and the 1975-
1978 Health Interview Surveys (VA, 1982). Both of these
monographs report that "in general, health characteristics
of the male veterans and non-veterans are very similar"(p.
IV). This summary applies to the elderly male veterans
and non-veterans as well as other age groups.

In addition to these efforts, the VA has sponsored
three national surveys of veterans (the first in 1977, the
second in 1979, and the third in 1983) to learn more about
the knowledge and use of benefits available to veterans.
The methodology took a step backward and precluded a comparison between veterans and non-veterans on medical care
issues. During the screening of households for veterans,
a small subsample of non-veterans could easily have been
asked the medical care items for comparison. This proce-
dure was not employed, and simple descriptive findings
without reference to comparison groups are presented.

There is no consensus concerning whether veterans consistently and significantly differ from non-veterans either in the characteristics associated with utilization or
in actual service utilization. Therefore, there is no
agreement about whether the VA needs to collect special
data for its health planning purposes.

Problem 2. Among elderly veterans, in what ways does
age influence utilization? Many of the previously published analyses of aging veterans have treated those aged
65 years and older as a unitary and homogeneous subgroup,
and have not examined age-specific relationships among
those aged 65 years or over (National Survey of Veterans I
and II did not, III is not yet available; the analyses of
Health Interview Surveys of 1971-1974 and 1975-1978 did
not). A recent VA monograph, however, did articulately

outline the rationale for examining age-specific relationships among those over age 65 years and presented some
preliminary analyses. This report titled The Aging Veteran, Present and Future Medical Needs (VA, 1977) clearly
set the stage for age-specific analyses among the elderly
veterans:

> An important aspect of geriatric care is the need
> to recognize that there are at least three stages
> of life after age 65. [sic] The first 10 years
> most individuals show little age-change and nor-
> mal activities continue unless there is a specif-
> ic illness. Between ages 75 and 85 most persons
> can continue normal activities, but many, even
> without an overt disease, begin to show the ef-
> fects of age. After age 85 there are few who can
> maintain full normal activity without some assis-
> tance (p. 17).

Though one could argue whether "many" between ages 75
and 85 "show the effects of age" (presumably this means a
functional decline, but we would prefer a less ageist expression), or that "few" over age 85 are fully independent, the general implications are important and can be
substantiated by data. The challenge issued by this monograph of presenting age-specific information about the
various age groups among elderly veterans has not resulted
in an overwhelming response, however. The challenge has
been reissued in the recent monograph Health Care of the
Aging Veteran: A Report of the Geriatrics and Gerontology
Advisory Committee (VA, 1983).

Problem 3. In what ways does functional status influence health care utilization among aging veterans? The
vast majority of multivariate prediction studies of health
care utilization among general populations (i.e., veteran
and non-veteran combined) consistently have demonstrated
that functional status has a significant and important association with subsequent medical care utilization. Nonetheless, none of the published reports from the National
Surveys of Veterans or the re-analyses of HIS data have
incorporated a thorough examination of the influence of
the functional status on utilization. In the case of the
re-analysis of HIS data, the data are insufficient to support this kind of analysis even though the analysts may
have desired to do so. To date, the HIS data only indicate a "limitation in major activities," and the concept
of "major activity" is undefined for retired people. How-

263

ever, the 1977 aging veteran monograph previously mentioned did indeed suggest that functional status information would be particularly useful for purposes of program development. Following their own suggestion, the authors presented nine hypothetical levels of disability or patient care needs which could influence the development of VA health care services, but the conceptual treatment of differential disability had no empirical basis. Therefore empirical investigations are still warranted.

Problem 4. Are we asking the right questions about the differences between elderly users of veteran health care services compared to elderly non-users of health care services? There are some published studies which examine the antecedents of VA medical care utilization among veterans which provide valuable insights into this area of how the decision to seek care from VA facilities is made (Page, 1982; Schneider and Dove, 1983). Page's analysis indicated that health insurance coverage was the predominant factor influencing a veteran's choice of facility for hospitalization, with age, income, and service-connected disability status secondary influences on the utilization decision. Page's analysis was limited to acute hospitalization episodes, however, and not the utilization of other components of the VA health service system. Admittedly the costs incurred by the 162 VA medical centers (VAMCs) dwarf the costs incurred by the 226 outpatient clinics or its 108 nursing home and domiciliary facilities then available, therefore this analysis was certainly an appropriate beginning to the investigation of why veterans choose VA facilities for health care.

Schneider and Dove (1983) attempted to clarify the antecedents associated with the utilization of another VA health care service -- VA emergency room facilities. This important analysis underscored that "although some patients may be abusing the system, the problem is difficult to correct because of Congressional legislation that deters the VA from providing primary care" (p. 57). Legislative prohibitions complicate the discussions of appropriate health policy options to more effectively and efficiently meet the needs of elderly veterans. Schneider and Dove's analysis might have been even more useful had it included an appropriate comparison group or even incorporated statistical controls, rather than simply providing a description of the characteristics of users.

264

The present analyses are preliminary and will not provide definitive results on any of the four preceding questions. Concerning the fourth question specifically, Page has reported that service-connected disability status exerts a secondary influence on the veteran's decision for a VA hospital. Unfortunately, the data available to us do not include information on this important factor. The analyses presented, however, should suggest which of these four very basic questions needs to be pursued with an appropriate commitment of resources.

Methods

The data available for the present analyses come from a total community survey effort of all people aged 65 years and over in East Boston, Massachusetts. This population study was sponsored by the National Institute on Aging (James O. Taylor, M.D., principal investigator; Denis A. Evans, M.D., Laurence G. Branch, Ph.D., and Edward H. Kass, M.D., co-investigators) as part of a three-site, prospective study of normal aging.

Threats to the generalizability of the East Boston data for VA health policy issues arise from the fact that the East Boston elderly population is almost exclusively Caucasian and predominantly of Italian descent. Since many veterans are neither Caucasian nor ethnically Italian, these data have limitations. Nevertheless, the total population enumeration and subsequent interviewing enabled us to identify the subset of males who were veterans (n = 372) and proceed with a series of analyses designed to clarify some of the questions raised in the previous section.

The East Boston Senior Health Project required a door-to-door census of the entire East Boston population to identify all people aged 65 years and over. This occurred in 1982. In the same year, a 45 to 60 minute personal interview was attempted with all people aged 65 years and over. With a response rate of 80%, 3764 East Boston elders enrolled in this prospective study and provided baseline information.

The baseline information included demographic items (including social security numbers); measured blood pressure, pulse, and peak expiratory flow rate; reported height and weight; health status indicators; medical histories (heart attacks, stroke, hip fracture, and diabetes);

medical symptoms (angina, dysporea, history of digitalis, history of blood pressure medications); smoking and alcohol histories; reported physical functional status including activities of daily living; measured cognitive functional status including recent and delayed memory skills; reported emotional functional status including a depression scale; social network assessment; and utilization of health and social services.

Results

Table 1 presents information bearing on the first issue: Are elderly male veterans different from elderly male non-veterans in ways or on dimensions which would influence VA geriatric health policy planning? Among the Caucasian, predominantly Italian community of East Boston, Massachusetts, elderly veterans are statistically significantly different from non-veterans on a variety of dimensions. Demographically, the elderly male veterans were significantly younger than elderly non-veterans, had significantly different marital status (more veterans were never married compared to non-veterans), had fewer living children (probably influenced by the larger percentage who had never married), had more formal education (probably influenced by the younger average age of these veterans), had greater income levels (probably related in part to their increased education and younger age), and fewer had their medical expenses covered by Medicaid (which has an income eligibility criterion and therefore probably is related to the greater income of elderly veterans).

There were no differences between elderly veterans and elderly non-veterans in either of two important risk factors, smoking history and alcohol consumption.

In terms of medical history, elderly veterans were more likely to have cancers and diabetes than non-veterans; no differences in rates were detected for angina, heart attacks, strokes, and hip fractures.

The self-perceived health status of the elderly veterans was significantly better than the elderly non-veterans, but self-perceptions of health are often influenced by age, and recall that the elderly veterans were younger on the average than the non-veterans.

There were no differences in emotional health status between elderly male veterans and elderly non-veterans.

On various measures of physical health status, the elderly veterans' self-reported levels of function were better than the elderly non-veterans. In three areas of activities of daily living (personal grooming, bathing, and dressing) elderly veterans were less dependent than non-veterans. Using an adaptation of Rosow–Breslau's Functional Health Scale, elderly veterans had fewer limitations. Elderly veterans also reported fewer difficulties with the performance of common tasks, and elderly veterans reported more frequent involvement in recreational activities. In none of the areas of physical health status did the male non-veterans report better function than the elderly male veterans.

The elderly veterans had significantly better cognitive function status in two out of the three tests of this dimension, including significantly fewer errors in both digit recall and immediate memory.

Although we have seen consistent differences between elderly veterans and elderly non-veterans in virtually every dimension which previous research suggests might be related to differential utilization of the health care and social service systems (with the exception of the risk factors of smoking history and alcohol consumption), there were no significant differences between elderly veterans and non-veterans in the primary utilization outcomes; namely the rates of hospital admissions and of nursing home admissions. Elderly veterans did report significantly more dental visits than non-veterans, probably related in part to the increased income and education of the elderly veterans relative to elderly non-veterans previously discussed.

In summary, elderly veterans were significantly different from elderly non-veterans on a wide range of variables usually associated with health and social service utilization, but did not differ in some primary utilization dimensions. However, age is one of the dimensions significantly differentiating elderly veterans from elderly non-veterans. Therefore, the bivariate relationships between veteran status and any second variable such as functional health or hospital utilization may be influenced predominantly by the third factor of age. Preliminary tests of these relationships controlling for age did not alter the pattern of findings. Nevertheless, it is clear that the initial question must be rephrased to ask whether elderly veterans differ from elderly non-veterans in their need and use of services after controlling for their age differences.

Table 2 presents information bearing on the second issue: <u>Among elderly male veterans, in what ways is age associated with utilization?</u> The demographic differences associated with age are few. The younger elderly male veterans are more likely to be married than older elderly veterans; younger elders are also more likely to have more formal education than older elders.

Younger elderly veterans were more likely to report being a current regular smoker than older elderly veterans, but there was no association with age in their reported medical history, their self-perception of general health, or their emotional health status.

There were significant differences associated with age in many of the physical health status areas. Assistance was required in six of these seven individual areas of activities of daily living (grooming, room walking, bathing, dressing, eating, using a toilet) for a significantly greater proportion of the older elderly veterans than the younger veterans. Furthermore, the younger elderly reported less limitations in the functional health scale. There was no association with age among elderly veterans in the reported difficulties with common tasks or recreational activities.

The cognitive functional status of these elderly male veterans was also significantly influenced by their age on all three dimensions; the younger elderly had significantly fewer errors in digit recall, immediate memory, and delayed memory.

Among these elderly male veterans, the four specific dimensions of health care utilization revealed a mixed pattern of association with age. Nursing home admissions were significantly more likely among older elderly veterans; dental visits were significantly more likely among younger elderly veterans; there were no differences associated with age in hospital admissions or the proportion with a regular source of medical care.

The data in Tables 6 through 30 present more specific information on the specific rates associated with various age subgroups. Although generalizations by their very definition minimize the richness of diversity, the data

nevertheless indicate that a greatly increased proportion
of elderly male veterans aged 85 years or more reported
dependencies and limitations on the various physical
health dimensions. The age group of 75 to 84 years was
more similar in functional status to those under age 75
than those over age 85. In the measurement of cognitive
functional status, however, those aged 75 to 84 were more
similar to those aged 85 and over. It bears emphasizing
that the age markers some health policy analysts continu-
ally look for probably vary depending on the domain of
consideration. None of these data support a contention
that any age below 75 is associated with dramatic increases in disability or functional decline. A decline in
physical function most likely occurs at a later age than
cognitive dysfunction.

It was interesting to note in Table 13 that none of
the male veterans aged 85 years or over reported currently
being a cigarette smoker.

These significant bivariate associations between age
and outcomes such as functional status among elderly male
veterans require a further word of caution before proceed-
ing to the next section. Because the primary purpose of
these analyses is to examine the bivariate relationships
between the primary predictors (the dimensions of veteran
status, veterans' age, veterans' functional status, and VA
utilization history) with utilization and characteristics
associated with utilization, we run the risk of misinter-
preting the underlying reason for an association. If age
is associated with utilization, and functional status is
also associated with utilization, only a multivariate
analysis (which is not the focus of the present study)
would indicate whether both age and functional status are
independent predictors, or whether one or the other is a
primary predictor and the other's influence is mediated
through the primary one.

Tables 3 and 4 present information bearing on the
third issue: In what ways does functional status influence health care utilization and the other factors associated with utilization among elderly veterans? The information summarized in Table 3 is based on the individual's responses to an adapted Rosow-Breslau Functional
Health Scale in which 57% of the respondents reported they
were able to do all three activities (heavy housework,
stair climbing, and walking 1/2 mile). Further informa-

269

tion on the distribution of the specific items of this functional health scale is contained in Table 20.

Those elderly male veterans with functional limitations of this type had significantly less formal education and less income. Curiously those without limitations reported greater alcohol consumption. In terms of past medical history, those without limitations had lower rates of angina, heart attacks, hip fractures, and diabetes; presumably these medical conditions contribute in part to the functional limitations reported. Not surprisingly, those without functional limitations reported better overall health status.

As one might expect, there was considerable concordance on the various measures of physical health status, though each measures a different dimension. Those without limitations in these functional health areas were significantly less likely to be dependent in all the activity of daily living areas with the sole exception of personal grooming, and were also less likely to report difficulties with common tasks. Those without limitations were significantly more likely to engage in regular recreational activities.

Those without functional limitations had fewer errors in immediate memory, but were not significantly different from those with limitations on the other two dimensions of cognitive functional status.

Those without functional limitations were also less likely to have a regular source of medical care and less likely to have had a hospital admission during the previous year.

Table 4 summarizes the differences associated with activities of daily living (ADL) functional status. From the information presented in Table 18, we identified the 40 elderly male veterans who reported dependency in one or more of the ADL areas (11%). Of those dependent in one or more ADL areas, two-thirds reported a dependency in walking across a small room; one-fourth to one-third reported dependency in bathing, dressing, and transferring from a bed to a chair; and less than one in five of those with dependencies was dependent in using a toilet, eating, or personal grooming.

Those ADL-independent elderly veterans had significantly fewer living children and significantly more income than the ADL-dependent elderly veterans.

ADL-independent veterans reported significantly more alcohol consumption than the ADL-dependent veterans, which is similar to what we observed previously, namely that those without functional limitations also reported more recreational alcohol consumption.

Among the medical history conditions, only stroke was significantly more likely among the ADL-dependent veterans.

The ADL-independent veterans were significantly more likely to rate their general health status better and have better emotional health status than ADL-dependent veterans.

As noted previously, there was concordance among our various measures of physical health status. Those elderly reporting ADL-independence were also more likely to report better functional health and less difficulty with common tasks.

ADL status among elderly male veterans was unrelated to any of the dimensions of cognitive functional status.

Elderly veterans who are ADL-dependent were significantly more likely to have hospital admissions than nursing home admissions than ADL-independent veterans.

It bears repeating that these associations with both measures of functional status and outcomes were not controlled for age, nor were the previous associations with age controlled for functional status.

Table 5 presents information bearing on the fourth issue: What are the characteristics of veterans associated with the decision to use VA facilities at least once during the previous five years? Although we did not examine directly the decision making process of an eligible elderly veteran concerning his decision to seek medical care within a VA medical facility or not, we were able to examine the characteristics of veterans which were significantly associated with this decision.

Table 29 indicates that 70% of the users of VA health care facilities did so during 1982, and only 13% had last

271

used VA facilities more than two years prior to the interview. For those interested, Table 30 indicates which VA facility was used most recently. Half (50%) had used the Court Street Outpatient Clinic in Boston, while over a third (36%) had last used the VAMC in Jamaica Plain.

None of the demographic characteristics were associated with VA health facility use.

Elderly veterans who used VA health care facilities had significantly less self-reported alcohol consumption.

There were no differences in the medical histories of elderly veterans who chose VA health care facilities versus those who did not, nor was there any difference in self-perceived health status.

The elderly users of VA facilities were also significantly more likely to have more depression than elderly non-users. Of all of the measures and dimensions of physical health status, only two areas of activities of daily living revealed significant differences between VA users and non-users: users were more dependent in eating and using the toilet, indicators of the most severe restrictions in activities of daily living.

There were no differences in the cognitive functional status of VA users versus non-users.

VA health facility users were significantly more likely to have a regular source of medical care and to have had a greater proportion of hospital admissions during the previous year.

Summary

Let us begin the summary by focusing on the primary outcome variables, namely the utilization of health care services. Elderly veterans differed from elderly non-veterans in the utilization of dental services only, not in having a regular source of medical care or number of hospital admissions or number of nursing home admissions. Among elderly veterans, their age was associated with nursing home use and dental care use, not with number of hospital admissions or having a regular source of medical care. For elderly veterans, the two measures of functional status were related to the most significant (in terms of costs and supply) health care utilization dimension,

272

namely hospitalization use. One measure of functional health status (the adapted Rosow-Breslau Scale) was also associated with having a regular source of medical care. The other functional status dimension (ADL-independence or dependence) was significantly related with nursing home utilization. A veteran's past decision to use a VA medical care facility was significantly related to having a regular source of medical care and increased hospital utilization. The obvious conclusion emerging from these findings is that functional status among elderly veterans is the most important variable associated with the most important health care utilization variable, hospital utilization. Any planning data base for VA health system architects should therefore include significant information on functional health status. Unfortunately, existing HIS data do not meet this requirement.

These population-based community data somewhat surprisingly indicate that users of VA medical facilities have higher rates of hospital utilization, but no significant differences in demographic characteristics, medical history, cognitive function, and virtually no difference in physical health status than elderly veterans who do not use VA medical facilities. The users of VA medical facilities did have significantly poorer emotional health status, however. One possible explanation for this configuration of findings might be that the users of VA facilities have increased hospitalization rates which are not otherwise related to factors usually associated with the need for increased hospitalization because increased hospitalizations are unintended byproducts of the congressional limitation to the VA from providing primary medical care. In the absence of primary medical care capabilities, perhaps unnecessary hospitalization episodes are the treatment of choice.

In terms of the original four questions posed, these data do not indicate substantial differences in health care utilization between elderly veterans and elderly non-veterans (thereby implying that perhaps the collection of special data is not necessary for planning VA health service systems). Among elderly veterans, age is a sensitive indicator of differential utilization of nursing homes and dental care, but not of hospital utilization or having a regular source of medical care. Functional status among elderly veterans is the most sensitive indicator of differences in health care utilization, particularly the most costly form (hospital utilization). Concerning the fourth

273

issue, there is some evidence to suggest that the veteran users of VA facilities are more likely to have been hospitalized than non-users, and this increased utilization is in the absence of any other differences between elderly VA users and non-users usually associated with increased hospital utilization rates.

Implications

The dimension of physical-functional status should be incorporated into any model or planning effort for the health service needs of elderly veterans. The sensitivity of this factor in differentiating more frequent users from less frequent users across a broad spectrum of health services is well established among civilian populations and now also among elderly veterans.

The VA planning models should pay particular attention to age. Its associations with nursing home admissions among elderly veterans as well as civilian populations has been established. Age-specific models rather than age-adjusted are preferable in this circumstance.

ACKNOWLEDGEMENTS

This chapter was sponsored in part by a contract from the National Institute on Aging (N01 AG 01027) under the Establishment of Populations for Epidemiological Studies, and in part by the Geriatric Research, Education and Clinical Center of the VA Medical Center in West Roxbury, Massachusetts. The role of the East Boston Neighborhood Health Center and its Board of Directors in sponsoring the research which collected these data, and the cooperation of the whole community of East Boston elders is gratefully acknowledged.

Table 1
SUMMARY OF DIFFERENCES BETWEEN ELDERLY MALE VETERANS AND ELDERLY MALE NON-VETERANS

	Statistical Significance	Elderly Veterans Relative to Non-Veterans
Demographic		
Age	.01	Younger
Living Arrangements	.01	Less "spouse only"
Marital Status	.001	More "never married"
Number of Living Children	.001	Less
Education	.001	More
Income	.001	More
Medicare Coverage	NS	
Medicaid Coverage	.01	Less
VA Coverage	Inappropriate	
Risk Factors		
Smoking History	NS	
Alcohol Consumption	NS	
Medical History		
Angina	NS	
Heart Attack	NS	
Stroke	NS	
Cancer	.05	More
Hip Fracture	NS	
Diabetes	.05	More
Self-Perceived Health Status	.01	More
Emotional Health Status	NS	

Table 1 (Cont.)
SUMMARY OF DIFFERENCES BETWEEN ELDERLY MALE VETERANS
AND ELDERLY MALE NON-VETERANS

	Statistical Significance	Elderly Veterans Relative to Non-Veterans
Physical Health Status		
ADL Areas: room walking, transferring, eating, using toilet	NS	
ADL Areas: grooming, bathing, dressing	.01 to .001	Less "dependent"
Functional Health Scale	.01	Less "limitations"
Difficulties with Common Tasks	.05	Less "difficulties"
Recreational Activities	.01	More
Cognitive Functional Status		
Digit Recall	.01	Less "errors"
Immediate Memory	.001	Less "errors"
Delayed Memory	NS	
Health Care Use		
Regular Source of Medical Care	NS	
Hospital Admissions	NS	
Nursing Home Admissions	NS	
Dental Visits	.01	More
Support Service Use		
Home Health Services	NS	
Social Services	NS	
Transportation Services	NS	

Table 2
SUMMARY OF DIFFERENCES ASSOCIATED WITH AGE
AMONG ELDERLY MALE VETERANS

	Statistical Significance	Younger Elderly Relative to Older Elderly
Demographic		
Age	Inappropriate	
Living Arrangements	NS	
Marital Status	.001	More "married"
Number of Living Children	NS	
Education	.001	More
Income	NS	
Medicare Coverage	NS	
Medicaid Coverage	NS	
VA Coverage	NS	
Risk Factors		
Smoking History	.01	More
Alcohol Consumption	NS	
Medical History		
Angina	NS	
Heart Attack	NS	
Stroke	NS	
Cancer	NS	
Hip Fracture	NS	
Diabetes	NS	
Self-Perceived Health Status	NS	
Emotional Health Status	NS	

Table 2 (Cont.)
SUMMARY OF DIFFERENCES ASSOCIATED WITH AGE
AMONG ELDERLY MALE VETERANS

	Statistical Significance	Younger Elderly Relative to Older Elderly
Physical Health Status		
ADL Areas: transferring	NS	
ADL Areas: grooming, room walking, bathing, dressing, eating, using toilet	.05 to .001	Less "dependent"
Functional Health Scale	.001	Less "limitations"
Difficulties with		
Common Tasks	NS	
Recreational Activities	NS	
Cognitive Functional Status		
Digit Recall	.05	Less "errors"
Immediate Memory	.001	Less "errors"
Delayed Memory	.01	Less "errors"
Health Care Use		
Regular Source of Medical Care	NS	
Hospital Admissions	NS	
Nursing Home Admissions	.01	Less
Dental Visits	.001	More
Support Service Use		
Home Health Services	.01	Less
Social Services	.001	Less
Transportation Services	.05	More

279

Table 3
SUMMARY OF DIFFERENCES
ASSOCIATED WITH FUNCTIONAL LIMITATIONS
AMONG ELDERLY MALE VETERANS

	Statistical Significance	Elderly Without Limitations Relative to Those With Limitations
Demographic		
Age	.001	Younger
Living Arrangements	NS	
Marital Status	NS	
Number of Living Children	NS	
Education	.01	More
Income	.001	More
Medicare Coverage	NS	
Medicaid Coverage	NS	
VA Coverage	NS	
Risk Factors		
Smoking History	NS	
Alcohol Consumption	.05	More
Medical History		
Angina	.01	Less
Heart Attack	.001	Less
Stroke	NS	
Cancer	NS	
Hip Fracture	.05	Less
Diabetes	.001	Less
Self-Perceived Health Status	.001	More
Emotional Health Status	.001	Less "depression"

Table 3 (Cont.)
SUMMARY OF DIFFERENCES
ASSOCIATED WITH FUNCTIONAL LIMITATIONS
AMONG ELDERLY MALE VETERANS

	Statistical Significance	Elderly Without Limitations Relative to Those With Limitations
Physical Health Status		
ADL Areas: grooming	NS	
ADL Areas: room walking, bathing, dressing, transferring, eating, using toilet	.01 to .001	Less "dependent"
Functional Health Scale	Inappropriate	
Difficulties with Common Tasks	.001	Less "difficulties"
Recreational Activities	.01	More
Cognitive Functional Status		
Digit Recall	NS	
Immediate Memory	.05	Less "errors"
Delayed Memory	NS	
Health Care Use		
Regular Source of Medical Care	.001	Less
Hospital Admissions	.001	Less
Nursing Home Admissions	NS	
Dental Visits	NS	
Support Service Use		
Home Health Services	.001	Less
Social Services	.001	Less
Transportation Services	.05	More

281

Table 4
SUMMARY OF DIFFERENCES ASSOCIATED WITH ADL STATUS
AMONG ELDERLY MALE VETERANS

	Statistical Significance	Elderly ADL-Independent Relative to ADL-Dependent
Demographic		
Age	.001	Younger
Living Arrangements	NS	
Marital Status	NS	
Number of Living Children	.05	Less
Education	NS	
Income	.01	More
Medicare Coverage	NS	
Medicaid Coverage	NS	
VA Coverage	.05	Less
Risk Factors		
Smoking History	NS	
Alcohol Consumption	.05	More
Medical History		
Angina	NS	
Heart Attack	NS	
Stroke	.01	Less
Cancer	NS	
Hip Fracture	NS	
Diabetes	NS	
Self-Perceived Health Status	.001	More
Emotional Health Status	.01	Less "depression"

Table 4 (Cont.)
SUMMARY OF DIFFERENCES ASSOCIATED WITH ADL STATUS
AMONG ELDERLY MALE VETERANS

	Statistical Significance	Elderly ADL–Independent Relative to ADL–Dependent
Physical Health Status		
ADL Areas	Inappropriate	
Functional Health Scale	.001	More
Difficulties with		
Common Tasks	.001	Less
Recreational Activities	NS	
Cognitive Functional Status		
Digit Recall	NS	
Immediate Memory	NS	
Delayed Memory	NS	
Health Care Use		
Regular Source of Medical Care	NS	
Hospital Admissions	.01	Less
Nursing Home Admissions	.05	Less
Dental Visits	NS	
Support Service Use		
Home Health Services	.001	Less
Social Services	.01	Less
Transportation Services	NS	

Table 5
SUMMARY OF DIFFERENCES
ASSOCIATED WITH VA HEALTH–USER STATUS
AMONG ELDERLY MALE VETERANS

	Statistical Significance	Elderly VA Health Care Users Relative to Non–Users
Demographic		
Age	NS	
Living Arrangements	NS	
Marital Status	NS	
Number of Living Children	NS	
Education	NS	
Income	NS	
Medicare Coverage	NS	
Medicaid Coverage	NS	
VA Coverage	.01	More
Risk Factors		
Smoking History	NS	
Alcohol Consumption	.01	Less
Medical History		
Angina	NS	
Heart Attack	NS	
Stroke	NS	
Cancer	NS	
Hip Fracture	NS	
Diabetes	NS	
Self-Perceived Health Status	NS	
Emotional Health Status	.05	More "depression"

Table 5 (Cont.)
SUMMARY OF DIFFERENCES
ASSOCIATED WITH VA HEALTH-USER STATUS
AMONG ELDERLY MALE VETERANS

	Statistical Significance	Elderly VA Health Care Users Relative to Non-Users
Physical Health Status		
ADL Areas: grooming, room walking, bathing, dressing, transferring	NS	
ADL Areas: eating, using toilet	.05	More "dependent"
Functional Health Scale	NS	
Difficulties with Common Tasks	NS	
Recreational Activities	NS	
Cognitive Functional Status		
Digit Recall	NS	
Immediate Memory	NS	
Delayed Memory	NS	
Health Care Use		
Regular Source of Medical Care	.01	More
Hospital Admissions	.05	More
Nursing Home Admissions	NS	
Dental Visits	NS	
Support Service Use		
Home Health Services	NS	
Social Services	NS	
Transportation Services	NS	

Table 6
AGE IN YEARS

	(n)	65-69	70-74	75-84	85+	Statistical Significance
Male Non-Veterans	(1037)	33%	30%	29%	8%	χ^2=11.49
Male Veterans	(372)	57%	23%	14%	6%	p < .01
For Male Veterans Only						
65-69 years	(213)	100%	–	–	–	χ^2: Inappro-
70-74 years	(86)	–	100%	–	–	priate
75-84 years	(50)	–	–	100%	–	
85+ years	(23)	–	–	–	100%	
Not Limited in Functional Health	(244)	63%	23%	12%	2%	χ^2=29.35
Limited in Functional Health	(127)	46%	22%	17%	15%	p < .001
Independent in ADL	(332)	59%	24%	13%	4%	χ^2=22.30
Dependent in ADL	(40)	45%	15%	18%	22%	p < .001
Users of VA Health Facilities	(80)	64%	21%	9%	6%	χ^2=2.41
Non-users of VA Health Facilities	(291)	56%	24%	14%	6%	p:NS

Table 7
LIVING ARRANGEMENTS

	(n)	Alone	With Spouse Only	With Spouse and/or Children Only	Other Arrangements	Statistical Significance
Male Non-Veterans	(1037)	20%	55%	15%	10%	$X^2=12.47$
Male Veterans	(372)	25%	46%	15%	14%	$p < .01$
For Male Veterans Only						
65-69 years	(213)	21%	47%	17%	15%	
70-74 years	(86)	25%	48%	13%	14%	$X^2=11.77$
75-84 years	(50)	42%	38%	6%	14%	p:NS
85+ years	(23)	26%	44%	17%	13%	
Not Limited in Functional Health	(244)	23%	47%	16%	14%	$X^2=2.03$
Limited in Functional Health	(127)	28%	43%	13%	16%	p:NS
Independent in ADL	(332)	24%	46%	15%	15%	$X^2=2.95$
Dependent in ADL	(40)	35%	45%	10%	10%	p:NS
Users of VA Health Facilities	(80)	20%	48%	17%	15%	$X^2=1.64$
Non-users of VA Health Facilities	(292)	27%	45%	14%	14%	p:NS

Table 8
MARITAL STATUS

	(n)	Never Married	Currently Married	Separated/ Divorced	Widowed	Statistical Significance
Male Non-Veterans	(1037)	7%	71%	5%	17%	X^2=31.87 p < .001
Male Veterans	(372)	15%	63%	7%	15%	
For Male Veterans Only						
65-69 years	(213)	13%	69%	9%	9%	X^2=36.69 p < .001
70-74 years	(86)	19%	64%	3%	14%	
75-84 years	(50)	20%	44%	4%	32%	
85+ years	(23)	13%	52%	0%	35%	
Not Limited in Functional Health	(244)	14%	66%	7%	13%	X^2=1.55
Limited in Functional Health	(127)	17%	59%	6%	18%	p:NS
Independent in ADL	(332)	16%	64%	6%	10%	X^2=2.29 p:NS
Dependent in ADL	(40)	8%	60%	10%	22%	
Users of VA Health Facilities	(80)	20%	61%	9%	10%	X^2=3.22
Non-users of VA Health Facilities	(291)	14%	64%	6%	16%	p:NS

Table 9
LIVING CHILDREN

	(n)	0	1	2	3	4 or more	Statistical Significance
Male Non-Veterans	(1033)	16%	14%	25%	18%	27%	X²=26.89
Male Veterans	(358)	28%	14%	22%	17%	19%	p < .001
For Male Veterans Only							
65-69 years	(212)	24%	14%	25%	20%	17%	X²=14.05
70-74 years	(34)	38%	15%	17%	13%	17%	p:NS
75-84 years	(49)	31%	16%	23%	10%	20%	
85+ years	(23)	22%	13%	17%	13%	35%	
Not Limited in Functional Health	(241)	29%	15%	24%	16%	16%	X²=4.68
Limited in Functional Health	(126)	27%	13%	18%	18%	24%	p:NS
Independent in ADL	(328)	30%	14%	23%	16%	17%	X²=9.79
Dependent in ADL	(40)	12%	15%	18%	22%	33%	p < .05
Users of VA Health Facilities	(30)	38%	10%	20%	16%	16%	X²=5.20
Non-users of VA Health Facilities	(237)	25%	16%	23%	17%	19%	p:NS

Table 10
FORMAL EDUCATION

	(n)	Seven Years or Less	Completed Elementary School	Some High School	Completed High School	Beyond High School	Statistical Significance
Male Non-Veterans	(968)	37%	19%	22%	15%	7%	$X^2=58.61$
Male Veterans	(364)	20%	17%	22%	30%	11%	$p < .001$
For Male Veterans Only							
65–69 years	(211)	14%	14%	23%	36%	13%	
70–74 years	(86)	15%	30%	20%	23%	12%	$X^2=61.66$
75–84 years	(49)	35%	12%	24%	27%	2%	$p < .001$
85+ years	(18)	74%	5%	11%	5%	5%	
Not Limited in Functional Health	(241)	14%	16%	25%	32%	13%	$X^2=18.19$
Limited in Functional Health	(122)	31%	19%	17%	26%	7%	$p < .01$
Independent in ADL	(327)	18%	17%	23%	30%	12%	$X^2=8.91$
Dependent in ADL	(37)	35%	16%	14%	32%	3%	p:NS
Users of VA Health Facilities	(79)	21%	18%	24%	29%	8%	$X^2=1.48$
Non-users of VA Health Facilities	(285)	19%	17%	21%	31%	12%	p:NS

Table 11
SELF-REPORTED INCOME OF RESPONDENT (AND SPOUSE)

	(n)	Less than $5,000	$5,000–6,999	$7,000–9,999	$10,000–14,999	$15,000 or More	Statistical Significance
Male Non-Veterans	(906)	18%	25%	33%	17%	8%	X^2=32.68
Male Veterans	(330)	9%	23%	29%	24%	15%	p < .001
For Male Veterans Only							
65–69 years	(189)	5%	21%	28%	25%	20%	X^2=18.56
70–74 years	(76)	9%	22%	34%	24%	11%	p:NS
75–84 years	(46)	17%	26%	26%	22%	9%	
85+ years	(19)	21%	37%	26%	11%	5%	
Not Limited in Functional Health	(221)	5%	18%	29%	27%	21%	X^2=35.28
Limited in Functional Health	(108)	17%	32%	30%	17%	4%	p < .001
Independent in ADL	(294)	9%	21%	28%	25%	17%	X^2=14.75
Dependent in ADL	(36)	14%	42%	30%	14%	0%	p < .01
Users of VA Health Facilities	(67)	13%	24%	32%	22%	9%	X^2=3.86
Non-users of VA Health Facilities	(263)	8%	23%	28%	24%	17%	p:NS

Table 12
INSURANCE COVERAGE

	(n)	With Medicare	Statistical Significance	With Medicaid	Statistical Significance	With VA Coverage	Statistical Significance
Male Non-Veterans	(1033)	92%	X^2=0.05 p:NS	22%	X^2=7.11 p < .01	--	X^2=Inappropriate
Male Veterans	(370)	92%		16%		2%	
For Male Veterans Only							
65-69 years	(212)	89%	X^2=4.99 p:NS	13%	X^2=3.55 p:NS	3%	X^2=12.54 p:NS
70-74 years	(86)	94%		19%		0%	
75-84 years	(49)	98%		23%		2%	
85+ years	(23)	91%		13%		4%	
Not Limited in Functional Health	(242)	93%	X^2=0.85 p:NS	14%	X^2=2.25 p:NS	2%	X^2=0.90 p:NS
Limited in Functional Health	(127)	90%		20%		3%	
Independent in ADL	(330)	91%	X^2=0.67 p:NS	15%	X^2=1.56 p:NS	2%	X^2=6.10 p < .05
Dependent in ADL	(40)	95%		22%		8%	
Users of VA Health Facilities	(79)	90%	X^2=0.39 p:NS	9%	X^2=3.38 p:NS	6%	X^2=8.10 p < .01
Non-users of VA Health Facilities	(290)	92%		17%		1%	

Table 13
SMOKING HISTORY

	(n)	Never Regular Smoker	Past Regular Smoker	Current Regular Smoker	Statistical Significance
Male Non-Veterans	(1037)	28%	47%	25%	X^2=0.17 p:NS
Male Veterans	(372)	27%	48%	25%	
For Male Veterans Only					
65-69 years	(213)	23%	46%	31%	X^2=21.83 p < .01
70-74 years	(86)	35%	43%	22%	
75-84 years	(50)	24%	62%	14%	
85+ years	(23)	48%	52%	0%	
Not Limited in Functional Health	(244)	28%	47%	25%	X^2=0.10
Limited in Functional Health	(127)	27%	49%	24%	p:NS
Independent in ADL	(332)	26%	48%	26%	X^2=3.45
Dependent in ADL	(40)	37%	48%	15%	p:NS
Users of VA Health Facilities	(80)	28%	50%	22%	X^2=0.38
Non-users of VA Health Facilities	(291)	27%	47%	26%	p:NS

293

Table 14

SELF-REPORTED ALCOHOL CONSUMPTION HISTORY

	(n)	Percent Having Had Beer within Month	Statistical Significance	Percent Having Had Wine within Month	Statistical Significance	Percent Having Had Liquor within Month	Statistical Significance	Percent Having Either Beer, Wine, Liquor within Month	Statistical Significance
Male Non-Veterans	(1037)	43%	$X^2=0.73$ p:NS	47%	$X^2=1.49$ p:NS	38%	$X^2=0.07$ p:NS	68%	$X^2=0.15$ p:NS
Male Veterans	(372)	47%		40%		40%		67%	
For Male Veterans Only									
65-69 years	(213)	53%	$X^2=1.32$ p:NS	39%	$X^2=1.86$ p:NS	46%	$X^2=1.63$ p:NS	72%	$X^2=2.27$ p:NS
70-74 years	(86)	47%		38%		33%		59%	
75-84 years	(50)	32%		46%		32%		66%	
85+ years	(23)	17%		35%		26%		57%	
Not Limited in Functional Health	(244)	54%	$X^2=4.01$ p < .05	43%	$X^2=1.19$ p:NS	49%	$X^2=30.00$ p < .001	75%	$X^2=4.78$ p < .05
Limited in Functional Health	(127)	32%		32%		22%		52%	
Independent in ADL	(332)	49%	$X^2=1.86$ p:NS	41%	$X^2=1.04$ p:NS	42%	$X^2=8.33$ p < .01	70%	$X^2=5.18$ p < .05
Dependent in ADL	(40)	28%		28%		20%		48%	
Users of VA Health Facilities	(80)	41%	$X^2=2.47$ p:NS	36%	$X^2=0.65$ p:NS	36%	$X^2=0.65$ p:NS	64%	$X^2=7.48$ p < .01
Non-users of VA Health Facilities	(291)	48%		41%		41%		69%	

Table 15
SELF-REPORTED MEDICAL HISTORY

	(n)	With Past Angina	Statistical Significance	With Past Heart Attack	Statistical Significance	With Past Stroke	Statistical Significance
Male Non-Veterans	(1034)	6%	$X^2=1.27$ p:NS	14%	$X^2=0.02$ p:NS	6%	$X^2=0.01$ p:NS
Male Veterans	(372)	8%		13%		6%	
For Male Veterans Only							
65-69 years	(213)	7%	$X^2=2.57$ p:NS	14%	$X^2=0.34$ p:NS	5%	$X^2=2.35$ p:NS
70-74 years	(86)	7%		12%		7%	
75-84 years	(50)	9%		14%		10%	
85+ years	(23)	15%		13%		4%	
Not Limited in Functional Health	(244)	5%	$X^2=7.90$ $p < .01$	9%	$X^2=12.16$ $p < .001$	5%	$X^2=2.58$ p:NS
Limited in Functional Health	(127)	14%		22%		9%	
Independent in ADL	(332)	7%	$X^2=2.02$ p:NS	13%	$X^2=0.64$ p:NS	5%	$X^2=6.65$ $p < .01$
Dependent in ADL	(40)	14%		18%		15%	
Users of VA Health Facilities	(80)	9%	$X^2=0.14$ p:NS	16%	$X^2=0.67$ p:NS	6%	$X^2=0.02$ p:NS
Non-users of VA Health Facilities	(291)	8%		13%		6%	

Table 15 (Cont.)
SELF-REPORTED MEDICAL HISTORY

	(n)	With Past Cancer	Statistical Significance	With Past Hip Fracture	Statistical Significance	With Past Diabetes	Statistical Significance
Male Non-Veterans	(1034)	9%	X^2=4.31	4%	X^2=2.68	15%	X^2=4.07
Male Veterans	(372)	13%	p < .05	2%	p:NS	19%	p < .05
For Male Veterans Only							
65-69 years	(213)	15%	X^2=3.29	2%	X^2=5.16	19%	X^2=1.04
70-74 years	(86)	7%	p:NS	1%	p:NS	20%	p:NS
75-84 years	(50)	14%		2%		16%	
85+ years	(23)	13%		9%		26%	
Not Limited in Functional Health	(244)	13%	X^2=0.13	1%	X^2=6.04	14%	X^2=11.68
Limited in Functional Health	(127)	12%	p:NS	5%	p < .05	29%	p < .001
Independent in ADL	(332)	13%	X^2=0.00	2%	X^2=1.73	18%	X^2=3.25
Dependent in ADL	(40)	12%	p:NS	5%	p:NS	30%	p:NS
Users of VA Health Facilities	(80)	11%	X^2=0.18	2%	X^2=0.06	22%	X^2=0.62
Non-users of VA Health Facilities	(291)	13%	p:NS	2%	p:NS	19%	p:NS

Table 16
SELF-PERCEIVED HEALTH STATUS

	(n)	Excellent	Good	Fair	Poor	Statistical Significance
Male Non-Veterans	(1026)	18%	44%	29%	9%	X^2=1.53
Male Veterans	(371)	20%	47%	29%	4%	p < .01
For Male Veterans Only						
65-69 years	(212)	20%	49%	27%	4%	X^2=4.92
70-74 years	(86)	23%	44%	29%	4%	p:NS
75-84 years	(50)	22%	40%	36%	2%	
85+ years	(23)	9%	52%	35%	4%	
Not Limited in Functional Health	(244)	25%	53%	21%	1/2%	X^2=50.33
Limited in Functional Health	(126)	10%	36%	44%	10%	p < .001
Independent in ADL	(331)	21%	50%	27%	2%	X^2=34.94
Dependent in ADL	(40)	10%	28%	45%	17%	p < .001
Users of VA Health Facilities	(79)	18%	41%	35%	6%	X^2=4.84
Non-users of VA Health Facilities	(291)	21%	49%	27%	3%	p:NS

Table 17
EMOTIONAL HEALTH STATUS

	Of Ten Items, Number Answered Suggesting Depression					
	(n)	None	One	Two	Three-Five	Six-Ten	Statistical Significance
Male Non-Veterans	(937)	36%	21%	16%	17%	10%	X^2=11.66
Male Veterans	(333)	44%	23%	14%	13%	6%	p:NS
For Male Veterans Only							
65-69 years	(200)	46%	20%	14%	16%	4%	X^2=35.91
70-74 years	(82)	46%	26%	13%	10%	5%	p:NS
75-84 years	(38)	39%	24%	13%	11%	13%	
85+ years	(13)	15%	39%	23%	15%	8%	
Not Limited in Functional Health	(229)	54%	21%	12%	9%	4%	X^2=41.61
Limited in Functional Health	(103)	22%	26%	18%	23%	11%	p < .001
Independent in ADL	(305)	47%	23%	13%	12%	5%	X^2=27.07
Dependent in ADL	(28)	18%	18%	18%	28%	18%	p < .01
Users of VA Health Facilities	(70)	27%	24%	21%	19%	9%	X^2=19.64
Non-users of VA Health Facilities	(263)	49%	22%	12%	12%	5%	p < .05

Table 18
DEPENDENCY IN INDIVIDUAL ACTIVITIES OF DAILY LIVING AREAS DURING PREVIOUS YEAR

Dependent on Person or Equipment or Unable Sometime during Previous Year

	(n)	Personal Grooming	Statistical Significance	Walking Across Small Room	Statistical Significance	Bathing	Statistical Significance
Male Non-Veterans	(1037)	3%	$X^2=8.03$ $p < .01$	9%	$X^2=0.82$ $p:NS$	12%	$X^2=19.40$ $p < .001$
Male Veterans	(372)	1/2%		7%		4%	
For Male Veterans Only							
65-69 years	(213)	0%	$X^2=15.22$ $p < .01$	5%	$X^2=23.23$ $p < .001$	2%	$X^2=13.00$ $p < .01$
70-74 years	(86)	0%		3%		3%	
75-84 years	(50)	0%		12%		4%	
85+ years	(23)	4%		30%		17%	
Not Limited in Functional Health	(244)	0%	$X^2=1.93$ $p:NS$	1%	$X^2=36.52$ $p < .001$	0%	$X^2=27.95$ $p < .001$
Limited in Functional Health	(127)	1%		18%		11%	
Independent in ADL	(332)	0%	$X^2=8.32$ $p < .01$	0%	$X^2=241.64$ $p < .001$	0%	$X^2=120.74$ $p < .001$
Dependent in ADL	(40)	2%		68%		35%	
Users of VA Health Facilities	(80)	0%	$X^2=0.28$ $p:NS$	10%	$X^2=1.12$ $p:NS$	6%	$X^2=1.72$ $p:NS$
Non-users of VA Health Facilities	(291)	1/2%		7%		3%	

Table 18 (Cont.)
DEPENDENCY IN INDIVIDUAL ACTIVITIES OF DAILY LIVING AREAS DURING PREVIOUS YEAR

	(n)	Dressing	Statistical Significance	Transferring	Statistical Significance	Eating	Statistical Significance
		Dependent on Person or Equipment or Unable Sometime during Previous Year					
Male Non-Veterans	(1037)	8%	$X^2=9.09$ p < .01	5%	$X^2=1.92$ p:NS	3%	$X^2=1.96$ p:NS
Male Veterans	(372)	4%		3%		1%	
For Male Veterans Only							
65-69 years	(213)	5%	$X^2=9.54$ p < .05	2%	$X^2=5.24$ p:NS	1/2%	$X^2=10.79$ p < .05
70-74 years	(86)	1%		2%		1%	
75-84 years	(50)	0%		6%		2%	
85+ years	(23)	13%		9%		9%	
Not Limited in Functional Health	(244)	1/2%	$X^2=22.21$ p < .001	1/2%	$X^2=16.18$ p < .001	0%	$X^2=9.74$ p < .01
Limited in Functional Health	(127)	10%		8%		4%	
Independent in ADL	(332)	0%	$X^2=120.74$ p < .001	0%	$X^2=94.08$ p < .001	0%	$X^2=42.06$ p < .001
Dependent in ADL	(40)	35%		28%		12%	
Users of VA Health Facilities	(80)	5%	$X^2=0.42$ p:NS	2%	$X^2=0.08$ p:NS	4%	$X^2=4.43$ p < .05
Non-users of VA Health Facilities	(291)	3%		3%		1%	

300

Table 18 (Cont.)
DEPENDENCY IN INDIVIDUAL ACTIVITIES OF DAILY LIVING AREAS DURING PREVIOUS YEAR

		Dependent on Person or Equipment or Unable Sometime during Previous Year	
	(n)	Using Toilet	Statistical Significance
Male Non-Veterans	(1037)	3%	$X^2=1.89$
Male Veterans	(372)	2%	p:NS
For Male Veterans Only			
65-69 years	(213)	1%	$X^2=8.26$
70-74 years	(86)	1%	$p < .05$
75-84 years	(50)	4%	
85+ years	(23)	9%	
Not Limited in Functional Health	(244)	1/2%	$X^2=8.40$
Limited in Functional Health	(127)	5%	$p < .01$
Independent in ADL	(332)	0%	$X^2=59.21$
Dependent in ADL	(40)	18%	$p < .001$
Users of VA Health Facilities	(80)	5%	$X^2=5.34$
Non-users of VA Health Facilities	(291)	1%	$p < .05$

301

Table 19

DEPENDENCY IN INDIVIDUAL ACTIVITIES OF DAILY LIVING AREAS AT TIME OF INTERVIEW

Dependent on Person or Equipment or Unable at Time of Interview

	(n)	Personal Grooming	Statistical Significance	Walking Across Small Room	Statistical Significance	Bathing	Statistical Significance
Male Non-Veterans	(1037)	3%	$X^2=8.03$	7%	$X^2=1.83$	11%	$X^2=16.31$
Male Veterans	(372)	1/2%	$p < .01$	5%	$p:NS$	4%	$p < .001$
For Male Veterans Only							
65-69 years	(213)	0%		3%		2%	
70-74 years	(86)	0%	$X^2=15.22$	1%	$X^2=37.98$	3%	$X^2=13.00$
75-84 years	(50)	0%	$p < .01$	10%	$p < .001$	4%	$p < .01$
85+ years	(23)	4%		30%		17%	
Not Limited in Functional Health	(244)	0%	$X^2=1.93$	1/2%	$X^2=32.56$	0%	$X^2=27.95$
Limited in Functional Health	(127)	1%	$p:NS$	14%	$p < .001$	11%	$p < .001$
Independent in ADL	(332)	0%	$X^2=8.32$	0%	$X^2=166.19$	0%	$X^2=120.74$
Dependent in ADL	(40)	2%	$p < .01$	48%	$p < .001$	35%	$p < .001$
Users of VA Health Facilities	(80)	0%	$X^2=0.28$	8%	$X^2=1.19$	6%	$X^2=1.72$
Non-users of VA Health Facilities	(291)	1/2%	$p:NS$	4%	$p:NS$	3%	$p:NS$

Table 19 (Cont.)
DEPENDENCY IN INDIVIDUAL ACTIVITIES OF DAILY LIVING AREAS AT TIME OF INTERVIEW

Dependent on Person or Equipment or Unable at Time of Interview

	(n)	Dressing	Statistical Significance	Transferring	Statistical Significance	Eating	Statistical Significance
Male Non-Veterans	(1037)	7%	$X^2=9.35$ $p<.01$	4%	$X^2=2.21$ $p:NS$	3%	$X^2=1.96$ $p:NS$
Male Veterans	(372)	3%		2%		1%	
For Male Veterans Only							
65-69 years	(213)	3%		1%		1/2%	
70-74 years	(86)	1%	$X^2=10.73$ $p<.05$	2%	$X^2=6.99$ $p:NS$	1%	$X^2=10.79$ $p<.05$
75-84 years	(50)	0%		4%		2%	
85+ years	(23)	13%		9%		9%	
Not Limited in Functional Health	(244)	0%		0%		1/2%	
Limited in Functional Health	(127)	9%	$X^2=21.78$ $p<.001$	4%	$X^2=9.74$ $p<.01$	6%	$X^2=10.30$ $p<.01$
Independent in ADL	(332)	0%		0%		0%	
Dependent in ADL	(40)	28%	$X^2=94.08$ $p<.001$	20%	$X^2=67.86$ $p<.001$	12%	$X^2=42.06$ $p<.001$
Users of VA Health Facilities	(80)	5%		1%		4%	
Non-users of VA Health Facilities	(291)	2%	$X^2=1.47$ $p:NS$	2%	$X^2=0.40$ $p:NS$	1%	$X^2=4.43$ $p<.05$

303

Table 19 (Cont.)
DEPENDENCY INDIVIDUAL ACTIVITIES OF DAILY LIVING
AREAS AT TIME OF INTERVIEW

| | (n) | Dependent on Person or Equipment or Unable at Time of Interview | |
		Using Toilet	Statistical Significance
Male Non-Veterans	(1037)	3%	$X^2=2.98$
Male Veterans	(372)	1%	p:NS
For Male Veterans Only			
65-69 years	(213)	1%	$X^2=10.97$
70-74 years	(86)	0%	$p < .05$
75-84 years	(50)	2%	
85+ years	(23)	9%	
Not Limited in Functional Health	(244)	0%	$X^2=9.74$
Limited in Functional Health	(127)	4%	$p < .01$
Independent in ADL	(332)	0%	$X^2=42.06$
Dependent in ADL	(40)	12%	$p < .001$
Users of VA Health Facilities	(80)	4%	$X^2=4.43$
Non-users of VA Health Facilities	(291)	1%	$p < .05$

Table 20

MODIFIED ROSOW-BRESLAU FUNCTIONAL HEALTH SCALE

	(n)	Able to Do Heavy Housework	Statistical Significance	Able to Walk Up and Down Stairs	Statistical Significance
Male Non-Veterans	(1033)	60%	$X^2=10.14$ $p < .01$	90%	$X^2=3.01$ $p:NS$
Male Veterans	(372)	69%		93%	
For Male Veterans Only					
65-69 years	(213)	75%	$X^2=32.60$ $p < .001$	95%	$X^2=28.18$ $p < .001$
70-74 years	(86)	72%		95%	
75-84 years	(50)	66%		92%	
85+ years	(23)	17%		65%	
Not Limited in Functional Health	(244)	100%	$X^2=316.18$ $p < .001$	100%	$X^2=55.95$ $p < .001$
Limited in Functional Health	(127)	10%		79%	
Independent in ADL	(332)	75%	$X^2=46.30$ $p < .001$	97%	$X^2=82.70$ $p < .001$
Dependent in ADL	(40)	22%		58%	
Users of VA Health Facilities	(80)	66%	$X^2=0.44$ $p:NS$	86%	$X^2=6.33$ $p < .05$
Non-users of VA Health Facilities	(291)	70%		94%	

Table 20 (Cont.)
MODIFIED ROSOW-BRESLAU FUNCTIONAL HEALTH SCALE

	(n)	Able to Walk Half Mile	Statistical Significance	Able to Do All Three	Statistical Significance
Male Non-Veterans	(1033)	80%	X^2=5.89	57%	X^2=9.23
Male Veterans	(372)	86%	p <.05	66%	p <.01
For Male Veterans Only					
65-69 years	(213)	89%		72%	
70-74 years	(86)	85%	X^2=9.68	67%	X^2=29.35
75-84 years	(50)	86%	p <.05	58%	p <.001
85+ years	(23)	65%		17%	
Not Limited in Functional Health	(244)	100%	X^2=116.19	100%	X^2=Inappropriate
Limited in Functional Health	(127)	59%	p <.001	0%	
Independent in ADL	(332)	91%	X^2=73.09	72%	X^2=59.65
Dependent in ADL	(40)	41%	p <.001	10%	p <.001
Users of VA Health Facilities	(80)	79%	X^2=4.38	59%	X^2=2.17
Non-users of VA Health Facilities	(291)	88%	p <.05	68%	p:NS

Table 21

DIFFICULTIES WITH COMMON TASKS

Percent with at Least a Little Difficulty with Common Tasks

	(n.)	Stooping, Crouching, Kneeling	Statistical Significance	Lifting Weights 10+ lbs.	Statistical Significance	Moving Large Objects	Statistical Significance
Male Non-Veterans	(1001)	38%	$X^2=4.18$ $p < .05$	35%	$X^2=7.58$ $p < .01$	35%	$X^2=3.67$ $p{:}NS$
Male Veterans	(355)	32%		27%		30%	
For Male Veterans Only							
65-69 years	(208)	31%	$X^2=.55$ $p{:}NS$	25%	$X^2=8.68$ $p < .05$	28%	$X^2=3.03$ $p{:}NS$
70-74 years	(84)	30%		24%		30%	
75-84 years	(45)	38%		31%		29%	
85+ years	(18)	41%		56%		47%	
Not Limited in Functional Health	(238)	18%	$X^2=57.25$ $p < .001$	10%	$X^2=98.67$ $p < .001$	15%	$X^2=72.40$ $p < .001$
Limited in Functional Health	(116)	59%		60%		59%	
Independent in ADL	(321)	28%	$X^2=29.26$ $p < .001$	22%	$X^2=36.14$ $p < .001$	25%	$X^2=39.20$ $p < .001$
Dependent in ADL	(34)	74%		71%		76%	
Users of VA Health Facilities	(80)	34%	$X^2=0.10$ $p{:}NS$	33%	$X^2=2.00$ $p{:}NS$	36%	$X^2=1.79$ $p{:}NS$
Non-users of VA Health Facilities	(291)	32%		25%		28%	

Table 21 (Cont.)
DIFFICULTIES WITH COMMON TASKS

	(n)	Extending Arms above Shoulders	Statistical Significance	Handling Small Objects	Statistical Significance	No Difficulty with Any of 5 Areas	Statistical Significance
		Percent with at Least a Little Difficulty with Common Tasks					
Male Non-Veterans	(1001)	14%	$X^2=2.74$	13%	$X^2=4.36$	44%	$X^2=6.21$
Male Veterans	(355)	11%	p:NS	9%	p < .05	52%	p < .05
For Male Veterans Only							
65-69 years	(208)	12%	$X^2=1.60$	6%	$X^2=7.08$	54%	$X^2=2.21$
70-74 years	(84)	7%	p:NS	12%	p:NS	51%	p:NS
75-84 years	(45)	13%		16%		49%	
85+ years	(18)	11%		17%		37%	
Not Limited in Functional Health	(238)	4%	$X^2=34.53$	4%	$X^2=20.96$	31%	$X^2=84.35$
Limited in Functional Health	(116)	24%	p < .001	19%	p < .001	83%	p < .001
Independent in ADL	(321)	7%	$X^2=43.92$	6%	$X^2=31.53$	56%	$X^2=27.66$
Dependent in ADL	(34)	44%	p < .001	35%	p < .001	9%	p < .001
Users of VA Health Facilities	(80)	18%	$X^2=5.49$	14%	$X^2=3.29$	47%	$X^2=0.72$
Non-users of VA Health Facilities	(291)	9%	p < .05	8%	p:NS	53%	p:NS

Table 22
RECREATIONAL PHYSICAL ACTIVITY

	(n)	Zero Times per Week	Once per Week	Two or More Times per Week	Statistical Significance
Male Non-Veterans	(1035)	84%	3%	13%	$X^2=12.77$
Male Veterans	(372)	76%	4%	20%	$p < .01$
For Male Veterans Only					
65-69 years	(213)	72%	5%	23%	$X^2=7.78$
70-74 years	(86)	83%	2%	15%	p:NS
75-84 years	(50)	78%	2%	20%	
85+ years	(23)	91%	0%	9%	
Not Limited in Functional Health	(244)	71%	4%	25%	$X^2=11.50$
Limited in Functional Health	(127)	87%	1%	12%	$p < .01$
Independent in ADL	(332)	75%	4%	21%	$X^2=4.96$
Dependent in ADL	(40)	90%	0%	10%	p:NS
Users of VA Health Facilities	(80)	78%	0%	22%	$X^2=3.86$
Non-users of VA Health Facilities	(291)	76%	4%	20%	p:NS

Table 23
COGNITIVE FUNCTION

	(n)	Able to Repeat 5 Numbers	Statistical Significance	Errors in Immediate Memory 0	1-2	3-6	Statistical Significance
Male Non-Veterans	(1002)	83%	$X^2=10.54$ $p < .01$	11%	45%	44%	$X^2=16.13$ $p < .001$
Male Veterans	(358)	90%		18%	47%	35%	
For Male Veterans Only							
65-69 years	(210)	92%	$X^2=8.46$ $p < .05$	22%	51%	27%	$X^2=33.70$ $p < .001$
70-74 years	(84)	90%		13%	54%	33%	
75-84 years	(45)	84%		9%	36%	55%	
85+ years	(19)	74%		11%	11%	78%	
Not Limited in Functional Health	(238)	92%	$X^2=2.68$ p:NS	20%	50%	30%	$X^2=6.89$ $p < .05$
Limited in Functional Health	(119)	87%		13%	43%	44%	
Independent in ADL	(321)	92%	$X^2=9.29$ $p < .01$	19%	47%	34%	$X^2=3.04$ p:NS
Dependent in ADL	(37)	76%		8%	49%	43%	
Users of VA Health Facilities	(79)	92%	$X^2=0.68$ p:NS	14%	51%	35%	$X^2=1.15$ p:NS
Non-users of VA Health Facilities	(279)	89%		19%	46%	35%	

Table 23 (Cont.)
COGNITIVE FUNCTION

	(n)	Errors in Delayed Memory			Statistical Significance
		Not Asked or 0	1-2	3-6	
Male Non-Veterans	(1002)	41%	19%	40%	$X^2=3.18$
Male Veterans	(358)	47%	19%	34%	p:NS
For Male Veterans Only					
65-69 years	(210)	51%	23%	26%	$X^2=14.31$
70-74 years	(84)	50%	17%	33%	
75-84 years	(45)	30%	12%	58%	p < .01
85+ years	(19)	35%	9%	56%	
Not Limited in Functional Health	(238)	50%	20%	30%	$X^2=2.24$
Limited in Functional Health	(119)	41%	17%	42%	p:NS
Independent in ADL	(321)	48%	19%	33%	$X^2=1.70$
Dependent in ADL	(37)	37%	15%	48%	p:NS
Users of VA Health Facilities	(80)	46%	20%	34%	$X^2=0.06$
Non-users of VA Health Facilities	(291)	46%	19%	35%	p:NS

Table 24
REGULAR SOURCE OF MEDICAL CARE

	(n)	Have Regular Source of Medical Care	Statistical Significance
Male Non-Veterans	(1036)	87%	$X^2=0.48$
Male Veterans	(371)	85%	p:NS
For Male Veterans Only			
65-69 years	(213)	84%	$X^2=2.75$
70-74 years	(86)	87%	p:NS
75-84 years	(49)	86%	
85+ years	(23)	96%	
Not Limited in Functional Health	(243)	81%	$X^2=12.24$
Limited in Functional Health	(127)	94%	p < .001
Independent in ADL	(331)	85%	$X^2=1.79$
Dependent in ADL	(40)	92%	p:NS
Users of VA Health Facilities	(80)	95%	$X^2=7.54$
Non-users of VA Health Facilities	(290)	83%	p < .01

Table 25

HOSPITAL ADMISSIONS DURING PREVIOUS YEAR

	(n)	None	One	Two	Three or More	Statistical Significance
Male Non-Veterans	(1022)	78%	14%	5%	3%	X^2=2.53
Male Veterans	(366)	77%	17%	4%	2%	p:NS
For Male Veterans Only						
65-69 years	(210)	79%	14%	5%	2%	X^2=9.52
70-74 years	(85)	79%	18%	2%	1%	p:NS
75-84 years	(49)	67%	25%	8%	0%	
85+ years	(22)	77%	23%	0%	0%	
Not Limited in Functional Health	(240)	84%	12%	3%	1%	X^2=17.50
Limited in Functional Health	(125)	65%	25%	7%	3%	p < .001
Independent in ADL	(327)	81%	14%	4%	1%	X^2=16.10
Dependent in ADL	(39)	54%	36%	5%	5%	p < .01
Users of VA Health Facilities	(78)	65%	24%	8%	3%	X^2=8.27
Non-users of VA Health Facilities	(287)	81%	15%	3%	1%	p < .05

Table 26
NURSING HOME HISTORY

	(n)	At Least Once during Lifetime	Statistical Significance	At Least Once during Previous Year	Statistical Significance
Male Non-Veterans	(1037)	1%	$X^2=0.57$ p:NS	1/2%	$X^2=1.40$ p:NS
Male Veterans	(372)	1%		0%	
For Male Veterans Only					
65-69 years	(213)	1/2%	$X^2=13.84$ p $<$ .01	0%	$X^2=$Inappropriate
70-74 years	(86)	1%		0%	
75-84 years	(50)	0%		0%	
85+ years	(23)	9%		0%	
Not Limited in Functional Health	(244)	1/2%	$X^2=2.98$ p:NS	0%	$X^2=$Inappropriate
Limited in Functional Health	(127)	2%		0%	
Independent in ADL	(332)	1%	$X^2=6.49$ p $<$ .05	0%	$X^2=$Inappropriate
Dependent in ADL	(40)	5%		0%	
Users of VA Health Facilities	(80)	1%	$X^2=0.03$ p:NS	0%	$X^2=$Inappropriate
Non-users of VA Health Facilities	(291)	1%		0%	

Table 27

LAST DENTAL VISIT

	(n)	Less than 6 Months	6 Months to 3 Years	3 Years to 5 Years	More than 5 Years	Never	Statistical Significance
Male Non-Veterans	(1020)	22%	25%	10%	41%	2%	X^2=20.22
Male Veterans	(366)	27%	33%	6%	33%	1%	p < .01
For Male Veterans Only							
65-69 years	(210)	30%	36%	9%	24%	1%	X^2=38.64
70-74 years	(85)	25%	28%	5%	42%	0%	p < .001
75-84 years	(48)	21%	31%	0%	48%	0%	
85+ years	(23)	17%	22%	0%	52%	9%	
Not Limited in Functional Health	(240)	29%	33%	6%	31%	1/2%	X^2=4.98
Limited in Functional Health	(125)	23%	31%	7%	37%	2%	p:NS
Independent in ADL	(327)	29%	33%	6%	31%	1%	X^2=9.33
Dependent in ADL	(39)	13%	30%	3%	51%	3%	p:NS
Users of VA Health Facilities	(79)	29%	34%	8%	28%	1%	X^2=5.07
Non-users of VA Health Facilities	(287)	26%	32%	6%	35%	1%	p:NS

Table 28
COMMUNITY SOCIAL SERVICE USE

	(n)	Percent Using Health Services in Past Year Such as Visiting Nurses, Public Health Nurse, Home Health Aid, or Medical Home Care	Statistical Significance	Percent Using Social Services in Past Year Such as Congregate Home Meals, or Homemaker	Statistical Significance
Male Non-Veterans	(1029)	9%	$X^2=0.69$	13%	$X^2=1.52$
Male Veterans	(369)	8%	p:NS	10%	p:NS
For Male Veterans Only					
65-69 years	(212)	5%		5%	
70-74 years	(86)	8%	$X^2=11.46$	8%	$X^2=35.48$
75-84 years	(48)	13%	$p < .01$	29%	$p < .001$
85+ years	(23)	23%		30%	
Not Limited in Functional Health	(242)	3%	$X^2=18.73$	5%	$X^2=22.13$
Limited in Functional Health	(126)	16%	$p < .001$	21%	$p < .001$
Independent in ADL	(329)	4%	$X^2=49.48$	8%	$X^2=10.56$
Dependent in ADL	(40)	36%	$p < .001$	25%	$p < .01$
Users of VA Health Facilities	(78)	5%	$X^2=0.88$	6%	$X^2=1.52$
Non-users of VA Health Facilities	(290)	8%	p:NS	11%	p:NS

Table 28 (Cont.)
COMMUNITY SOCIAL SERVICE USE

	(n)	Percent Using Transportation Services in Past Year Such as Senior Shuttle, MBTA Discount Passes, or MBTA Rides	Statistical Significance
Male Non-Veterans	(1030)	66%	X²=0.54
Male Veterans	(370)	68%	p:NS
For Male Veterans Only			
65-69 years	(212)	67%	X²=8.82
70-74 years	(86)	71%	p < .05
75-84 years	(49)	78%	
85+ years	(23)	43%	
Not Limited in Functional Health	(243)	72%	X²=5.22
Limited in Functional Health	(126)	60%	p < .05
Independent in ADL	(330)	69%	X²=2.20
Dependent in ADL	(40)	53%	p:NS
Users of VA Health Facilities	(79)	70%	X²=0.16
Non-users of VA Health Facilities	(290)	67%	p:NS

317

Table 29

YEAR VA FACILITY LAST USED

		1982	1981	1980	1979	1978	Statistical Significance
Male Non-Veterans	(1037)	---	---	---	---	---	X^2=Inappropriate
Male Veterans	(71)	70%	17%	9%	1%	3%	
For Male Veterans Only							
65-69 years	(47)	69%	19%	6%	2%	4%	X^2=7.12
70-74 years	(13)	77%	15%	8%	0%	0%	p:NS
75-84 years	(7)	57%	14%	29%	0%	0%	
85+ years	(4)	100%	0%	0%	0%	0%	
Not Limited in Functional Health	(44)	70%	20%	5%	0%	5%	X^2=5.81
Limited in Functional Health	(27)	70%	11%	15%	4%	0%	p:NS
Independent in ADL	(58)	74%	17%	5%	0%	4%	X^2=9.58
Dependent in ADL	(13)	54%	15%	23%	8%	0%	p < .05
Users of VA Health Facilities	(71)	71%	17%	8%	1%	3%	X^2=Inappropriate
Non-users of VA Health Facilities	(291)	---	---	---	---	---	

Table 30
VA FACILITY MOST RECENTLY USED

	(n)	Boston VAMC (Jamaica Plain)	West Roxbury VAMC	Court Street Clinic	Bedford VAMC	Other	Statistical Significance
Male Non-Veterans	(1037)	---	---	---	---	---	X^2=Inappropriate
Male Veterans	(82)	36%	6%	50%	1%	7%	
For Male Veterans Only							
65-69 years	(53)	40%	4%	47%	2%	7%	X^2=15.82
70-74 years	(17)	29%	12%	59%	0%	0%	p:NS
75-84 years	(7)	43%	0%	57%	0%	0%	
85+ years	(5)	0%	20%	40%	0%	40%	
Not Limited in Functional Health	(48)	33%	2%	55%	2%	8%	X^2=4.47
Limited in Functional Health	(34)	38%	12%	44%	0%	6%	p:NS
Independent in ADL	(68)	31%	6%	56%	1%	6%	X^2=6.38
Dependent in ADL	(14)	57%	7%	22%	0%	14%	p:NS
Users of VA Health Facilities	(80)	36%	6%	50%	1%	7%	X^2=Inappropriate
Non-users of VA Health Facilities	(291)	---	---	---	---	---	

REFERENCES

Freeman, H.E., Richardson, A.H., Cummins, J.F. and Schnaper, H.W. "Use of Medical Resources by Spancos: I. Extent and Sources of Medical Care in a Very Old Population." American Journal of Public Health, 56(9), pp. 1530-1539, 1966.

Page, W.F. "Why Veterans Choose Veterans Administration Hospitalization: A Multivariate Model." Medical Care, XX(3), pp. 308-320, 1982.

Richardson, A.H., Freeman, H.E., Cummins, J.F. and Schnaper, H.W. "Use of Medical Resources by Spancos: II. Social Factors in Medical Care Experience." Milbank Memorial Fund Quarterly, 45 (1), pp. 61-75, 1967.

Rosow, I. and Breslau, N. "A Guttman Health Scale for the Aged." Journal of Gerontology, 21, pp. 556-559, 1966.

Schneider, K.C. and Dove, H. "High Users of VA Emergency Room Facilities: Are Outpatients Abusing this System or Is the System Abusing Them?" Inquiry, 20, p. 5764, 1983.

Seiling, V. and Page, W.F. "Health Characteristics of Veterans and Non-Veterans: Health Interview Surveys, 1971-1974." Controller Monograph, No. 11, Veterans Administration, Washington, D.C., April, 1980.

U.S. Veterans Administration. The Aging Veteran, Present and Future Medical Needs. Washington, D.C., October, 1977.

U.S. Veterans Administration. Health Characteristics of Veterans and Non-Veterans: Health Interview Surveys, 1975-1978. Controller Monograph, Washington, D.C., October, 1982.

U.S. Veterans Administration. Health Care of the Aging Veteran: A Report of the Geriatrics and Gerontology Advisory Committee. Washington, D.C., April, 1983.

10. Utilization of the VA by Elder Veterans: An Empirical Analysis

Mark Schlesinger
Ann Moran, Dr.P.H.
Linda Zangwill, M.S.

Introduction

The Veterans Administration is actively developing plans for sharing and coordination with the non-VA health system for care of elder veterans. The extent and success of these arrangements are affected by factors beyond formal affiliations between the two systems. Veterans move between VA and non-VA health care systems in response to a series of decisions. Some of these are made by the veteran, others by physicians or other providers of care. Plans for sharing and coordination must reflect an understanding of the factors which influence these decisions.

The choices which channel veterans between VA and non-VA systems can be outlined schematically as in Figure 1. The initial decision to seek care is made by the older veteran and reflects a variety of considerations, including the cost of non-VA care, perceptions of the quality of care in both systems, and awareness of the options for care under VA and non-VA auspices. Once under care, placement of patients is influenced to a much greater degree by the decisions and perceptions of providers. Decisions to transfer veterans between VA and non-VA systems or place them in community settings are affected by the availability of services in each system, the veteran's

321

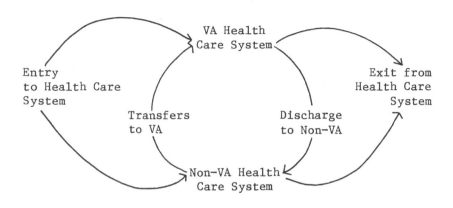

Figure 1

health care needs and the provider's perceptions of the veteran's ability to prosper in a non-institutional environment.

This chapter contains an empirical analysis of the factors affecting these decisions. This analysis is divided into two parts: 1) the factors which lead older veterans to seek care under VA auspices are examined, and 2) the impact of the changing availability of non-VA health care resources on the care of elder veterans within the VA is explored. In each case, decisions affecting care of veterans will be shown to reflect a number of factors external to the VA, factors which are often altered by changes in public policy involving health and social programs. Future planning by the VA and policy-making by other government bodies must reflect these interactions.

I. Characteristics of Veterans and Use of the VA Health Care System

There has been relatively little analysis of the determinants of utilization of VA health care facilities. Page (1982) studied a small set of factors believed to be determinants of hospital utilization. He examined the relationship between the probability of hospitalization in the VA and age, entitlement, income and insurance coverage. He concluded that the probability of hospitalization under

VA auspices was increased by service-connected disability (SCD) status, low income and lack of insurance. Age was found to have little effect on hospitalization.

Functional status in VA nursing homes was studied by Geoghegan (1982). Married residents were found on average to have a lower level of function than unmarried residents, controlling for age and diagnostic group. This was taken to indicate a selection process in which less impaired, unmarried elders are institutionalized because there is no spouse to provide care at home.

These studies have provided important insights into the utilization of the VA health care system. However, they do leave a number of questions unanswered. It is not apparent, given the unique health seeking behavior of the elderly, that the factors which influence the utilization of VA facilities among younger veterans also apply to elders. Each study, moreover, covers only certain determinants of utilization. For example, the influence of income, insurance and entitlement on hospitalization has been studied, but not the influence of these factors on placement in a nursing home. Marital status seems to affect the use of extended care in the VA, but its influence on hospitalization is unstudied. No examination has been made of outpatient utilization by the elderly, although this is the fastest growing component of the VA health care system (VA, Annual Report 1982).

A. Factors Affecting VA Utilization

To analyze the decision by elder veterans to use VA facilities, it is important to identify those factors which affect health care utilization by the elderly in general. The literature on health care utilization by the elderly suggests that five sets of factors influence utilization decisions. These are:

1. Socioeconomic Factors. Economic well-being seems to have a limited direct impact on the health utilization of the elderly, but may be a determinant of access to certain health services, such as ambulatory care (Link, et al., 1982) and nursing home care (McCoy and Edwards, 1981).

2. Demographic Factors. Demographic factors influence health care utilization among the elderly in a variety of ways. As noted earlier, health seeking behavior is influenced in part by age itself. Family relationships

323

and living arrangements determine the availability of informal social support. A social support network can directly influence health status and may act as a substitute for formal health care services (Atchley, 1972; Katz and Akpom, 1976). Education often facilitates maneuvers through the complex health care system, while minority status may erect barriers to access (Wan, 1982). Location of residence also has an influence. An urban location may facilitate access -- health care utilization by the elderly appears to be particularly sensitive to the amount of travel required to the site of care (Wan and Odell, 1981; Stoller, 1982).

3. <u>Availability of Health Services</u>. A larger capacity among VA-operated facilities increases the opportunities for access, particularly among veterans without service-connected disabilities. Studies suggest, however, that the VA is often the last choice of the veteran. Hence, the availability of other sources of care can strongly influence utilization within the VA.

4. <u>Health Status</u>. Health care utilization by the elderly has been linked to their perceived health status (Stoller, 1982; Coulton and Frost, 1982). Health status may have a particularly pronounced influence on use of VA facilities. Studies have shown that the VA system disproportionately serves veterans in very poor health (Horgan, et al., 1983). This may result from conscious efforts of administrators in the VA to serve particularly disabled veterans or may reflect the inability of disabled veterans to obtain adequate quality care elsewhere (Demkovich, 1980).

5. <u>Perceptions of Quality and Availability of Care</u>. Studies have documented that perceptions among the elderly may have an important effect on utilization, independent of the objective quality and availability of care (Stoller, 1982).

The analysis of utilization presented here draws on data from the 1979 Survey of Veterans (Hammond, 1980). Variables constructed from this survey cover four of the five areas identified above; the survey contained little useful information on health status. The specific variables included in the utilization regressions are listed in Table 1.

Type of Variable	Type of Regression	
	Decisions Made by Veterans	Admission/Discharge Decisions Made by Providers
SOCIOECONOMIC	Income Employment	Income Unemployment Rates
DEMOGRAPHIC	Age Education Marital Status Race Population Density # of Dependents	Age Marital Status Race Population Density

VA SYSTEM CHARACTERISTICS	Eligibility
	VA as Regular
	  Source of Care
		Eligibility
		Medical School
		  Affiliation
		Hospital Beds/Veteran
		Outpatient Visits/
		  Veteran
		Nursing Home Beds/
		  Veteran

NON-VA SYSTEM CHARACTERISTICS	Insurance
	Non-VA Regular
	  Source of Care
		Hospital Beds/Capita
		Nursing Home Beds/
		  Capita
		% Private Nursing
		  Home Beds
		Physicians/Capita
		Nurse Practitioners/
		  Capita
		Hospice Units/Elder
		Measures of Unmet
		  Need: Services Un-
		  available, Payment
		  Unavailable

PERCEPTIONS BY VETERAN	Quality of Care
	Awareness of
	  Benefits
	Perception of
	  Access
		Attitude of Providers

HEALTH STATUS		Length of Stay Diagnosis Level of Care

Table 1
VARIABLES IN UTILIZATION
AND ADMISSION/DISCHARGE REGRESSIONS

B. The Analysis of Utilization

The analysis presented here expands the scope of past studies in two ways. First, it controls for a broader set of independent variables than has past research. Second, it focuses on three separate types of utilization: (1) hospitalization in VA facilities, (2) use of VA outpatient clinics, and (3) use of VA physicians as a "regular source of care." Understanding each type of utilization is important for comprehending the interaction of VA and non-VA health care systems. Hospitalization is the single most expensive aspect of care; outpatient care is the fastest growing. The choice of a regular source of care can shape other types of utilization and reflects to some extent the degree of dependence of the veteran on services provided by the VA.

These three aspects of utilization are measured in the following manner. The propensity to use VA hospitals is measured by the proportion of all hospitalizations of veterans that occurred in the past year which were in facilities under VA auspices. Outpatient utilization is measured in the same fashion (visits to non-VA physicians which have been authorized by the VA on a fee-basis are treated as care under VA auspices). For both types of care, regressions relate the proportion of care occurring under VA auspices to the explanatory variables defined in the last sections. The decision to use the VA as a regular source of care is quantified as a binary variable.[1] In this case, regression coefficients measure the impact of a change in an explanatory variable on the probability of using the VA as a regular source of care.[2]

1. Data

The 1979 Survey of Veterans (Hammond, 1980) collected information on health care utilization of veterans, 1121 of whom were over the age of 65. Unfortunately, hospitalization, even among the elderly, is a sufficiently scarce event that a sample of this size is not sufficiently large for reliable estimates of the coefficients in a regression model. For this reason, hospital utilization regressions have estimated the utilization data of all veterans aged 45 and over, a sample of over 6500 veterans. The regressions on outpatient utilization and regular source of care are estimated on data from veterans over the age of 65. Results using data from veterans 45+ are also presented for ready comparison with the estimates for hospital utilization.[3]

326

2. Results – The Determinants of Utilization of the VA by Elders

The estimated relationships between utilization and characteristics of the veteran are presented in Table 2. The findings are reviewed by category of explanatory variable. For ease of presentation, only the estimated signs of relationships are included in this table. Complete regression results are included in Appendix II A–C. The regression coefficients represent the change in dependent variable for a given change in the independent variable, controlling for the other factors included as explanatory variables.[4]

(a) Socioeconomic Factors. The use of VA hospitals and the selection of the VA as a regular source of care is greatest for elderly veterans with below average incomes. These findings match those by Page (1982). Interestingly, however, this does not apply to the utilization of outpatient services. Older veterans in the middle income ranges seem to use a higher proportion of VA outpatient services than those with higher or lower incomes. These findings are only suggestive, however, since for only one of the six coefficients on income was the difference statistically significant at a 5% confidence level.

If the elder veteran is employed, he is less likely to seek care under VA auspices. This may be due to several factors. First, employment may be an indicator of functional status. Second, insurance provided to employees is often subsidized by employers, so that it is likely that the insured veterans who are employed have more extensive coverage than those who are not. Third, those who are employed may view their time as more valuable than do the unemployed or retired. If veterans perceive that using the VA is costly in terms of their time, they would seek other sources of care (Thompson, 1981).

(b) Demographic Factors. For all three types of utilization, the more educated the veteran, controlling for level of income, the lower the use of VA services. This may reflect an inability of less educated elders to negotiate the complexities of the non-VA health care system. Veterans who are white, located in urban settings and who are older also appear to turn to providers other than the VA for hospitalization and regular sources of care. All these factors may well be related to access considerations. Black veterans may live in neighborhoods underserved by non-VA physicians forcing them to turn to the VA (Wan, 1982). Urban settings

Table 2

RELATIONSHIP BETWEEN EXPLANATORY VARIABLE AND PROPORTION OF CARE UNDER VA AUSPICES

Explanatory Variables	Hospitalization	Outpatient Visits		Utilization of the VA as a Regular Source of Care	
	Aged 45+	Aged 45+	Aged 65+	Aged 45+	Aged 65+
Socioeconomic					
Income below poverty line	+ *	–	– *	+ *	+
Near poor (150% of poverty line)	+	+	–	+ *	+
High income ($25,000)	–	–	–	– *	–
Employment	– *	– *	–	– *	–
Demographic					
Education (years)	–	–	–	– *	– *
Married	+	– *	–	– *	–
Never married	+ *	+	+	– *	–
Dependents (no.)	–	+	+	– *	–
Caucasian	–	–	+	– *	– *
Urban setting	–	+	+	– *	– *
Age (years)	–	– *	NA	–	NA
VA System Characteristics					
Service-connected disability	+ *	+ *	+ *	+ *	+ *
Regular source of care	+ *	+ *	+ *	– *	– *

Non-VA System Characteristics

Medicare coverage	– *	– *	– *	– *	– *
Medicare plus private insurance	+ *	+	+	+	+
Private hospital insurance	–	–	– *	– *	–
Medicaid coverage	–	– *	–	– *	+
Other insurance	– *	– *	– *	– *	– *
M.D. as regular source of care	– *	– *	–	NA	NA
Clinic as regular source of care	– *	– *	–	NA	NA
Admission did not give choice to veteran	– *	NA	NA	NA	NA

Perceptions of Veteran

VA cares about veterans	–	–	–	– *	–
VA provides high quality care	–	+ *	–	+ *	+ *
Aware of hospital benefits	+ *	+ *	+ *	+ *	+ *
Problems with access	– *	+ *	– *	– *	– *

* Statistically significant at a 5% confidence level

329

often provide more choice among non-VA providers and, therefore, more alternatives to using the VA. Older veterans may be particularly sensitive to the need to travel and thus less inclined to use VA facilities which are inconvenient for them to reach.[5]

It is generally expected that greater informal support, in the form of a spouse or family member, reduces the need for formal health care (Pihlbland and Adams, 1972). Whether this makes the veteran more or less likely to seek professional care within the VA, however, is unclear. The coefficients on the variables representing marital status and number of dependents are not consistent on this issue. Veterans who have been divorced, widowed or separated are more likely to view the VA as a regular source of care, as are elder veterans who have few dependents. Curiously, though, veterans who have never been married are no more likely to view the VA as a regular source of care than are those who are married. This suggests that it may be discontinuity of social support more than isolation which stimulates the identification of the VA as a regular source of care.

The complexity of the relationship between social support and VA utilization is further illustrated by the regression analysis of hospitalizations and outpatient visits. Married veterans receive a smaller proportion of their outpatient care from the VA, but a greater fraction of hospital services. Veterans who never married are more likely to be hospitalized in VA facilities than are veterans who are either married, widowed, divorced or separated.

This reversal of relationships between inpatient and outpatient care is puzzling. It may reflect different attitudes held by veterans toward the two types of services or may reflect subtle differences in the interaction of social support and help seeking behavior.

(c) Health System Characteristics. The variables in this group have the predicted impact on utilization of the VA. As expected, veterans with service-connected disabilities were more likely to use VA inpatient and outpatient facilities. Insurance generally reduces the use of VA facilities. This suggests that if alternative sources of care can be obtained at reasonably low cost, VA utilization will decrease. The sole exception is for veterans who supplement Medicare with private insurance -- so-called Medigap policies. One explanation of the positive sign on this coefficient is that a selection process is occurring. Veterans who have below average health may be more inclined to purchase Medigap policies to supplement Medicare and may also be more likely to use the VA to fill in the "gaps" in both Medicare and Medigap coverages.[6]

The choice of a regular source of care has a significant influence on outpatient and inpatient utilization. Physicians who are not employed by the VA tend not to recommend patients for hospitalization within the VA system. Patterns of hospitalization are therefore indirectly determined by choices made by veterans when initially seeking care.

(d) Perceptions Held by Elder Veterans. Perceptions of the VA do appear to be systematically related to utilization. The direction of causality, however, is unclear. Utilization is clearly higher among those who are aware of benefits; however, using the VA may in itself have produced that awareness. The sign of the coefficient on the access variable varies from one model to the other. For both hospitalization and selection of a regular source of care, reported problems of access are associated with less use of the VA. For outpatient care, however, the reverse is true.

To interpret this relationship correctly it is important to consider how this variable was constructed. Veterans were asked to select the issue which represented the most serious obstacle to their use of the VA. The findings presented above suggest that those who are most concerned with access -- as opposed to, say, quality of care -- tend to use VA hospitals less, but that outpatient utilization is more sensitive to perceptions of quality of care or related issues. The greater sensitivity of hospital care to perceptions of access may be related to the more complete coverage provided by Medicare for inpatient as opposed to outpatient services; that is, given the opportunity to seek care elsewhere, the veteran becomes more sensitive to the travel costs of seeking care within the VA. Insurance may therefore reduce use of VA facilities in two ways: by increasing access to alternative sources of care and by increasing sensitivity to the costs of time of obtaining care from the VA.[7]

C. Conclusion – Characteristics of Veterans and Utilization of the VA

Overall it is apparent that characteristics of elder veterans do alter the propensity to use the VA as a source of health care. Particularly important for planning purposes are the influence on utilization of insurance coverage, the average income of the elder veteran, the use of non-VA regular sources of care and the awareness of VA benefits.

The regression models estimated in this section of the chapter suggest that the availability of Medicare and Medicaid alter the behavior of elder veterans in several ways: by increasing access to alternative sources of care, by increasing veterans' sensitivity to the costs of access to VA facilities and by causing veterans to seek care from the VA for those services not covered due to "gaps" in these public-financed insurance programs. As the extent of eligibility or coverage under Medicare and Medicaid changes in response to political ideologies or limited government budgets, a variety of effects may be felt within the VA health care system.

The socioeconomic status of the veteran was shown to exert an influence on use of the VA independent of the effects of insurance coverage. As the income of elder veterans rises or falls in response to changes in private pensions or the Social Security system, the number and type of veterans seeking care from the VA will also change. For elder veterans, the effect of changing income is apparently very different on the utilization of outpatient and inpatient services.

Finally, it is apparent that lack of information may play an important role in limiting the number of veterans who seek care from the VA. The 1979 Survey of Veterans (Hammond, 1980) revealed that roughly 20% of elder veterans were not aware that the VA offered inpatient care and over 60% were not aware of the availability of outpatient services. Increasing awareness could obviously significantly increase the demands for care under VA auspices. Equally important, the difference in awareness of inpatient and outpatient care may well hinder the delivery of high quality care and increase costs. To the extent that elder veterans, unaware of VA-provided outpatient services, fail to seek care elsewhere, a variety of illnesses and disabilities may go undiagnosed and untreated until the veteran believes that he is in need of hospitalization. Treatment at that point may often be less effective and more costly than earlier intervention.

II. The Interaction of VA and Non-VA Services

There have been few studies of the interaction between the VA and general health care sectors. Generally these fall into two categories: analyses of the veteran's choice of care setting and studies of the extent to which admissions to and lengths of stay in VA facilities are affected by the availability of non-VA providers.

The earliest study of choice of care setting was produced by the Congressional Budget Office in the course of evaluating the prospects for national health insurance. The results of this analysis indicate that if access to non-VA facilities is increased by the passage of national health insurance, utilization within the VA would decrease 20-40% (Congressional Budget Office, 1976). A more recent study, based on data collected by the VA, revealed that veterans with insurance and higher income -- those most likely to have access to non-VA care -- were substantially less likely to be hospitalized within the VA system (Page, 1982). A third analysis used data from the 1977 National Medical Care Expenditure Survey. It found that veterans who were either uninsured or in poor health were substantially more likely to use VA facilities than was the average veteran (Horgan, et al., 1982).

Two studies have examined the link between non-VA health services and utilization of VA facilities. Seitz (1981a and 1982) demonstrated that a substantial number of admissions to the VA system come from other health care institutions. Moran (1980) examined the relationship between length of stay in VA psychiatric hospitals and the purchase of outpatient services from community based providers. VA hospitals that more extensively purchased services from non-VA professionals had significantly shorter average lengths of stay, suggesting that these purchased services substituted for care which otherwise would have been provided directly by the VA.

This literature provides some glimpse of the ways in which VA and non-VA health care systems interact. Many important questions, however, are left unanswered. There has been no systematic analysis focusing specifically on the elderly veteran, for whom the potential for interaction would seem to be the greatest. No study has identified which types of non-VA facilities have the largest impact on the VA system or estimated the magnitude of this influence. With an aging veteran population, the answers to these questions are important for directing public policy dealing with both the VA and non-VA health care systems.

A. A Model of the Interaction of VA and Non-VA Health Care Systems

The availability of non-VA health care services can be expected to have a direct impact on the delivery of care within the VA. The direction of the effect depends on whether the non-VA service acts to channel veterans into the VA, to draw potential users away, or to facilitate or impede discharges from VA facilities. Scarce non-VA services and manpower, for example, may make it more difficult for discharge planners within the VA to appropriately place veterans in community settings. Formal contracting between the VA and non-VA providers may also be affected. With limited alternatives for care outside the VA, veterans can also be expected to turn in increasing numbers to the VA. The combination of increased admissions and reduced options for discharge will lead to greater numbers of inappropriately placed veterans in VA facilities.

The regression models presented in this chapter analyze each of these three interaction effects: admissions from non-VA settings, utilization of care within the VA and discharges to community settings. Using data from the VA's Annual One-Day Census, four measures are employed to examine the effect of non-VA health care resources on VA services. These are summarized schematically in Figure 2 and described below.

Changing Patterns of Admission. Admissions to VA facilities come from three sources: referrals within the VA system, transfers from non-VA facilities and decisions by veterans to seek care from the VA. Previous studies have analyzed the utilization decisions of veterans (Page, 1982; Horgan, et al., 1983). This study examines the effects of changing the supply of non-VA services on admissions from non-VA sources. Past research indicates that 60% of the veterans admitted to VA hospitals and 30% of the veterans admitted to nursing homes under VA auspices are transferred or referred from non-VA sources (VA, 1983).

Figure 2

A SCHEMATIC PRESENTATION OF MEASURES OF VA/NON-VA INTERACTION

Patient Flows

Admission from
Non-VA Settings

Care Provided
Auspices of VA

Discharge to Community
Non-VA Provider

Measured in Terms of:

Probability Veteran
Admitted from Non-
VA Facility

Match between Needs
of Patient and Care
Provided in VA

Probability
Discharge Blocked
by Lack of Services

Probability Patient
or Family Resists
Discharge

335

Altered Utilization within the VA. Supply limitations
in the non-VA sector may be reflected in longer lengths of
stay in VA facilities and in greater numbers of inappropriately placed patients in VA facilities. The magnitude
of this influence will depend on the extent of discretion
in treatment -- and thus on the diagnosis -- and on the
type of services required for care. Past research has
identified comparatively longer lengths of stay as a principle source of excess costs within the VA system, making
this a particularly important variable for purposes of
policy (National Academy of Sciences, 1977; Lindsay,
1976). Unfortunately, sample sizes for particular diagnostic groups in the one-day census were not sufficiently
large to reliably estimate the effects of non-VA resources.

Constrained availability of non-VA services reduces
the options for discharges and increases the likelihood
that veterans will remain hospitalized when they would be
more appropriately placed in a nursing home or other setting. In this analysis, the extent of mismatch between
needs and services is measured by determining whether the
current treatment facility matched the "most appropriate
setting for care" identified by VA providers in the annual
census.[8] By this criteria, 47.6% of elder veterans in
VA hospitals are "mismatched" to services, 10.6% in VA
domiciliaries and 13.9% in VA nursing homes.

Changing Opportunities for Discharge. Barriers to
discharge are measured in this study in two ways: (1) reports by providers that a patient "could have been discharged" if appropriate services were available and (2)
reports of patient or family resistance to discharge. According to the VA's 1981 annual census, 29.8% of the veterans over the age of 65 in VA hospitals could have been
discharged if needed services were available. 25.6% of
the elder veterans in domiciliaries and 27.7% of those in
nursing homes reportedly could have been discharged if
services were available. Insufficient services may also
influence the willingness of families to care for elder
veterans at home, further decreasing the opportunities for
appropriate placement.

The influence of non-VA resources on the VA health
care system is measured here using four different dependent variables: (1) tranfers from non-VA facilities, (2)
reports of "mismatched" services, (3) reports of inappropriately delayed discharges from VA institutions, and (4)
reports of resistance to discharge. Separate regressions

are estimated for hospitals and extended care (nursing home and domiciliary) facilities.[9] The independent variables used in these eight regressions are described in more detail below.

Availability of Non-VA Health Care. Using data contained in the Area Resource File maintained by the National Technical Information Service and data available from the VA's one-day census, the availability of non-VA health resources is described in terms of seven services which measure the capacity of the local community to supply health care to the elderly. These are: short term hospital beds, long term hospital beds, nursing home beds, physicians involved in direct patient care, geriatric nurse practitioners, hospice units in hospitals and home support services.[10]

The "community" surrounding a VA medical center (VAMC) is defined as the Primary Service Area (PSA) calculated by the VA. Each PSA is constructed by aggregating counties from which the majority of veterans using a particular medical center originate. Community resources, for all services except social services, will be measured by the per capita supply in the counties making up the PSA. The availability of social services will be estimated from information contained in the VA's annual one-day census. A full description of variables is included in Appendix I.

As indicated above, the expected effect of increasing or decreasing a specific community service depends on the way in which that service influences admissions to and discharges from VA facilities. The seven services included in this study have been grouped into three categories based on predictions of their effects on these patient flows. These groupings are presented in Figure 3. The predicted impact of these three groups of services on the four dependent variables defined above is presented in Figure 4.

A greater availability of Chronic Care (CC) is expected to decrease transfers to VA facilities and increase the ease with which elder veterans can be discharged to the community. The combination of these two effects reduces the demand for beds within the VA, thus reducing the amount of misplacement created by excess demand for one form of service or another.

<table>
<tr><td colspan="3">===</td></tr>
<tr><td colspan="3" align="center">Figure 3
CATEGORIZING COMMUNITY SERVICES
BY THEIR EFFECT ON PATIENT FLOWS</td></tr>
</table>

Effect of Greater Availability of Community Resources on:

Admissions	Discharges	
	Positive	No Effect
Services that Reduce Admissions to the VA	Chronic Care Long Term Beds Nursing Home Beds	Acute Care Physicians Short Term Hospital Beds
Services that Increase Admissions to the VA	Home Support Services Social Services Hospice Units Nurse Practitioners	

===

Figure 4
PREDICTED EFFECTS OF INCREASED COMMUNITY SERVICES
ON THE VA

Type of Service	Impact On:		
	Admissions	Discharges	Misplacement
Chronic Care	Negative	Positive	Negative
Acute Care	Negative	None	Negative
Home Support Services	Ambiguous [Positive?]	Positive	Ambiguous

===

Acute Care (AC) services, represented by short term hospital beds and physicians, are predicted to act as substitutes for VA inpatient care and outpatient clinics. Increasing the availability of these services will not necessarily facilitate discharges following care in VA facilities, but may draw away potential patients from the VA system. Again, because this would reduce the demand for beds, there should be a consequent reduction in misplacement produced when there is an inadequate supply of appropriate services.

Increased availability of Home Support Services (HSS) can be expected to facilitate discharges from the VA and to facilitate placement in community settings for elder patients. These services affect admissions in two ways. On one hand, the availability of support services may allow the impaired or ill elder veteran to maintain his community-dwelling arrangements. This would reduce admissions to the VA. On the other hand, home support services have been shown to act as "case-finders," identifying patients with previously unmet needs and routing them into the formal health care system (Stasson and Holakan, 1981). It is impossible to predict, a priori, which of these effects will prove more significant. Studies of the delivery of various types of home care in other settings, however, suggest that case-finding may significantly increase the amount of care sought in the VA (General Accounting Office, 1982). It therefore seems likely that these home support services would increase admissions to the VA. The predicted effect on misplacement is ambiguous. By facilitating discharge, HSS should reduce misplacement. If, however, these services produce significant increases in admissions to the VA, the resulting pressure to place veterans in VA facilities may induce additional misplacement.

B. Controlling for Other Factors

Two additional sets of factors may influence health care utilization within the VA system: characteristics of VA-operated facilities in the geographic area and characteristics of the elder veterans seeking care. To identify the effects of the availability of community health care resources it is necessary to control for these other influences.

In this study, the facilities in an area operating under VA auspices are characterized by four variables. The first three are measures of capacity:

    (1) The number of VA hospital beds per veteran in the PSA;

(2) The number of beds in VA nursing homes and domiciliaries, including the number of beds in nursing homes operated by states for the use of veterans and beds supplied by private facilities to the VA on a contract basis; and

(3) The number of visits to the outpatient clinic at the VAMC.

A dummy variable is also included to represent the affiliation of the VAMC with a medical school. Such affiliations may affect the flow of patients between the VA and facilities in the community. They may also lead to increases in the quality of care (Thompson, 1981), which may reduce the amount of misplacement or lead to more expeditious discharges from VA facilities.

Patients are characterized in this study by a variety of variables including: extent of VA eligibility, socioeconomic status, demographic attributes and health status. Eligibility is measured by the veteran's service-connected disability status. Demographic variables include the veteran's age, marital status and race. An additional variable records whether the veteran's county of residence was primarily urban or rural. Average income and unemployment rates in the county of residence were used as proxy variables because socioeconomic data for the individual veteran were not available. Health status is characterized by primary diagnosis (grouped into broad categories), length of stay in the institution, and the level of care that providers report that the veteran required at the time of the annual census. A more complete description of these variables is included in Appendix I.

C. Regression Specification and Source of Data

Eight regressions are estimated to relate the availability of non-VA health care resources to a number of measures of performance within the VA system. This statistical analysis is based on data from the 1981 Annual One-Day Census conducted by the VA and the 1980 Area Resource File (ARF). The one-day census is based on medical records and information collected from providers of care. The census consists of a 20% sample of all inpatients in VA hospitals and domiciliaries (including those operated by state governments for use of veterans) and a 100% sample of all patients in nursing homes under VA auspices. The 1981 census tallied roughly 13,000 hospital patients,

7,000 residents of nursing homes and 1,800 veterans residing in domiciliaries. Approximately one-half of the hospital patients and four-fifths of the residents of extended care facilities were over the age of 65. The actual number of observations varies with the regression, since there was a varying amount of non-response to specific questions in the census.

The ARF data-base consolidates information from a number of sources on a county-by-county basis. As mentioned above, county-specific data were used to estimate socioeconomic and some demographic characteristics of the elder veterans. Counties were aggregated into roughly 140 PSAs to establish the boundaries of the area served by each VAMC. These aggregates were then used to calculate the availability of community based health care resources.

Many of the dependent variables (e.g., mismatch of services, failure to appropriately discharge) are dichotomous. Regression coefficients estimated by ordinary least squares (OLS), while unbiased, tend to have inflated standard errors. Re-estimating equations using either LOGIT or PROBIT techniques produced only minimal reductions in the estimated standard errors and did not change calculations of statistical significance. OLS estimates are therefore presented here as these allow calculation of the fraction of variance explained by the regression.

D. Results

The eight sets of regression coefficients relating the availability of non-VA health care resources to care delivered within the VA are presented in Appendix II D-G. To simplify these tables, the explanatory variables are presented in mnemonic form. The mnemonics are defined in Table 3.

The discussion of results is divided into several sections. The first three examine the impact of characteristics of veterans on the interactions between VA and non-VA health care systems. The fourth examines the effects of characteristics of VA facilities. The final section examines the impact of the availability of non-VA health care resources.

341

Table 3
DEFINITION OF MNEMONIC VARIABLES
FOR ADMISSION/DISCHARGE REGRESSIONS

Mnemonic	Definition
AGE	Age of veteran in years
MARRIED	Veteran is married
SPSABSNT	Spouse Absent: Divorced/Separated/Widowed ("Never Married" is standard of comparison)
CAUCASIAN	Veteran is Caucasian (all other races aggregated for comparison)
METRO	Veteran lives in county in metropolitan area
NEARMETRO	Veteran lives in county contiguous to metropolitan area (rural areas are the standard of comparison)
INCOME	Mean income of county of veteran's residence
UNEMPLOYMENT	Percent unemployed in county of veteran's residence
LOSDAYS	Length of stay in days in VA facility
DXCHEM	Primary diagnosis is alcohol- or drug-related disorder
DXPSYCH	Primary diagnosis involves psychiatric disorder
LEVEL OF CARE	Appropriate level of care for veteran
LOCPSY	Appropriate care involves psychiatric treatment
NHSTAT	Veteran is in VA nursing home
HOSTAT	Veteran is in VA hospital (domiciliaries are the standard of comparison)
STBEDS/C	Non-VA short term hospital beds per capita in PSA
LTBEDS/E	Non-VA long term hospital beds per elder in PSA
NHBEDS/E	Non-VA nursing home beds per elder in PSA
NHPCTPRIV	Percent private nursing home beds in PSA
MD/C	Physicians active in patient care per capita in PSA
HSPC/E	Hospital based hospices per elder in PSA
NPGER/E	Nurse practitioners (geriatric specialty) per elder in PSA
UNMETSER	Veteran unable to obtain needed outpatient services
UNMETPAY	Veteran unable to pay for needed outpatient services
VAAFF	VAMC in PSA affiliated with medical school
VABED/V	VA-operated hospital beds per veteran in PSA
VANURS/V	VA-operated nursing home beds and beds in state homes for veterans per veteran in PSA
VAOUT/V	Visits to VA-operated outpatient clinics per veteran in PSA

1. Demographic Factors

In the regression models estimated here, marital status appears to be a determinant of admissions and discharges within the VA system. Married elder veterans who are divorced, separated or widowed are more likely to be "misplaced" for care than are married elder veterans. These findings fit widely-held beliefs that informal support networks lead to more appropriate matching of elders' needs to the setting for care. Some implications of marital status, however, are more surprising. Efforts to discharge older married veterans are _more_ likely to lead to resistance by the patient or family. The very fact that the patient is married may raise fears of burdening others, and this in turn may inhibit appropriate placements. If this is the case, the results presented here underscore the fact that informal social supports cannot be taken for granted. In the absence of needed formal services, spouses who could potentially provide care may lack the personal, economic or social resources to carry the full burden of necessary care.

2. Socioeconomic Factors

It is often argued that the VA primarily serves veterans who lack resources to seek care elsewhere. It is, therefore, not surprising that the regressions presented here indicate that in counties with below-average income and above-average unemployment, an increased proportion of elder veterans seek care from the VA. One surprising finding is that in areas with higher income, it appears that there is _more_ likely to be resistance to discharge by either patients or their families. This suggests that one cannot assume that greater financial resources make families more willing or able to care for elders at home. Although more money may indeed facilitate purchasing formal support services, families in areas with above-average income may have less access to various types of informal support. Families with above average incomes may be those in which husband and wife both work, limiting the amount of time available to care for an older spouse or parent. In addition, families with lower incomes may qualify for a variety of non-VA, means-tested support services, for which other families would not qualify.

343

3. Health Status

The ability of the VA health care system to match settings to needs and the probability that a veteran can be expeditiously discharged are linked to the type of illness besetting the patient. This is reflected in the very broad diagnostic categories included in the regressions here. Elder veterans with a primary psychiatric diagnosis were more likely to be misplaced than were patients with somatic disorders. Veterans with alcohol and drug addictions are more likely than other patients to be misplaced in nursing homes and have a higher probability of being transferred to the VA from a non-VA provider.

Movement of patients among settings also appears to be related to the level of care required. Elder veterans requiring less intensive care are more likely to be mismatched to a setting for care and are more often associated with resistance to discharge. This finding suggests that as the number of elder veterans who are more likely to have chronic problems than their younger counterparts increases, the problems created by mismatch of services will grow. Thus, the need to develop service to reduce resistance to discharge from VA facilities will grow in importance.

4. Characteristics of the VA System

The availability of beds in VA facilities appears to significantly affect the extent of misplacement and the probability that a patient will be expeditiously discharged. In some cases, adding capacity to VA facilities apparently produces some undesirable by-products. Additional nursing home beds, for example, increase the number of misplaced veterans in nursing home facilities, perhaps reflecting the incentives facing VA administrators to ensure that their facilities operate near full capacity.

The effect of other characteristics of the VA system was less predictable. It appears, for instance, the relationship between structure and performance in the VA system is often quite complex. Expeditious discharges from VA hospitals, for example, were affected by the capacity of VA nursing homes and vice versa. A second unexpected finding was that while affiliations with medical schools did not appear to significantly alter the delivery of care in VA hospitals, it did alter care in VA nursing homes. Extended care facilities associated with "affiliated" VAMCs displayed lower levels of misplacement and more expeditious discharge of patients.

5. Interactions with Community Services

As hypothesized, the availability of health care resources in the community significantly affects care delivered within the VA health care system. In general, the greater the availability of community based services, the more expeditiously patients are discharged from VA facilities and the less misplacement there is in VA-operated institutions.

It was also hypothesized that different types of community services would affect the VA health care system in different ways. In particular, community based services were divided here into three groups, each thought to produce a different combination of effects on VA facilities.

A number of the hypothesized effects were borne out in the regressions (see Table 4). As predicted, the availability of home support services apparently increases casefinding and channeling of additional patients to the VA. In contrast, chronic institutional care and acute care, at least to some extent, draw patients away from the VA. The exact nature of this interaction depends on the specific type of non-VA facility in question. For example, increased numbers of community nursing home beds per elder are associated with fewer admissions to VA nursing homes but greater numbers of admissions to VA hospitals. Similarly, the increased availability of long term care beds in community hospitals is associated with reduced numbers of veterans admitted to VA hospitals but increased admissions to VA nursing homes. Some sort of substitution is clearly occurring between the two types of VA facilities.

Also as predicted, acute care resources have an ambiguous impact on discharges from VA-operated facilities. This contrasted sharply with the effect of both chronic institutional care and home support services; for these two groups, greater availability of community services facilitated discharge from the VA.

Some of the findings involving VA and non-VA interactions are unexpected. This is most clearly reflected in the regression estimates of the impact of increasing the supply of physicians in an area. In regions with high physician-to-population ratios, the results indicate that

Table 4
RELATIONSHIP BETWEEN ADDED COMMUNITY RESOURCES AND IMPACT ON THE VA

Type of Community Service	Type of Interaction			
	Admissions	Resistance	Discharge	Misplacement
Acute Care				
Predicted	**Reduced**	**No effect**	**No effect**	**Reduced**
Short Term Hospital Beds	Increased	Reduced # Increased *	No effect	Reduced
Physicians	Reduced #*	Increased # Reduced *	Reduced # Increased *	Increased #*
Chronic Care				
Predicted	**Reduced**	**Reduced**	**Increased**	**Reduced**
Nursing Homes	Increased # Reduced *	Reduced #	No effect	Reduced #*
Long Term Hospital Beds	Reduced # Increased *	Reduced *	Increased *	Reduced *

346

Home Support Services

Predicted	Increased(?)	Reduced	Increased	Ambiguous
Home Services	Increased #	Reduced #*	Increased #*	Reduced *
Hospice Unit	Increased *	Reduced #*	Increased *	Reduced *
Nurse Practitioners	Increased #*	Reduced # Increased *	No effect	Reduced *

Notes: (1) When two findings are reported for a variable, the top finding represents the relationship for VA hospitals, the bottom for VA extended care facilities. When only one finding is shown the signs on the coefficients were the same for both types of VA facilities.

(2) # = Finding for VA hospitals statistically significant at 5% confidence level.

* = Finding for VA extended care facilities significant at 5% confidence level.

there are greater resistance and more barriers to discharge than in other areas. Similarly, VA facilities located in areas with many physicians evidence greater misplacement than those in regions with fewer physicians. The cause of this relationship is difficult to determine. One might speculate that in areas in which physicians are abundant, the community health care system tends to have an acute care orientation. Given available data, there is no way of testing this hypothesis. It is apparent that more research is required to understand this evidently complex interaction between VA and non-VA health care providers.

E. Conclusion - The Interaction of VA and Non-VA Services

The regression results described above suggest that there are extensive and complex interactions between services within the VA and the non-VA health care systems. Many of these results are predictable; others are surprising. These findings illustrate two general conclusions. First, while non-VA resources affect the delivery of care within the VA, this influence is greater for certain types of resources and particular kinds of care than for others. Second, although past discussions have described the relationship between VA and non-VA systems almost entirely in terms of one substituting for the other, this analysis indicates that non-VA providers can act as either substitutes or complements for care within the VA system. In the former case they reduce the need for services within the VA, in the latter case they can lead to increased demand for care.

These findings also provide a better understanding of the extent of the interactions between VA and non-VA systems and the spill-over effects that are likely to be produced by changing policies. Future federal policies directed at both the VA and non-VA health care systems must reflect these interactions.

FOOTNOTES

1. The variable is set equal to one if the veteran has designated the VA as a regular source of care, otherwise it is zero.

2. In the outpatient and hospitalization regressions, the dependent variable is a proportion. The models will therefore be estimated using a PROBIT regression technique. The probability of choosing the VA as a regular source of care will be analyzed in a LOGIT regression model. For a discussion of the rationale behind the use of these techniques, see Neter and Wasserman (1974).

3. We recognize that the number of observations, even for the sample aged 45+, is small relative to the number of variables used in the regressions. The coefficients estimated here may therefore not be stable. To test the robustness of our findings, we re-estimated the regressions using a smaller set of independent variables. In general, only small changes in the coefficients were observed under these re-specifications.

4. When the independent variable is categorical, all but one of the categories are presented in the table. The omitted variable serves as the standard of comparison. For marital status, for instance, the separated/divorced/widowed category is omitted. The results in the hospitalization regression indicate that both married and never-married veterans have a greater proportion of hospitalization in VA facilities than do those who are separated, divorced or widowed.

5. Outpatient care represents an exception to this pattern. Access may be a less important determinant of the choice of VA facilities for this type of care.

6. Medicare, for instance, provides only very limited coverage for outpatient mental health care.

7. The prediction that hospitalization and choice of regular source of care are more sensitive to considerations of access matches the findings on demographic characteristics which may be related to access.

8. In the 1981 Annual One-Day Census providers were requested to identify the most appropriate setting for
care for all patients. If this response did not match
the type of facility in which the patient currently
resided, there was considered to be a "mismatch" of
services and needs. This may overstate the true level
of misplacement since undoubtedly some patients who
were labeled as inappropriately placed with this pro-
cedure might have been transferred or discharged
shortly after the census was completed.

9. We recognize that, in general, the residents of VA
domiciliaries tend to be younger and to have more psychiatric disorders than do veterans in nursing homes.
Since the analysis in this chapter is restricted to
veterans over the age of 65, however, these population
differences are largely eliminated, making it reasonable to group the data from these two types of extended care facilities.

10. The Annual One-Day Census identified a range of services of this sort, including basic subsistence (living quarters, transportation and food), aid in activities of daily living, continuous non-medical supervision, homemaking, outpatient medical and mental health
services, rehabilitation therapies and adaptive housing.

Definition of Independent Variables
for Utilization Regressions

Source: 1979 National Survey of Veterans
(Hammond, 1980)

All missing values were randomized into categories by the proportion of variables in that category without adjusting for age.

Socioeconomic

Income: Adjusted the combined family income information into four income categories based on the number of dependents. The four categories are:

1) Poverty — based on 1980 poverty levels adjusted for the number of dependents taken from the Current Population Report Series P-60, No. 134.
2) Near Poverty — 150% of poverty level.
3) Upper Income — above $25,000.
4) Middle Income — all others.

Employment: The employment variable was created from the survey question: "What were you doing most of last week?" Employment was defined as working or having a job but not at work.

Demographic

Education: Years of education.

Marital Status: Classified as married or never married. Absence of spouse, whether widowed, divorced or separated was the standard for comparison.

Dependents: The number of total dependents is a continuous variable in the regressions.

Race: Categorized as white and non-white.

Urban Setting: Classification from the current population survey assessment of urban and rural status.

Age: Each regression analysis included veterans over the age of 45. In addition, the outpatient and regular source of care regressions were performed with veterans over the age of 65.

VA System Characteristics

Service-Connected Disability Status: Applied to a veteran with any degree of service-connected disability.

Regular Source of Care: Veterans were classified as either utilizing the VA or a non-VA physician or service as their regular source of care. No regular source of care was the standard for comparison.

Non-VA System Characteristics

Insurance: There are four insurance variables: Medicare A and/or B Coverage, Medicare B plus Private Insurance, Private Hospital and/or Outpatient Insurance, and Medicaid Coverage. No insurance is the standard for comparison. Private insurance included HMO, employer, group or private insurance. The type of Medicare or Private Insurance used in the regression depended on whether inpatient or outpatient care was being analyzed. Medicare A and Private Hospital Insurance were used in the regression of the proportion of hospitalization under VA auspices. Medicare B and Private Outpatient Insurance were used in the regressions of outpatient utilization and regular source of care.

Admission Did Not Give Choice to Veteran: If the veteran's reason for non-VA utilization was reported as: the VA didn't offer care needed, a doctor arranged the admission, not entitled to care, or care needed was an accident or emergency, then the veteran was classified as not having a choice to use the VA system.

Perception of Veteran

VA Cares about Veterans: This variable is based on the survey question "Do you agree that officials in the VA really don't care much about what people like you think?" Answers are scored as 1-agree, -1-disagree, and 0-don't know.

VA Provides High Quality of Care: Constructed a three-point index based on the veteran's rating of VA effectiveness in providing health benefits to disabled veterans, treating alcohol problems and treating drug prob-

352

lems. Points were allocated as follows: 1 for an answer
of effectiveness, 0 for an answer of don't know or in-be-
tween, and −1 for an answer of ineffectiveness. The index
is an average across the three responses.

Awareness of Medical Care: Awareness of VA hospitalization benefits and of VA outpatient care were treated as
separate variables.

Problems with Access: If "lived too far" or "too long
a wait to get in" were reported reasons for using a non-VA
facility, then the veteran was classified as having access
problems to VA facilities.

Definition of Independent Variables
for Admission/Discharge Regressions

Variable   Definition

DEMOGRAPHIC

Age   Age of veteran in years. Source: 1981 VA
                 Census.

Marital
Status   Source: 1981 VA Census.

  MARRIED   Veteran is married.
  SPSABSNT   Spouse Absent: Divorced/Separated/Widowed.
                 ("Never Married" is the standard of compari-
                 son.)

Race   Source: 1981 VA Census.

  CAUCASIAN   Veteran is Caucasian. (All other races ag-
                 gregated for comparison.)

Population Density

  METRO   Veteran lives in county in metropolitan area
                 with a county population greater than 50,000.
  NEARMETRO   Veteran lives in county contiguous to metro
                 area. (Rural areas are the standard for com-
                 parison.)

VA Region   Source: 1980 Area Resource File. Informa-
                 tion was provided by the VA.

353

REGION 1   Veteran lives in VA Region 1. Similar for
            Regions 2 through 5. (Region 6 is standard
            for comparison.)

SOCIOECONOMIC

INCOME   Per capita income of county of veteran's
            residence.
            Source: 1980 Area Resource File. Infor-
            mation provided by the 1977 Population Es-
            timates and Projections of the Bureau of the
            Census, Series P-25.

UNEMPLOYMENT
            Percent unemployed in county of veteran's
            residence.
            Source: Area Resource File. Information
            provided by the Bureau of Labor Statistics
            Annual Average.

HEALTH STATUS

LOSDAYS   Length of stay in days in VA facility.
            Source: 1981 VA Census.

Diagnosis   Source: 1981 VA Census.

DXCHEM   Primary diagnosis is alcohol- or drug-
            related.
DXPSYCH   Primary diagnosis involves psychiatric
            disorder. (Other diagnoses are the stan-
            dard of comparison.)

HEALTH SYSTEM CHARACTERISTICS

Appropriate Source: 1981 VA Census special question
Care   on the appropriate level of care for the
            patient.

LEVEL OF CARE
            A scale of 0 to 7 measured the intensity of
            the level of medical, surgical or psy-
            chiatric care needed. Outpatient or other
            care was designated as 0. Intensive care
            was classified as 7.
LOCPSY   Appropriate care involves psychiatric
            treatment.

<u>Station Type</u>   Source: 1981 VA Census.

   NHSTAT   Veteran is in VA nursing home.
   HOSTAT   Veteran is in VA hospital. (Domiciliaries
                 are the standard of comparison.)

<u>Non-VA Supply</u> Source: 1980 Area Resource File. Hospi-
tal information was provided by the 1980
County Hospital File created from the
American Hospital Association Annual Survey of Hospitals. Nursing home data were
provided by the 1978 County Hospital File.
Total active non-federal physician data were
from the American Medical Association
surveys. Nurse practitioner data were obtained from the 1980 National Center for
Health Services Research Nurse Practitioner Tape. All supply variables were constructed at the county level. An average by
PSA was calculated and assigned to each
county in the PSA. This average was used in
the analysis. All variables defined as a
ratio were constructed at the PSA level. The
numerators and denominators were treated as
separate variables before the PSA average
was constructed.

   STBEDS/C   Non-VA short term hospital beds per capita
            in PSA includes short term hospital beds and
            long term care swing beds.
   LTBEDS/E   Non-VA long term hospital beds per elder in
            PSA includes long term hospital beds and
            skilled nursing, chronic care and swing beds
            in short term hospitals.
   NHBEDS/E   Non-VA nursing home beds per elder in PSA.
   NHPCTPRIV Percent private nursing home beds in PSA.
   MD/C   Physicians active in patient care per cap-
            ita in PSA.
   HSPC/E   Hospital based hospices per elder in PSA.
   NPGER/E   Nurse practitioners (geriatric specialty)
            per elder in PSA.

<u>Unmet Need</u>   Source: 1981 VA Census special questions on
services needed by patient.

   UNMETSER   Veteran unable to obtain needed outpatient
            services.

UNMETPAY   Veteran unable to pay for needed outpa-
            tient services.

VA Supply   Source: 1980 Area Resource File except for
            nursing home data which were obtained from
            the 1980 VA Annual Report.

   VAAFF   VAMC in PSA affiliated with medical school.
   VABED/V VA-operated hospital beds per veteran in PSA.
   VANURS/V VA-operated nursing home beds and beds in
            state homes for veterans per veteran in PSA.
   VAOUT/V Visits to VA-operated outpatient clinics per
            veteran in PSA.

PROBIT Regression Coefficients

Proportion of Hospitalization under VA Auspices in Past Year

Veterans Aged 45+

Coefficient	Maximum Likelihood Estimates	T Statistics
1. CONSTANT	-1.48	-2.86
2. INCPOV	0.33	2.53
3. INCNPOV	0.049	0.37
4. INCUP	-0.22	-1.28
5. EDUC	-0.02	-1.27
6. INSURTMA	-0.14	-0.97
7. INSURTMD	0.11	0.44
8. INSURCHO	0.061	0.20
9. INSRPROT	0.37	-1.22
10. INSRFRMH	0.11	0.46
11. SCD	0.23	1.99
12. WHITE	-0.16	-1.23
13. EMPL	-0.37	-2.94
14. MARRIED	0.26	1.74
15. NEVMARRD	0.35	1.85
16. DEP	-0.034	-0.70
17. URBAN	-0.062	-0.60
18. SCOO8	-0.0069	-0.98
19. QUALITY	0.051	1.35
20. CARE	-0.56	-1.03
21. REGVA	0.87	5.38
22. REGNVAMD	-0.46	-2.85
23. REGNVAOT	-0.39	-1.72
24. ACSSHOS	0.054	0.19
25. AWAREH	0.35	1.88
26. NDISCHOS	0.17	0.78

n = 6605

Source: 1979 National Survey of Veterans (Hammond, 1980)

PROBIT Regression Coefficients

Proportion of Outpatient Visits under VA Auspices in Past Year

| | Aged 45+ | | Aged 65+ | |
Coefficient	Maximum Likelihood Estimates	T Statistics	Maximum Likelihood Estimates	T Statistics
1. CONSTANT	−0.91	−2.69	−1.80	−3.70
2. INCPOV	0.076	0.79	−0.47	−2.31
3. INCNPOV	0.11	1.28	−0.30	1.70
4. INCUP	−0.094	−1.11	−0.17	−0.59
5. EDUC	−0.098	−1.33	0.00073	0.024
6. INSURCOF	−0.098	−1.33	−0.051	−0.26
7. INSURTMB	0.03	0.26	0.036	0.18
8. INSURTMD	0.18	−0.88	−0.10	−0.31
9. INSRPROT	−0.34	−3.68	−0.28	−1.08
10. INSRPRMO	0.057	0.37	−0.036	−0.12
11. SCD	0.75	10.43	0.96	6.00
12. WHITE	−0.17	−1.86	−0.10	−0.43
13. EMPL	−0.31	−4.02	−0.26	−1.19
14. MARRIED	−0.17	−1.79	−0.20	−0.81
15. NEVMARRD	−0.10	−0.70	−0.20	−0.73
16. DEP	0.06	2.27	0.097	0.55
17. URBAN	0.088	1.32	0.32	1.92
18. QUALITY	0.0085	0.35	0.0041	0.067
19. CARE	0.125	−0.70	0.02	0.25
20. REGVA	1.25	10.82	1.18	4.54
21. REGNVAMD	−0.28	−2.50	−0.70	−2.62
22. REGNVAOT	−0.23	−1.72	−0.86	−2.40
23. ACCESS	0.32	4.28	0.44	2.32
24. AWAREO	0.69	9.44	0.96	5.30
25. AGE	0.0091	−2.08		

n = 6485   n = 1107

Source: 1979 National Survey of Veterans (Hammond, 1980)

PROBIT Regression Coefficients

Utilization of the VA as a Regular Source of Care

Coefficient	Aged 45+ Maximum Likelihood Estimates	T Statistics	Aged 65+ Maximum Likelihood Estimates	T Statistics
1. CONSTANT	1.39	4.16	0.93	1.98
2. INCPOV	0.13	1.26	0.14	0.73
3. INCNPOV	0.27	2.97	0.11	0.65
4. INCUP	-0.44	-4.61	-0.35	-1.06
5. EDUC	-0.058	-5.38	-0.067	-2.89
6. INSURCOF	-0.29	-3.65	-0.089	-0.43
7. INSURTMB	-0.34	-2.84	-0.44	-2.38
8. INSURTMD	-0.047	-0.24	0.21	0.79
9. INSRPROT	-0.85	-9.48	-0.89	-3.59
10. INSRPRMO	0.14	0.84	0.12	0.39
11. SCD	0.84	10.00	0.75	4.21
12. WHITE	-0.55	-5.89	-0.58	-2.68
13. EMPL	-0.24	-2.97	-0.19	-0.84
14. MARRIED	-0.21	-2.25	-0.01	-0.036
15. NEVMARRD	-0.39	-2.79	-0.34	-1.36
16. DEP	-0.12	-3.68	-0.20	-0.80
17. URBAN	-0.40	-5.90	-0.65	-4.19
18. QUALITY	0.15	5.97	-0.097	-1.19
19. CARE	-0.087	-2.38	-4.22	-2.83
20. ACCESS	-0.405	-5.44	-4.22	-2.83
21. AWAREO	0.62	9.37		
22. AGE	-0.0072	-1.59		

n = 6485   n = 1107

Source: 1979 National Survey of Veterans (Hammond, 1980)

Ordinary Least Squares Regression Coefficients

Proportion of Patients in VA Facilities
Whose Needs Are Mismatched to Care Provided

Veterans Aged 65+

Variable	Hospitals		Nursing Homes & Domiciliaries	
	Parameter Estimate	T Ratio	Parameter Estimate	T Ratio
1. INTERCEPT	0.90	5.70	0.83	10.10
2. LOSDAYS	−0.0000069	−1.02	−0.00002	−5.83
3. AGE	0.0048	4.65	−0.0021	−3.89
4. MARRIED	−0.02	−0.85	−0.0082	−0.66
5. ISOLATED	−0.0098	0.37	0.03	2.30
6. WHITE	−0.03	−1.33	0.02	1.12
7. DX1CHEM	0.09	1.70	0.05	2.06
8. DX1PSY	0.10	3.81	−0.04	−4.03
9. LOCREG	−0.16	−29.99	−0.03	−5.10
10. UNMETSER	0.11	1.29	0.40	8.72
11. UNMETPAY	0.15	1.94	0.17	4.92
12. LOCPSY	0.04	1.07	0.06	4.25
13. METRO	−0.02	−0.49	0.05	2.83
14. NEARMETRO	−0.08	−2.07	0.0097	0.50
15. INCOME	−0.0000077	−0.67	−0.000069	−4.05
16. UNEMP	−0.0036	−0.83	−0.0066	−2.83
17. STBED−P	−10.46	−0.85	−11.21	−1.59
18. LTBED−E	−0.03	−0.03	−3.81	−7.18
19. NHBED−E	−0.11	−3.83	−0.07	−0.28
20. NGPOTPRV	−0.07	−0.78	−0.34	−6.90
21. MD−P	113.18	4.21	74.96	4.79
22. HSPC−E	−996.91	−1.65	−944.37	−3.20
23. NPGER−E	910.44	0.90	−1665.08	−3.94
24. VAAFF	−0.05	−1.84	−0.02	−1.89
25. VABED−V	−3.82	−1.60	−1.43	−1.02
26. VANURS−V	−4.97	−0.42	12.90	2.28

n = 2640
r^2 = .328

n = 5481
r^2 = .069

Source: VA Census 1981 and Area Resource File 1980

Ordinary Least Squares Regression Coefficients

Proportion of Patients in VA Facilities
Who Report a Resistance to Discharge

Veterans Aged 65+

Variable	Hospitals		Nursing Homes & Domiciliaries	
	Parameter Estimate	T Ratio	Parameter Estimate	T Ratio
1. INTERCEPT	0.29	3.28	-0.19	-0.36
2. LOSDAYS	0.0000061	1.57	0.0000021	0.63
3. AGE	0.000981	1.61	-0.00049	-0.96
4. MARRIED	0.00987	0.68	0.02	2.13
5. ISOLATED	0.00096	0.06	0.00947	0.85
6. WHITE	0.00114	0.05	0.06	3.41
7. DX1CHEM	-0.02	-0.61	0.01	0.51
8. DX1PSY	-0.0039	-0.25	-0.03	-2.58
9. LOCREG	-0.03	-8.46	-0.02	-4.59
10. UNMETSER	0.35	7.04	0.26	5.88
11. UNMETPAY	0.33	7.31	0.37	11.13
12. LOCPSY	0.05	2.57	0.00867	0.62
13. METRO	-0.03	-1.50	0.06	2.96
14. NRMETRO	0.00335	0.15	-0.01	-0.58
15. INCOME	0.0000073	1.11	0.0000283	4.50
16. UNEMP	-0.0013	-0.56	0.02	7.54
17. STBED-P	-14.73	-2.13	40.22	6.23
18. LTBED-E	-0.67	-1.23	-2.86	-5.74
19. NHBED-E	-0.04	-2.37	-0.25	-1.14
20. NHPCTPRV	-0.24	-4.96	-0.02	0.40
21. MD-P	54.90	3.61	-57.126	-3.90
22. HSPC-E	-835.49	-2.39	-1223.72	-4.37
23. NPGER-E	-972.29	-1.71	852.22	2.20
24. VAAFF	0.02	1.06	-0.02	-1.32

$$n = 2642 \qquad\qquad n = 5483$$
$$r^2 = .098 \qquad\qquad r^2 = .080$$

Source: VA Census 1981 and Area Resource File 1980

APPENDIX II-F

Ordinary Least Squares Regression Coefficients

Proportion of Patients in VA Facilities
Who Were Admitted from Non-VA Sources

Veterans Aged 65+

	Hospitals		Nursing Homes & Domiciliaries	
Variable	Parameter Estimate	T Ratio	Parameter Estimate	T Ratio
1. INTERCEPT	0.28	1.50	−0.23	−2.12
2. LOCDAYS	0.0000077	1.00	−3.06	−0.07
3. AGE	0.00301	2.51	−0.000046	−0.02
4. MARRIED	−0.0083	−0.29	0.05	3.09
5. ISOLATED	0.01	0.33	0.04	2.54
6. WHITE	−0.07	−2.55	−0.0048	−0.23
7. DX1CHEM	0.17	2.82	−0.0087	−0.31
8. DX1PSY	0.03	1.02	−0.02	−1.33
9. UNMETSER	−0.20	−2.00	0.06	1.04
10. UNMETPAY	0.02	0.23	0.07	1.59
11. SEX1	−0.03	−0.54	0.01	0.49
12. METRO	0.16	3.59	−0.06	−2.39
13. NRMETRO	−0.08	−1.75	−0.05	−2.13
14. INCOME	−0.000056	−4.25	0.000034	3.71
15. UNEMP	0.02	2.29	0.004	1.37
16. STBED-P	21.01	1.48	0.45	0.05
17. LTBED-E	−3.86	−3.36	2.11	3.19
18. NHBED-E	0.21	5.95	−2.90	−8.25
19. NHPCTPRV	0.47	4.79	0.52	8.39
20. MD-P	−59.46	−1.91	−51.25	−2.65
21. HSPC-E	364.96	0.52	1073.32	2.92
22. NPGER-E	3825.46	3.27	1633.61	3.18
23. VAAFF	−0.04	−1.18	−0.02	−0.94
24. VABED-V	7.50	1.70	−6.71	−3.12
25. VANURS-V	−46.34	−3.37	−18.33	−2.56
26. VAOUT-V	−0.11	−2.02	−0.08	4.22

$$n = 2640 \qquad n = 5481$$
$$r^2 = .055 \qquad r^2 = .050$$

Source: VA Census 1981 and Area Resource File 1980

Ordinary Least Squares Regression Coefficients

Proportion of Patients in VA Facilities
Who Could Be Discharged If Resources Were Available

Veterans Aged 65+

Variable	Hospitals		Nursing Homes & Domiciliaries	
	Parameter Estimate	T Ratio	Parameter Estimate	T Ratio
1. INTERCEPT	0.60	3.89	0.40	3.81
2. LOSDAYS	0.0000074	1.11	0.000075	−1.75
3. AGE	0.00208	2.04	−0.00	−1.55
4. MARRIED	−0.02	−1.03	0.02	1.26
5. ISOLATED	−0.0074	−0.28	0.02	1.60
6. WHITE	−0.03	−1.48	0.01	0.52
7. DX1CHEM	0.04	0.80	0.03	0.94
8. DX1PSY	0.12	4.58	−0.04	−3.27
9. LOCREG	−0.08	−14.94	−0.05	−8.50
10. UNMETSER	0.63	7.53	0.51	8.96
11. UNMETPAY	0.04	1.01	0.03	1.87
12. METRO	0.03	0.43	0.01	0.52
13. NRMETRO	0.04	1.00	−0.08	−3.52
14. INCOME	0.0000072	0.64	0.000037	4.45
15. UNEMP	−0.01	−2.65	0.03	11.27
16. STBED-P	−19.14	−1.59	10.09	1.16
17. LTBED-E	0.08	0.09	−5.82	−8.87
18. NHBED-E	0.01	0.49	−0.33	−1.14
19. NHPCTRPRV	−0.19	−2.26	−0.07	−1.21
20. MD-P	53.29	2.02	−84.89	−4.39
21. HSPC-E	1049.02	−1.77	−2717.40	−7.45
22. NPGER-E	−3.09	0.00	496.85	0.96
23. VAAFF	0.05	1.81	−0.06	−3.65
24. VABED-V	−2.65	−1.13	−6.07	−3.52
25. VANURS-V	31.86	2.73	1.98	0.28

n = 2640
r^2 = .168

n = 5481
r^2 = .146

Source: VA Census 1981 and Area Resource File 1980

REFERENCES

Atchley, R. The Social Forces in Later Life. Belmont, California: Wadsworth Publishing Co., 1972.

Black, G. "Pennsylvania Department of Aging Perspective: Planning Services for Aging Veterans and Their Spouses." Presented at the 7th National Association of Social Workers Professional Symposium – "Social Work Practice in a Turbulent World" for the symposium "The Aging Veteran Population: Interorganizational Relations." Philadelphia, Pennsylvania, November 21, 1981.

Congressional Budget Office. "Projected Acute-Care Bed Needs of Veterans Administration Hospitals." Staff Working Paper, Washington, D.C., April, 1977.

Coulton, C. and Frost, A. "Use of Social and Health Services by the Elderly." Journal of Health and Social Behavior, 23, pp. 330-339, December, 1982.

Cromwell, J. and Kanak, J. "The Effects of Prospective Reimbursement Programs on Hospital Adoption and Service Sharing." Health Care Financing Review, 4, pp. 67-88, December, 1982.

Custis, D. Testimony at hearing on oversight of the VA's Extended Care and Geriatric Program, U.S. House of Representatives Subcommittee on Hospitals and Health Care, Washington, D.C., July 14, 1982.

Demkovich, L. "When It Comes to Planning Hospitals, the VA Marches to Its Own Beat." National Journal, 35, pp. 1428-1433, August 30, 1980.

General Accounting Office. State Veterans Homes: Opportunities to Reduce VA and State Costs and Improve Program Management. GAO/HRD-82-7, Washington, D.C., October 22, 1981.

General Accounting Office. The Elderly Should Benefit from Expanded Home Health Care But Increasing these Services Will Not Insure Cost Reductions. GAO/IPE-83-1, Washington, D.C.: U.S. Government Printing Office, December 7, 1982.

Geoghegan, G. Activities of Daily Living in VA Nursing Home Patients: A Multivariate Model. Veterans Administration Biometrics Monograph, No. 16, Washington, D.C., November, 1982.

Hammond, D. 1979 National Survey of Veterans: Summary Report. Veterans Administration, Reports and Statistics Service of the Office of the Comptroller, Washington, D.C., December, 1980.

Horgan C., Taylor, A. and Wilensky, G. "Aging Veterans: Will They Overwhelm the VA Medical Care System?" Health Affairs, 2, pp. 77-86, Fall, 1983.

Joskow, P. Controlling Hospital Costs: The Role of Government Regulation. Cambridge, Massachusetts: The MIT Press, 1981.

Katz, S. and Akpom, A. "A Measure of Primary Socio-Biologic Functions." International Journal of Health Services, 6, pp. 518-526, 1976.

Lindsay, C. "A Theory of Government Enterprise." Journal of Political Economy, 87, pp. 1061-1077, October, 1976.

Link, C., Long, S. and Settle, R. "Equity and the Utilization of Health Care Services by the Medicare Elderly." The Journal of Human Resources, 17, pp. 195-212, 1982.

McCoy, J. and Edwards, B. "Contextual and Socio-demographic Antecedents of Institutionalization Among Aged Welfare Recipients." Medical Care, 19, pp. 907-921, September, 1981.

Moran, A. "Psychiatric Bed Needs: Quantifying the Impact of Alternative Services." Journal of Medical Systems, 4, pp. 9-26, 1980.

National Academy of Sciences. Health Care for American Veterans. National Academy of Sciences, Washington, D.C., 1977.

Neter, J. and Wasserman, W. Applied Linear Statistical Models. Homewood, Illinois: Richard D. Irwin, 1974.

Page, W. "Why Veterans Choose Veterans Administration Hospitalization." Medical Care, 20(3), pp. 308-320, March, 1982.

Pihlbland, C. and Adams, D. "Widowhood, Social Participation and Life Satisfaction." Aging and Human Development, 3, pp. 323-330, 1972.

Seitz, L. Multiple Facility Visits within the VA Health Care Delivery System. Veterans Administration, MSS Report No. 81-6, Washington, D.C., August, 1981a.

Seitz, L. The Impact upon the VA Health Care Delivery System of Treating a Higher Proportion of Older Veterans. Veterans Administration, HSIS Report No. 81-8, Washington, D.C., October, 1981b.

Seitz, L. Multiple Program Utilization: The Number of Individuals Discharged from More than One Inpatient Health Care Setting. Veterans Administration, HSIS Report No. 82-2, Washington, D.C., January, 1982.

Special Medical Advisory Group, Task Force on the VA Geriatrics Plan. Caring for the Older Veteran. Veterans Administration, Washington, D.C., July 18, 1983.

Stasson, M. and Holakan, J. Long Term Care Demonstration Projects: A Review of Recent Evaluations. Working Paper No. 1227-2, Washington, D.C.: Urban Institute, February, 1981.

Stoller, E. "Patterns of Physician Utilization by the Elderly: A Multivariate Analysis." Medical Care, 20, pp. 1080-1089, November, 1982.

Thompson, F. Health Policy and Bureaucracy. Cambridge, Massachusetts: The MIT Press, 1981.

U.S. Department of Health and Human Services. Health United States, 1981. PHS 82-1232, Washington, D.C., December, 1981.

U.S. Veterans Administration, Administrator of Veterans Affairs. Annual Report 1982. Washington, D.C., April, 1983.

U.S. Veterans Administration. Health Care of the Aging Veteran: A Report of the Geriatrics and Gerontology Advisory Committee. Washington, D.C., April, 1983.

Wan, T. "Use of Health Services by the Elderly in Low-Income Communities." Milbank Memorial Fund Quarterly, 60, pp. 82-107, 1982.

Wan, T. and Odell, B. "Factors Affecting the Use of Social and Health Services Among the Elderly." Aging and Society, 1, pp. 95-113, March, 1981.

11. Meeting the Oral Health Needs of the Aging Veteran

Linda Niessen, D.M.D., M.P.P.
Harry A. Dunlevy, B.A.

Introduction

As the proportion of elderly veterans increases, the Veterans Administration will need to make significant changes in the present system of health care delivery (VA, 1977, 1983a, 1983c). The VA's Office of Dentistry, as part of the Department of Medicine and Surgery, will be faced with new challenges as a result of this demographic shift. The purpose of this chapter is to examine the effect of this demographic shift on the VA's dental service and to discuss strategies for altering the current dental care delivery system to meet the changing dental needs of the aging veteran. This analysis examines: (1) the mission of the VA regarding dental care for eligible veterans, (2) dental care utilization including a comparison of future dental needs with present needs, (3) cost projections to meet the needs, (4) organizational strategies to assist the VA dental service in meeting the future dental needs of this population, and (5) recommendations based on the analysis of these options.

369

Importance of Oral Health to the Elderly

The oral cavity has many functions including being the main entry for nutrients, enabling the communication of thoughts and emotions, and contributing to one's overall self-image. Alterations in any of the oral functions, though not of a life-threatening nature, do have considerable influence on the quality of one's life. Tooth loss is not a normal age-related change. Oral diseases can contribute to inadequate nutrition and lead to deterioration in various medical conditions.

Infection from any source can be debilitating to an elder. Untreated, oral infection particularly in a medically compromised elder will result in loss of oral function and will affect one's overall health.

Comprehensive health care includes oral health care. With aging comes an increase in the number of chronic diseases. The goal of medical intervention is to control or slow the rate of progression of the disease process. However, restoration of function is often not possible. In the case of dental diseases, however, not only does oral health care aim to diagnose, control and prevent the further progression of dental diseases, but dental treatment can in fact restore oral function. Thus, at a time when an elder is coping with various functional declines, oral health status should not and does not have to decline as a function of aging.

I. VA Dental Service

A. Mission

Since its establishment over 50 years ago, the VA health care system's primary mission has been to provide comprehensive health care to veterans with service-connected disabilities. Its secondary mission has been to provide health care to veterans with non-service-connected disabilities who are unable to pay for care from private providers, but only to the extent that facilities and staff are available (General Accounting Office, 1981).

The VA operates dental services in 172 VA medical centers (VAMCs), 18 satellite outpatient medical centers and eight independently operated outpatient clinics with dental services. As of September 30, 1982, the VA employed

940 dentists, 167 hygienists and 1063 dental assistants. The dental service not only provides patient care, but also engages in research activities and dental education through affiliations with dental schools and residency programs with over 300 dental residents.

In FY 1979, the VA reported that about 840,000 veterans were provided dental examinations and/or treatments at VA clinics at a cost of approximately $77 million (General Accounting Office, 1981). An additional 90,000 veterans were authorized care from private dentists on a fee-for-service basis at a cost of $52 million in FY 1979. For FY 1982, the VA dental expenditure was approximately $110 million, of which $79 million was for dental staff salaries and $31 million was the fee program.

B. Eligibility

Although the veteran with a service-connected dental disability has the highest priority for dental care, a veteran may be eligible for dental care while an inpatient at a VA hospital, domiciliary, or nursing home. Title 38 U.S.C. 610(a) authorized the VA to furnish hospital, domiciliary, or nursing home care, including dental services, to any veteran for: (1) a service-connected disability or (2) a non-service-connected disability if the veteran is unable to pay for the care. Under Section 610(c), the VA is authorized, within the limits of VA facilities:

> ...to furnish medical services (including dental) to correct or treat any non-service-connected disability of such veteran, in addition to treatment incident to the disability for which such veteran is hospitalized, if...the Administrator finds such services to be reasonably necessary to protect the health of such veteran.

Outpatient dental services are available to: (1) veterans with service-connected dental conditions, (2) veterans with non-service-connected dental conditions if treatment was initiated while the veteran was an inpatient at a VA facility and it is professionally determined to be necessary to complete the treatment, and (3) both veterans and non-veterans in cases of dental emergencies. Eligibility for outpatient dental care is fairly complex. A veteran must fall into one of six categories in order to receive dental care on an outpatient basis. Table 1 lists the six classes of eligibility and the extent of dental

371

Table 1

OUTPATIENT DENTAL ELIGIBILITY BY CLASS

Class	Description	Extent of Treatment
I	Compensable service-connected dental condition or disability.	Comprehensive. Repeat Basis.
II	Service-connected noncompensable condition shown to be in existence at time of discharge from at least six months of creditable service, if application is made within 90 days of discharge.	Restorative. Missing teeth may need adjudication before replacement. One episode of care only.
IIA	Service-connected noncompensable dental condition or disability adjudicated as resulting from combat wounds or service trauma.	Treatment linked to specific teeth, as rated. Repeat Basis.
IIB	Former prisoners of war (POW) who were prisoners less than six months and have a service-connected dental condition or disability.	Repeat care for service-connected condition.

IIC	Former prisoners of war for six months or more.	Comprehensive. Repeat Basis.
III	Dental condition professionally determined by VA to be currently aggravating a service-connected medical condition.	Treatment to satisfactorily resolve the problem. Each episode of care must be medically approved.
IV	In receipt of 100% compensation for service-connected disability.	Comprehensive. Repeat Basis.
V	Service-connected disabled veteran approved by VA for vocational rehabilitation training, objective has been selected, or is pursuing this training.	Sufficient care to prevent the interruption of training or goal achievement.
VI	Service in wars prior to World War I.	Comprehensive. Repeat Basis.

373

treatment by category. Not all veterans eligible for dental care receive comprehensive dental care on a continuing basis. For example, veterans applying for dental care under the Class II eligibility will receive only one episode of dental care. (An episode is defined as the amount of care needed to restore them to dental health.) Veterans who fall into the Class IV category receive comprehensive care on a regular basis.

The VA does not know what proportion of those presently receiving dental care is over 65 as the VA's current automated management information system (AMIS) does not collect data on the patient's age. A recent survey of veterans receiving care at the Boston VA Outpatient Clinic found that 36% of the service-connected outpatients receiving care are over 60, while 57% of the outpatients are over 50. In addition, 60% of the Class III and IV categories of outpatients are over age 50 while 71% of Class II and V categories are between the ages of 20-29 years.

For the acute care patient population, a dental exam is considered part of the medical exam. While the dental service attempts to provide a dental examination on all acute care patients, the nature of the patient's illness or a short length of stay sometimes prohibits this. In a VA Nursing Home Care Unit (NHCU), it is estimated that over 60% of the residents are over 65. For these residents, the VA is responsible for providing any needed dental treatment. For veterans in community nursing homes under VA auspices, unless service-connected, these veterans have no legal entitlement to dental care.

C. Dental Needs

An Institute of Medicine Report on Public Policy Options for Better Dental Health (1980) concluded that:

> ...Americans have a substantial unmet need for dental care as indicated by surveys employing objective professional examinations of persons to determine their dental health. At the same time, proven methods exist for preventing and reducing dental diseases which if untreated are important causes of pain, discomfort and disfigurement and can contribute to nutritional deficits or impaired social function (p. 1).

Since dental diseases are predominantly chronic and progressive, the patient's age and the backlog of treatment needed will influence the nature of required dental care treatment.

Documentation of the oral health needs of the elderly has received considerable attention during recent years. Certain demographic variables have been shown to be associated with dental needs, particularly income, race, and sex. Data from the National Center for Health Statistics (NCHS) show that the need for dental care varies with income; low income people have a greater need for dental care than higher income people (Institute of Medicine, 1980). Elderly blacks demonstrate greater unmet need than elderly whites and 68% of elderly males need dental treatment as compared to 56% of elderly females.

Surveys by the NCHS (1974a) also show that the elderly are keeping their teeth longer than previous generations of elders. In 1960-1962, 55% of adults aged 65-74 were edentulous, while in 1971-1974, the percentage of edentulous persons decreased to 45%. Of the elderly retaining some teeth, approximately 50% of the women and 72% of the men have periodontal disease which can lead to tooth loss (NCHS, 1974b).

Gustafsson, et al., (1954), identified a positive correlation between increased age and the frequency of root surface caries. More recent studies on root caries reported that the prevalence of root caries increases with age (Hazen, et al., 1972; Sumney, et al., 1973). In fact, Sumney, et al., (1973), found that in the over 60 age group examined, 70% of the population studied showed evidence of root surface caries. In addition, the prevalence and severity of periodontal diseases and oral cancer are known to increase with age (U.S. DHEW, 1981; Douglass, et al., 1983). The detection of malignant tumors of the oral cavity is of particular concern to the veteran population, since men who smoke and drink are known to be at higher risk of developing oral cancer than the general population (Douglass, et al., in press). Thus, with greater longevity comes an increase in the relative risk of the major oral and dental diseases.

Large unmet dental needs have been documented in institutionalized populations (Bernhardt, 1971; Clark and Vergeen, 1975; Feld, 1971; Drake, 1970). In Vermont, Milton, et al., (1981), found that over 70% of the residents surveyed were edentulous. Seventy-five percent of the residents had not visited a dentist in the last 12 months. In a survey of North Carolina nursing homes, Drake (1970) found that among the 274 residents examined with a mean age of 76.8 years, the patients with remaining natural teeth had a high rate of periodontal disease and poor oral hygiene.

D. Utilization

Although the elderly have substantial unmet dental needs, data from NCHS show that the elderly have the lowest rates of dental care utilization (American Dental Association, 1980). Of a group of non-institutionalized elders surveyed in 1975, only 21.4% visited a dentist annually, while approximately 50% of the general population saw a dentist annually. For the 50% of the elderly who were edentulous only 8% saw a dentist at least once a year. For those elders receiving dental care, 90% of the dental expenses were paid by the family, compared to 73% of dental expenses for 25-54 year olds (National Center for Health Services Research, 1982).

Institutionalized elders have greater unmet dental needs than community dwelling elders since they have increased difficulty in getting to the dental office to receive care. In 1975, the Massachusetts Dental Society in cooperation with the Massachusetts Federation of Nursing Homes surveyed 400 member nursing homes (Reinhalter, 1975). Of the 41% of the nursing homes responding, only 30% had a dental treatment room available, although 47% of the residents were felt to be unable to leave the facility to obtain dental care. Although only 33% of the 11,617 residents in these 164 nursing homes had remaining natural teeth, 27% of the homes responding felt that routine dental care for residents was a major problem. Carlson (1982) found that over half of the 207 Massachusetts dentists surveyed reported that 75% of the residents were unable to leave the facility to obtain dental care.

Previous generations believed tooth loss was a natural part of the aging process. It is now recognized that edentulous old people are edentulous because they had dental disease, not because they are old. The data show that the percentage of edentulism in all age groups is decreasing. Widespread use of fluoride, improved patient oral hygiene, increased dental education, and higher educational and income levels are thought to contribute to the decline of edentulism. As a result of the changing needs, the distribution of services used by the elderly has also changed from 1964 to 1971. While dental visits for denture services are decreasing, dental visits for preventive and maintenance services are increasing (American Dental Association, 1980).

This changing trend in utilization of dental services by the elderly suggests that new cohorts of elderly may view dentistry in a more preventive oriented light and may be more concerned with preserving their natural teeth. As a result, this group may demonstrate a greater demand for dental services. Recent work by Ettinger and Beck (1982) supports this view. This survey found that when the elderly are categorized in 60-64, 65-74, and 75+ age groups, the 60-64 group had higher utilization rates as well as more positive dental attitudes than the 75+ age group. These findings are supported by a survey by Yellowitz, et al., (1982), on the users and non-users of a dental care program for senior citizens. This survey found that the 60-64 year old group had a higher utilization rate than the 75+ age group. This difference suggests that not only will the number of elderly veterans be increasing, but the demand for dental services among this group will also be increasing.

Behavioral models have been developed in order to determine which factors are more prominent in determining if the elderly will visit a dentist in a given year (Wan and Odell, 1981; Evashwick, et al., 1982; Conrad, 1983). Wan and Odell (1981) reported that the most significant predisposing factors affecting the use of dental services among the elderly were economic dependency, age, and educational level. Evashwick, et al., (1982) reported that the three factors significantly related to visiting the dentist were: education, the presence of a regular source of dental care, and the individual's perception of the extent of his or her oral health problems. This study further suggests that the demand for dental care among the elderly, although lower than the demand by younger age groups, is responsive to many of the same factors which influence the utilization of dental services by persons of all age groups.

The VA Survey of Veterans (1979) found that 50% of veterans received dental care in 1978. Five percent of this care was provided under VA auspices. Almost half of

377

the veterans who did not receive dental care in 1978 needed care.

To receive dental care, veterans must apply for care and be eligible for care. Unfortunately, it is not known what percentage of those eligible for dental services actually demand care. The VA dental service is a patient-initiated system. As a result, it has data only on the veterans who utilize the dental program. However, it is believed that if the veterans presently using the VA dental service were declared ineligible for VA dental care, most would not seek care in the private sector. Further, it is likely that some private dentists would be uncomfortable treating those who did seek care because of their various medical, physical and psychiatric conditions.

These data have several implications for the VA dental service. First, the private dental sector is not adequately meeting the needs of the community-dwelling or the institutionalized elderly. Thus, shifting the burden of care from the VA to the private sector does not seem viable given the physical, medical and psychiatric problems of the VA population. Second, in addition to the increasing numbers of elderly veterans, needs for dental services increase additionally due to the increased prevalence and severity of certain oral diseases with age. Third, it is likely that new cohorts of elderly will be more concerned about preserving their dentition and will therefore make greater demands for dental services. Fourth, as the numbers of veterans in VA nursing homes and domiciliaries increase, the dental service must address the question of how to provide dental treatment to these residents both in terms of personnel and facilities since residents are often unable to leave the facility to obtain dental care. For veterans in a VA nursing home who are likely to be closer to the VA dental service, this question may be easier to address than for veterans who reside in community nursing homes. Since few private sector dentists provide care in nursing homes, veterans in community nursing homes will not have access to needed dental care. Fifth, as the VA expands hospital based home care programs in an effort to reduce the need for hospital and/or nursing home care, the question of meeting the dental needs of this homebound population must be addressed.

378

The inability of the private sector to meet the dental needs of the elderly, the changing pattern of need and demand for dental care by the elderly, and the VA's projected increase in long term care patients suggest that the VA dental service will need to adjust its supply of dental personnel in order to meet the oral health needs of the aging veteran.

II. Current Services Provided Versus Future Need

Over the next 10 years, the VA anticipates an increase of about 10,000 inpatients based on the estimated growth in nursing home beds. An increased need for outpatient dental services is more difficult to project. However, as the number of elderly eligible veterans with dental needs increases, an increase in the demand for dental services is anticipated. The purpose of this section is to compare the mix of services provided by the VA dental service to the projected needs of the veteran population in order to appropriately plan to meet the needs of this aging population. A comparison of services provided today with services needed in the future will enable the VA to identify areas of change necessary to meet future needs.

A needs-based model was used to project the future treatment needs. Data from the 1971-74 NCHS were used as baseline estimates for dental treatment needs. The Health and Nutrition Examination Survey (HANES) data have been shown to yield valid and reliable estimates of the actual dental treatment needs in a population (Gillings, et al., 1983). Modifications to the HANES data were made to account for: 1) the changing patterns of dental practice, 2) the elderly nature of the population, and 3) the institutionalized nature of a portion of this aging population.

Current services provided were taken from the VA Office of Dentistry AMIS Reports for FY 1983 (VA, 1983b). Table 2 represents the percentage of all dental services delivered by the VA in FY 1983 (inpatient and outpatient) and the future treatment needs, as predicted by the model. It is evident that the VA provides dental care in proportions which closely approximate those projected to be needed by future cohorts of elders. The most obvious difference occurs in the delivery of preventive services. Whereas the model projects that 25% of services needed by the elderly will be preventive, only 7.6% of present VA

379

services provided are preventive services. The VA provides more restorative and prosthetic services compared to model projections. The VA also performs a higher proportion of oral surgical procedures than the model predicts future cohorts of elders will need.

Table 2

PERCENT DISTRIBUTION OF SERVICES PROVIDED AND FUTURE NEEDS

	Presently Provided	Future Needs
Diagnosis	39.1	31.3
Prevention	7.6	25.0
Restorative	17.2	13.9
Periodontics	11.4	14.5
Prosthodontics	12.6	11.7
Oral Surgery	11.2	3.5
Endodontics	0.9	0.1
TOTAL	100.0	100.0

Figure 1 illustrates the relationship of the proportion of specific services provided to VA nursing home residents, domiciliary residents and outpatients as they relate to the overall model projections. Prosthetic and restorative care are presently provided to outpatients in higher proportions than estimates project will be needed in the future. Nursing home and domiciliary residents receive more diagnostic services than estimates project will be needed in the future.

The estimates of future needs suggest that certain services provided parallel the needs of the present elderly population while other services may need to be increased to meet future estimates. In particular, future elders will require more preventive care and less oral surgical and prosthetic services. As seen in Figure 1, a higher proportion of preventive care is provided to residents in NHCUs than to veterans in domiciliaries, VAMCs or outpatient clinics. This suggests that there may be a more coordinated effort to meet the preventive needs of the NHCU population than other categories of veterans. Such preventive efforts should be expanded.

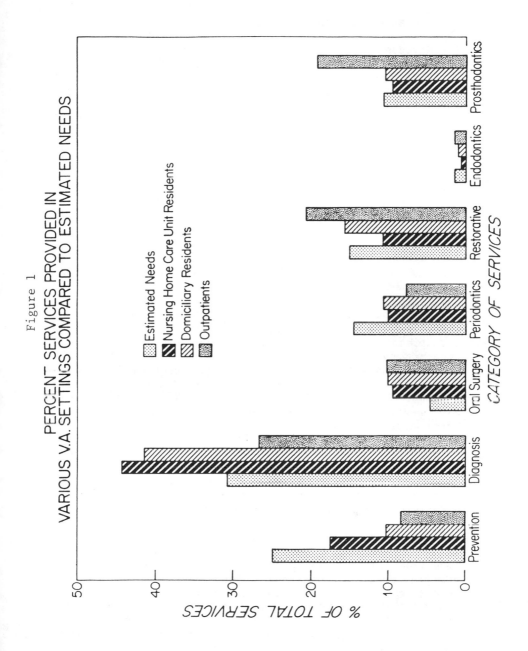

Figure 1

PERCENT SERVICES PROVIDED IN
VARIOUS V.A. SETTINGS COMPARED TO ESTIMATED NEEDS

III. Cost Projections

A. Methods

A needs-based model was used to estimate the costs of providing dental care to the increasing elderly veteran population. The model was developed by the Institute of Medicine to estimate the costs of various components of a dental plan for national health insurance (Institute of Medicine, 1980). The model was shown to give valid estimates when compared with a demand-based model. Needs-based estimates are possible when there are valid and reliable measures of needs for services available. While these data are often unavailable for medical care, specific needs for dental services can be determined more objectively.

Figure 2 shows the five sets of variables used to project the cost of providing dental services to the increased demand of the elderly veterans. The model is a multiplicative model with four variables for the outpatient cost component and five variables for the inpatient cost component. Cost components for inpatient and outpatient care are calculated separately and then added together to arrive at a total cost for the program. The model examines the costs of patient care providers only. Costs for dental laboratory technicians and supplies are not included in the model. To the extent that these costs represent a certain percentage of the provider costs, these costs can be derived from the model estimates. It is assumed that no new dental operatories will be constructed. All costs are projected in constant 1982 dollars. This model assumes no major wars in the next ten years and no large increases in the number of military personnel. A brief description of each variable and its underlying assumptions follows.

One recognizes that as the VA population ages and the VA shifts beds from acute care to long term care, the amount of health care provided to the elderly will increase. However, cost projections will not be made for providing dental care for all the elderly who utilize dental services since the resources of the current budget provide a portion of that care. Rather the model is used to examine the costs of providing care to veterans newly demanding care. In other words, the model calculates additional costs over present operating costs. These costs

Figure 2

MODEL FOR PROJECTING VA DENTAL PROVIDER EXPENDITURES
TO MEET THE INCREASED DEMAND FOR DENTAL SERVICES
BY THE ELDERLY VETERAN

1	2	3	4	5

Cost of
Component =
$\begin{bmatrix} \text{Increased} \\ \text{number} \\ \text{of veterans} \end{bmatrix}$ X $\begin{bmatrix} \text{Age specific} \\ \text{estimate for} \\ \text{need for} \\ \text{dental care} \end{bmatrix}$ X $\begin{bmatrix} \text{Time needed} \\ \text{for services} \end{bmatrix}$ X $\begin{bmatrix} \text{Cost of} \\ \text{provider} \\ \text{time} \end{bmatrix}$ X $\begin{bmatrix} \text{Inpatient} \\ \text{adjustment} \\ \text{factor} \end{bmatrix}$

Component =
inpatient or
outpatient

For
inpatient
component
only

Total Cost – Cost of Inpatient Component and Cost of Outpatient Component

For a more complete discussion of the model see: "Application of a Needs-Based Model for
Planning Geriatric Dental Services in the VA." Special Care in Dentistry, in press.

383

will result from elderly veterans "new" to the VA dental services.

Variable One. The first variable in the model reflects the potential for increased demand among the aging veteran population. Presently there are 30 million veterans in the United States. The VA provides medical care to about three million of these. In FY 1979, the VA dental service provided care to approximately 930,000 veterans through VA staff dental clinics and the VA fee program (GAO, 1981).

Demand increases will result from newly entering inpatients and outpatients. The increased demand for inpatient dental care results from a planned increase in 10,000 long term care beds over ten years.

There is a degree of uncertainty associated with the increased demand for dental care by outpatients. VA officials anticipate that as the veteran population ages and their medical conditions worsen, dental treatment may be needed to improve their overall health. Also it is known that certain veterans eligible for dental care do not seek dental care at all or seek it from sources other than the VA. If economic conditions worsen and/or Medicaid and Medicare benefits change, this group could begin to avail themselves of the dental care to which they are entitled.

As a result of the uncertainty associated with the increased number of elderly who will seek care as outpatients, three estimates of increased demand are made. Costs are projected for each demand level. These estimates of increased demand over the next ten years will be 20%, 35%, and 50%, representing a low, mid and high level of increased demand. These increases correspond to 32,113, 56,197, and 80,282 veterans, respectively. The estimated increases in demand are assumed to occur evenly on a straight line basis over the ten-year period.

Variable Two. The second variable in the model is the age specific estimate of need. HANES data were used to estimate the treatment needs.

Specific treatment needs were taken from the HANES data (NCHS, 1979). The Health and Nutrition Examination Survey of the NCHS conducted during 1971-74 included direct measurements of dental treatment needs. The national survey documented dental treatment needs for each

384

age category based on standardized dental examinations for a stratified random sample of approximately 20,000 persons. The examinations were performed by dentists hired solely for the survey, not by dentists who actually would perform the needed treatment. For this reason, the HANES data were considered to be free of a treatment planning bias (often an overestimate of treatment needs) and an accurate representation of the sample population's dental treatment needs.

The sample reflects the United States population of non-institutionalized individuals who are under age 75. HANES data used in these projections are for males aged 65 to 74. Although the number of women treated by the VA is growing, it is still less than 3% and is not included in this analysis. Since there are no national data on the treatment needs of the population over 75, these data will be applied to project costs of treatment to the over 75 population. While it is recognized that the treatment needs of the over 75 group will differ somewhat from those aged 65-74, the HANES data provide a reasonable approximation of their needs in the absence of other national needs data.

Variable Three. The third variable in the model is the provider time required to perform the dental service. It is assumed that the dental treatment will be provided by the VA dental service rather than the fee program. For this reason the cost of providing specific dental services will be estimated based on the costs of dental personnel. In these calculations, the time needed to provide various services is multiplied by the cost of the time of each dental staff member to provide the service. The estimates of time needed for dental treatment are averages which have been generated by an Indian Health Survey (IHS) (Wolford, 1983). Since the IHS provides services to an ambulatory, younger and healthier population than the VA, these time estimates were increased by 30% to account for the older, often medically compromised VA population. This 30% adjustment also incorporates an adjustment for non-clinical office time to account for the different dental assistant to dentist ratios in the IHS and the VA. Since this ratio is approximately 2:1 in the IHS as compared to 1.2:1 in the VA, time necessary to complete each service is higher in the VA delivery system.

Variable Four. The cost of the dental personnel time is the fourth variable in the model. These costs are calculated based on current VA average salaries of $52,967 per year for dentists, $15,850 per year for dental hygienists and $12,256 for dental assistants (Fischer, 1982). Since the VA now employs only a few expanded-function dental assistants, the costs will not include services provided using an expanded-function dental assistant. Fringe benefits were calculated at 25% of the wage rate and added to the total annual cost of all services.

Dental prophylaxis was considered to be performed by dental hygienists only. Dental radiographs were assumed to be taken solely by dental assistants. All other dental services were considered to be performed by dentists working with dental assistants. Thus the cost per minute of these services include the cost of the dental assistants' time. Table 3 lists the services and provider or provider combination assumed to deliver each service. The cost of the providers' time per minute was multiplied by the number of minutes needed to perform the service to arrive at an average cost per service. The actual cost per service is the product of variable three (the time necessary to perform each service) and four (the cost of providing each service) in the model.

Variable Five. The fifth variable is an adjustment factor for the inpatient cost estimates only. In calculating costs for inpatients, the HANES data present a more difficult problem since these data are for a noninstitutionalized population. Studies have shown that the dental needs as well as the medical needs of this population are greater than those of the non-institutionalized and thus the upward adjustment factor for the institutionalized will be 20% (Drake, 1970; Feld, 1971; Milton, et al., 1981). HANES data found approximately 60% of the 65-74 year old group in need of some dental treatment. Adjusting this upward by 20% would result in 72% of the institutionalized needing dental treatment, which is consistent with previous work on the needs of the institutionalized.

B. Results

Table 4 shows the annual costs of various services to inpatients and outpatients with an increased demand of 20, 35, and 50 percent, respectively. These annual first year

Table 3
COSTS OF PERSONNEL NEEDED TO PROVIDE SERVICES

		Provider/s	Provider Cost/min.	Time of Service (in minutes)	Cost/ Service ($)
A)	Examination	DMD + DA	$.42+.10= .52/min.	15.6 min.	$ 8.11
B)	Prophylaxis	RHD	.13	58.5	7.61
C)	Radiographic 1 complete set	DA	.10	28.6	2.86
D)	Extractions	DMD + DA	.52	19.5	10.14
E)	Periodontal Treatment				
	—Gingival curettage/ quadrant	DMD + DA	.52	58.5	30.42
	—Periodontal scaling and root planing	DMD	.42	58.5	24.57
	—Perio surgery/quadrant	DMD + DA	.52	97.5	50.70
F)	Restorations				
	—1 surface	DMD + DA	.52	15.6	8.11
	—2 surface	DMD + DA	.52	23.4	12.17
	—3 or more	DMD + DA	.52	31.2	16.22
G)	Crowns	DMD + DA	.52	149.5	77.74
H)	Endo-root canal therapy (1 canal)	DMD + DA	.52	78	40.56
I)	Replacement Services				
	—Full dentures				
	—Upper denture	DMD + DA	.52	208	108.16
	—Lower denture	DMD + DA	.52	208	108.16
	—Partial denture	DMD + DA	.52	195	101.40
	—Repair bridges	DMD + DA	.52	26	13.52
	—Repair denture	DMD	.42	26	10.92
	—Reline denture	DMD + DA	.52	61.1	31.77

Table 4

COST CALCULATIONS FOR INPATIENT AND OUTPATIENT DEMAND INCREASES*
FOR YEAR ONE (in dollars)

| DENTAL TREATMENT | OUTPATIENT INCREASES | | | INPATIENT |
	20%	35%	50%	
A) Examination	$ 26,041	$ 45,578	$ 65,107	$ 9,732
B) Prophylaxis	7,233	12,659	18,084	2,702
C) Radiographs	9,183	16,073	22,960	3,432
D) Extractions	4,982	8,719	12,455	1,861
E) Periodontal Rx				
-Gingival curettage/ quadrant	27,252	47,698	68,135	10,191
-Periodontal scaling & root planing (entire mouth)	27,929	48,882	69,826	10,443
-Periodontal surgery/ quadrant	27,350	47,869	68,379	10,191

388

F) Restorations				
-1 surface	8,167	14,290	20,418	3,114
-2 surfaces	9,200	16,089	22,982	3,505
-3 surfaces or more	4,087	7,153	10,205	1,557
G) Crowns	3,187	5,597	8,007	2,318
H) Endodontic Rx				
-1 canal	2,231	3,875	5,535	832
I) Replacement Services				
-Full dentures	139,616	244,359	349,060	52,133
-Upper denture	18,754	32,824	46,889	7,031
-Lower denture	12,156	21,275	30,391	4,541
-Partial denture	31,908	55,847	79,776	11,925
-Repair bridges	1,650	2,887	4,124	615
-Repair dentures	386	675	964	142
-Reline dentures	3,672	6,428	9,182	1,366
SUBTOTAL	$364,984	$638,777	$912,479	$137,631
+25% fringe benefits	91,246	159,694	228,120	34,408
TOTAL	$456,230	$798,471	$1,140,599	$172,039

*(Assume straight line increase in demand over a ten-year period and based on inpatient increases of 10,000 and outpatient increases of 32,110, 56,200, and 80,280, respectively, over ten years).

costs for new patients in the system range from $172,039 for the inpatient's increased demand, to $1,140,599 for the 50% outpatient demand increase. Replacement services account for over 50% of the costs.

Table 5 shows the cost estimates for low, mid and high demand increases projected over a ten-year period. The cost of providing care increases as the number of patients in the system increases. The cost of recall visits for patients in the following years was calculated to be 17% of the total new costs, which is the ratio of the cost of examinations, prophylaxis and periodontal scaling and root planing to the total costs of treatment needed to provide care to the increased inpatient demand and are costs over current budget costs. Initially, the cost of providing care to the new patients is greater than the cost for the recall patients. By year seven, the cost to provide care to the recall patients is greater than the cost for the new patients.

In the first year, the costs range (in constant 1982 dollars) from $628,269 for the low demand to $1,312,638 for the high demand level. The low demand level cost estimates represent less than 1% of the VA Office of Dentistry's FY 1982 expenditures. For the high demand level, the costs in year one are less than 2% of the VA FY 1982 dental expenditure for dental staff salaries. By year ten, these costs increase to $1,589,523 and $3,320,979 (in 1982 dollars) for the low and high demand levels, respectively. The average annual cost per person in year one is approximately $150. This decreases each year to approximately $40 per person (in 1982 dollars) by year ten. This decline reflects the fact that the cost to provide care to first time demanders who may have a backlog of untreated need is greater than the cost to provide maintenance care.

This model illustrates that the cost to provide dental care to elderly veterans new to the VA system may not be overwhelming. However, these ranges of estimates may vary over time for several reasons. First, these estimates assume that the dentist is working with an assistant in most cases. Frequently, due to constraints in staffing patterns the dentist works without an assistant and the time needed to provide the service is usually greater than the offsetting decrease in cost per minute to provide the time without the dental assistant. The model also assumes

Table 5

DIRECT PERSONNEL COST ESTIMATES FOR
LOW, MID AND HIGH LEVEL DEMAND INCREASES
OVER A TEN-YEAR PERIOD (in constant 1982 dollars)

DEMAND LEVEL*

Year	LOW	MID	HIGH
1	$ 628,269	$ 970,510	$1,312,638
2	735,075	1,135,497	1,535,787
3	841,881	1,300,484	1,758,936
4	948,687	1,465,471	1,982,085
5	1,055,493	1,630,458	2,205,234
6	1,162,299	1,795,445	2,428,383
7	1,269,105	1,960,432	2,651,532
8	1,375,911	2,125,419	2,874,681
9	1,482,717	2,290,406	3,097,830
10	1,589,523	2,455,393	3,320,979

*Low demand corresponds to 20% outpatient demand increase
plus the projected 10,000 inpatient increase over ten
years. Moderate demand corresponds to 35% outpatient demand increase plus projected 10,000 inpatient increase.
High demand corresponds to 50% outpatient demand increase
plus projected 10,000 inpatient increase.

that the dental hygienist provides all prophylaxis. Studies have found that dentists do perform prophylaxis some
of the time depending on the availability of the dental
hygienist. Since 40% of the dental facilities do not have
a dental hygienist on staff, at these facilities the dentists perform the prophylaxis routinely. This model did
not include the cost of additional supplies generated by
increased personnel providing services. Also, it is assumed that there will be no increase in office space,
therefore capital costs for increased facilities are not
included in any of these cost estimates. However, since
studies on various nursing home populations have found at
least 50% of the residents unable to leave the nursing
home to receive dental care, the purchase of portable dental equipment may be necessary in the provision of care to

the long term care residents. Portable equipment costs approximately $6,000 for a complete unit (ADEC self-contained unit or ASEPTICO Unit with necessary instruments and supplies). If each of the 172 VAMCs purchased portable equipment the costs incurred would be only $1,032,000 for the entire VA system. However, while the purchase cost is a one-time cost, replacement, maintenance and repair costs would add to overhead costs of each VAMC.

IV. Strategies for Meeting Future Needs

A. Organizational Strategies

The factors which act as barriers to elder veterans receiving needed dental care can be summarized as:

1) Attitudinal barriers on the part of dental staff;
2) Attitudinal barriers on the part of the veteran;
3) Institutional factors, (i.e., factors which prevent the dental service from functioning as cost-effectively as possible);
4) Access/eligibility factors, (i.e., which elderly veterans will be eligible for dental care); and
5) Resource availability.

The most obvious model of VA/community sharing is the existing fee-basis program. However, because of the political concerns regarding this program, specific options for sharing resources are not discussed in this chapter. Rather, a variety of options for improving the delivery of dental care within the VA is provided.

The organizational strategies which the VA can employ to remove these barriers fall into two basic categories: 1) strategies related to the supply of services, and 2) strategies related to the demand for services. The supply strategies focus on measures which enable the VA dental service to improve the quality and quantity of dental care available to the aging veteran. Strategies for increasing supply include: 1) increased VA dental staff, 2) education of dental staff, and 3) increased productivity of the dental service. Demand strategies include: 1) clarifying access and eligibility for various categories of elderly veterans, 2) altering the encounter system from a patient-initiated system to a dental service-initiated system, and 3) changing the attitudes and knowledge base of veterans (potential users).

B. Supply Strategies

1. Increased Personnel

It is difficult to predict the increase in the number of dentists needed to meet the dental care needs of the veteran population. However, it is clear that there will be a need for dental staff, particularly dental hygienists, with skills in geriatric dentistry. Increased dental staff would certainly depend upon increased appropriations and an increase in the number of positions available to the dental service. In the last five years, in terms of real dollars, the VA Office of Dentistry budget has been deflationary. It is clear that meeting the dental needs of an increased number of veterans will increase costs. However, shifting the ratio of dentists to dental hygienists may enable the VA to meet the hygiene needs of veterans more cost-effectively (see Section IV.B.3. Improve Productivity).

2. Educational Resource Programs

Dental staff attitudes play a significant role in the quality of dental care provided. As the need for dental staff with skills in geriatric dentistry increases, continuing dental education programs should be developed to train current dental staff in aspects of geriatric dentistry. In addition, the VA should develop educational programs for nursing staff caring for institutionalized veterans.

In considering educational programs, one cannot ignore the role of dental residents. The VA recently has been re-evaluating the role of residency training programs and in general, affiliation with medical and dental schools. Marcus and Drabek (1976) found that as a result of the presence of dental residents, VA staff dentists stay current with the new and changing technologies of dentistry, thus contributing to improved quality of dental care. Integrating gerontology and geriatric dentistry into the curriculum of the residency training programs would enable residents, as well as dental staff conducting the programs, to develop skills in these areas.

The VA also has initiated a Geriatric Dentistry Fellowship Program to provide training for dentists to become teachers, clinicians and/or researchers in the area of geriatric dentistry. The VA may wish to retain some or all of these fellows to assist in meeting the oral health needs of the aging veteran, specifically to design and conduct educational programs, provide clinical care and/or conduct research in geriatric dentistry.

The Dental Longitudinal Study of the Normative Aging Study has contributed to our understanding of age-related oral changes and dental disease patterns over time (Chauncey and Wayler, 1981; Chauncey, et al., 1981). Such research efforts should be continued and supported. In addition, the VA has a potential to be a leader in the area of dental care delivery to the elderly. In the past, dental health services research and delivery programs have not had as much support as biomedical research. With the increasing number of elderly veterans, the VA has an opportunity to develop and evaluate innovative and cost effective delivery systems.

3. Improve Productivity

Improved productivity can result from several initiatives including: a) altering the mix of dental personnel to increase efficiency in the delivery of dental services, b) improving the management and patient scheduling to decrease underutilization of dental resources, and c) providing more cost effective services.

Alter the Mix of Dental Personnel. Several studies (General Accounting Office, 1981; Marcus and Drabek, 1976) have identified a lack of sufficient dental auxiliaries as a barrier to efficient dental service delivery. In 1981, the General Accounting Office found that over 40% of VA dental clinics did not have even one hygienist on staff. Since 1981, the VA has increased the number of hygienists in the dental program. However, there are still facilities without a dental hygienist.

Marcus and Drabek (1976) found that the shortage of dental hygienists in the VA resulted in dentists performing hygienists' tasks thus preventing them from providing other needed services (i.e., preventive care). As more dentulous elderly seek dental care from the VA, the need for preventive dental services will increase. Since dental hygienists can provide similar services at one-third the costs of a dentist, it is to the VA's advantage to increase the number of dental hygienists on staff.

In the case of providing dental care to the VA nursing home population, studies have shown that dental hygienists can play a significant role in providing dental care to long term care residents (Fontana-Smith and Bennett, 1980; Ayers, 1965). One VAMC Dental Chief interviewed recently has a dental hygienist performing initial screening and oral hygiene to the long term care residents on the wards. Such a program demonstrates that dental hygienists in the VA system can assume a greater responsibility for patient care within the scope of their training. The use of dental hygienists to provide such services should be expanded.

Additionally, studies have noted that the employment of Expanded-Function Dental Auxiliaries (EFDAs) could increase the amount of restorative care dentists could provide (Douglass, et al., 1976; Redig, et al., 1974; Abramowitz and Berg, 1973; Soricelli, 1972; General Accounting Office, 1980). A recent evaluation of the EFDA program in the VA found that EFDAs performed expanded functions about 50% of the time (VA, 1983d). While the EFDA is trained for predominantly restorative dental tasks, the needs of the VA population are often prosthetic in nature. This difference in dental needs primarily accounted for the EFDAs underutilization. If modifications are made in EFDA training to account for the different treatment needs of the VA population, and in particular the elderly veteran, employment of EFDAs could aid in improving productivity of the dental program and in meeting the needs of the elderly veteran.

Improve Management of the Dental Clinics. Cancelled and broken appointments lead to underutilization of chair time and the associated decreased productivity in dental clinics (Marcus and Drabek, 1976). Previous recommendations addressing this problem include improving the clinic management procedures such as initiating a patient appointment reminder system. In his study of the health and social needs of the elderly, Branch (1977) found that one-third of the elderly surveyed reported that they did not have reliable transportation. Transportation to dental clinics and the initiation of a patient reminder system will aid in decreasing appointment cancellation.

For homebound residents of VA nursing homes, dental care could be provided in nursing home facilities using portable dental equipment. One Boston area VA dental service has found that the availability of portable equipment has resulted in patients no longer needing to be scheduled at the convenience of the nursing staff. The availability of portable equipment has been shown to increase the efficiency of dental clinic staff by decreasing the need for transportation of homebound patients, thus enabling institutional staff who were previously required to transport patients to the dental clinic to devote more time to ward duties. It is recommended that the VA make available portable equipment and provide dental services in facilities with NHCUs or large numbers of long term care residents.

Provide Cost Effective Services. Preventive services have been shown to be more cost effective than restorative or prosthetic services (Burt, 1978). Topical and systemic fluorides have been shown to be effective in reducing root caries and xerostomia-related dental caries in adults (Banting and Stamm, 1982; Dreizen, et al., 1977; Westcott, et al., 1975; Johansen, et al., 1979; Stamm and Banting, 1980). Frequent oral prophylaxis has been shown to be effective in controlling the progression of periodontal disease in the elderly (Gron, 1981).

The VA should play a more assertive role in the delivery of preventive dental care to both inpatients and outpatients. Such efforts will preserve the veteran's dental health as well as provide more cost effective care. A strong emphasis on preventive dental services will eliminate the need for more expensive dental procedures (such as the need for restorative procedures due to secondary decay and root surface caries, endodontic treatment due to decay, periodontal treatment due to the lack of adequate oral hygiene skills, and various prosthetic services due to unnecessary loss of teeth). As the number of elderly increase, the ratio of preventive services provided versus the more expensive procedures should be altered so that providing comprehensive dental care to the eligible elderly veteran population is not prohibitively expensive.

As Hospital Based Home Care (HBHC) programs expand, the VA may need to consider developing a dental component to the program. The HBHC program attempts to provide health care to homebound veterans to prevent their re-hospitalization in acute or chronic care facilities. VA dental service staff could train HBHC staff in routine oral hygiene care and oral examinations. The need for dental treatment could be coordinated by the HBHC team with the dental service.

Presently, veterans in community nursing homes and those who are homebound who are eligible for dental care must be transported to the VAMC to receive dental care. Often they are transported at the expense of the VA. Portable dental equipment purchased for use in VA nursing homes could also be used in providing care to the homebound. By taking the dental personnel to the homebound, the VA could eliminate the transportation of frail elderly patients. Current legislation does not permit such activity by dental personnel. Thus, if the VA is to fulfill its Congressional mandate to plan for the health needs of the elderly veteran, legislation similar to that which allows VA physicians to make home visits, should be requested for VA dental personnel.

Improve Delivery of Preventive Services. Specific improvements on the current method of delivering preventive dental care include the following:

1) Decrease the time interval between recall visits to reflect the patient's need, taking into consideration one's physical, mental and dental status. For those veterans with severe limitations in oral hygiene skills, monthly or bimonthly visits with the dental hygienist may be necessary rather than the usual annual or semiannual visits.

2) Develop a standard protocol for the dispensing of tin-gel and other preventive chemotherapeutic agents. Although various preventive agents are readily available to VA dental services, standard protocols for dispensing them to patients do not exist. Such protocols would standardize the use of these preventive agents throughout the VA.

3) Increase the number of dental hygienists on dental service staff to allow efficient utilization of dentist's time. Currently, dentists perform prophylaxis treatments on about 25% of all patients receiving prophylaxis. Although there are some instances where a hygienist cannot perform the task alone (such as cases of severely debilitated or anxious patients), in general, dental services could operate more efficiently if more hygienists were available to perform the necessary preventive services.

4) Develop ward preventive dental programs for VAMCs with sizeable chronic care populations, nursing home care units or domiciliaries. Ward prevention programs can effectively provide oral hygiene care to non-ambulatory patients.

5) Purchase portable dental equipment to enable dental care to be provided to non-ambulatory veterans on the ward or to veterans in community nursing homes.

6) Develop oral hygiene and preventive dental education programs for nurses, patients, their families and VA dental personnel.

Thus, increased emphasis on preventive dentistry should become a major goal of the VA dental service as it prepares to care for the increasing numbers of elderly veterans.

C. Demand Strategies

1. Access

With few exceptions, the private sector is not meeting the dental needs of homebound and institutionalized elders. In order to prevent further deterioration in nutrition and health status, the array of services available to homebound and institutionalized veterans should include dental care. Similarly, elderly veterans with various physical, medical or psychiatric problems are best treated in a hospital environment accustomed to dealing with such problems.

2. Eligibility

Eligibility for VA dental care has become very complicated and difficult to understand even for those working in the VA and, as a result, often acts as a barrier to receiving needed dental care. This occurs for several reasons. First, the vagueness regarding eligibility for outpatient treatment as an adjunct to medical treatment makes it difficult to predict how many Class III veterans will be eligible for dental care as a result of their worsening medical condition. While the law is specific regarding which veterans are eligible for outpatient dental care, there is some variability among professionals in the interpretation of the law. Different medical centers seem to have differing views regarding the types of medical conditions that will be aggravated by various dental diseases. Second, while veterans in VA NHCUs have access to the VA dental service, veterans residing in community nursing homes unless service-connected are not eligible for dental care. Thus, eligibility for dental care for the elderly veteran varies depending upon one's medical condition and one's location of institutionalization.

To eliminate the barrier caused by eligibility complexity and to meet the dental needs of aging veterans, legislation regarding eligibility for dental care should be simplified. An example would be to extend dental benefits to all veterans over age 75. Another option would be to consider providing certain types of services such as diagnosis, prevention and restorative care to all veterans over a certain age. This would allow a large number of elderly veterans to receive some care as opposed to the present system which provides extensive care to a limited number of veterans.

3. Patient Identification

In order to receive dental care, an outpatient must initiate contact with the VA system. This is in contrast to the system for inpatients, particularly VA nursing home residents, where by virtue of their residence in the NHCU, the dental service usually intiates the encounter. Unfortunately, outpatient veterans often seek care only when an emergency arises. As a result, more expensive secondary and tertiary care is needed. To avoid more costly and painful emergency care episodes and to stimulate preventive health behaviors, the VA should actively identify eligible veterans and initiate the encounter rather than wait for the patient to do so. Such action would serve to maintain and preserve the oral health of all eligible veterans and improve the quality of life for older veterans.

4. Change Attitudes of Potential Users

Patient education programs should be developed to 1) enable the veteran to recognize the importance of preventive dental care, and 2) assist the veteran in making appropriate use of both the VA and non-VA dental care systems. It has been suggested that the Office of Dentistry and the Department of Veterans Benefits could develop a pamphlet specific to VA dental benefits. Veterans benefits counselors could distribute this pamphlet, fulfilling a much needed role in public education.

V. Recommendations

In light of this analysis and discussion of organizational strategies, several recommendations are offered in summary.

A. The array of services available to the older veteran should include dental care. The VA Office of Dentistry should develop its potential as a leader in the field of geriatric dentistry.

B. The VA dental service should integrate gerontology into the dental training programs and recruit dental personnel with skills in geriatric dentistry.

C. The VA should continue support of research efforts in the areas of age-related and disease-related changes and expand dental health services research programs in the area of geriatric oral health care.

D. The VA should increase the number of dental hygienists on staff in an effort to meet the preventive needs of an increasingly elderly veteran population. At the minimum, each VAMC should have one dental hygienist on staff.

E. The VA dental service should be a strong advocate for preventive dentistry for the older veteran.

F. To meet the dental needs of the increasing VA nursing home population, the VA should develop a standardized model for delivering dental care to this population, with the dental hygienist as the primary care provider.

G. The VA dental service should make available portable dental equipment to meet the dental needs of non-ambulatory nursing home residents and the homebound.

H. The VA Office of Dentistry should develop a dental component to integrate dentistry into the hospital based home care program and demonstrate its effectiveness in providing oral hygiene care to this population.

I. Congress should provide legislation to allow VA dental personnel to provide dental care to homebound veterans and non-ambulatory residents of community nursing homes in their respective homes.

J. Congress should simplify legislation to allow elderly veterans to receive needed dental care.

REFERENCES

Abramowitz, A. and Berg, L.E. "A Four-Year Study of the Utilization of Dental Assistants with Expanded Functions." Journal of the American Dental Association, 87, p. 623, 1973.

American Dental Association, Bureau of Economic Research and Statistics. "Utilization of Dental Services by the Elderly Population." Chicago, Illinois, 1980.

Ayers, P. Dental Services for Chronically Ill and Aged Patients. Final Report. Community Health Services Grant CH01-1, Birmingham, Alabama, Jefferson County Department of Health, 1965.

Banting, D. and Stamm, J. "Effects of Age and Length of Exposure to Fluoridated Water on Root Surface Fluoride Concentration." Clinical Preventive Dentistry, 4, pp. 3-7, 1982.

Bernhardt, M. "The Dental Problem in Nursing Homes." Pennsylvania Dental Journal, 38, p. 10, 1971.

Branch, L.G. Understanding the Health and Social Needs of People Over Age 65. Center for Survey Research, University of Massachusetts and Joint Center for Urban Studies of Massachusetts Institute of Technology and Harvard University, 1977.

Burt, B. The Relative Efficiency of Methods of Caries Prevention in Dental Public Health. Ann Arbor, Michigan: University of Michigan, 1978.

Carlson, H. "Survey of Massachusetts Nursing Home Dental Consultants." Senior thesis. Harvard School of Dental Medicine, Boston, Massachusetts, 1982.

Chauncey, H. and Wayler, A. "The Modifying Influence of Age on Taste Perception." Special Care in Dentistry, 1, pp. 68-74, 1981.

Chauncey, H., Borkan, G., Wayler, A., et al. "Parotid Fluid Composition in Healthy Aging Males." Advances in Physical Sciences, 28, pp. 323-328, 1981.

Clark, C.R. and Vergeen, S. "Dental Hygiene and Dental Neglect in Nursing Homes in America." Journal of the Oregon Dental Association, 44, pp. 21-41, February, 1975.

Conrad, D. "Dental Care Demand: Age-Specific Estimates for the Population 65 Years of Age and Over." Health Care Financing Review, 4(4), Summer 1983.

Douglass, C.W., Gillings, D.B., Lindahl, R.L. and Moore, S. "Expanded Duty Dental Assistants in Solo Private Practice." Journal of the American College of Dentistry, 43, p. 44, 1976.

Douglass, C., Gillings, D., Sollicito, W. and Gammon, M. "The Potential for Increase in the Periodontal Diseases of the Aged Population." Journal of Periodontology, 54, pp. 721-730, 1983.

Douglass, C., Gammon, M. and Horgan, W. "Epidemiology of Oral Cancer." In Oral Cancer, Sklar, G. (Ed.). Philadelphia: Saunders Company, in press.

Drake, C.W. "Dental Needs of the Chronically Ill and Aged." Journal of Public Health Dentistry, 30, p. 239, 1970.

Dreizen, S., Brown, L., Daly, T. and Drone, J. "Prevention of Xerostomia-Related Dental Caries in Irradiated Cancer Patients." Journal of Dental Research, 56, pp. 99-104, 1977.

Ettinger, R. and Beck, J. "The New Elderly: What Can the Dental Profession Expect?" Special Care in Dentistry, 2(2), March-April, 1982.

Evashwick, C., Conrad, D. and Lee, F. "Factors Related to Utilization of Dental Services by the Elderly." American Journal of Public Health, 72(10), 1982.

Feld, R. "Dental Needs of Nursing Home Patients." Pennsylvania Dental Journal, 38, pp. 7-9, 1971.

Fischer, E. Director, Dental Planning and Analysis Service, VA Office of Dentistry. Personal communication, 1982.

Fontana-Smith, D. and Bennett, J. "Preliminary Report on a Dental Program in a Long-Term Care Facility." University of Oregon, Health Sciences Center. Personal communication, December, 1980.

General Accounting Office. Increased Use of Expanded Function Dental Auxiliaries Would Benefit Consumers, Dentists, and Taxpayers. Washington, D.C.: USGAO, March, 1980.

General Accounting Office. Providing Veterans with Service-Connected Dental Problems Higher Priority at VA Clinics Could Reduce Fee-Program Costs. Report to the Honorable Alan Cranston, U.S. Senate. Washington, D.C.: USGAO, June, 1981.

Gillings, D., Sollicito, W. and Douglass, C.W. "A Needs-Based Model to Project National Dental Expenditures." Journal of Public Health Dentistry, 43, pp. 8-24, 1983.

Gron, P. "Preventive Dental Health Program for the Elderly: Rationale and Preliminary Findings." Special Care, 1, pp. 129-132, 1981.

Gustafsson, B.E., Quensel, C.E., Lanke, L.S., Lundquist, C., Grahnen, H., Bonow, B.E. and Krasse, B. "The Vepeholm Dental Caries Study: The Effect of Different Levels of Carbohydrate Intake on Caries Activity in 436 Individuals Observed for Five Years." Acta Odontologica Scandinavica, 11, p. 232, 1954.

Hazen, S.P., Chilton, N.W. and Mumma, R.D. "The Problem of Root Caries. 3. A Clinical Study." International Association of Dental Research Abstract, 50, p. 219, 1972.

Institute of Medicine. Public Policy Options for Better Dental Health. Report of a Study. IOM 80-06. Washington, D.C.: National Academy Press, December, 1980.

Johansen, E., Taves, D. and Olsen, T. (Eds.) Continuing Evaluation of the Use of Fluorides. American Association for the Advancement of Science, pp. 61-110, 1979.

Marcus, M. and Drabek, L. Study of VA Dental Manpower Requirements. Los Angeles: UCLA School of Dentistry, 1976.

Milton, B., Donohue, M. and Gregory, J. "Oral Health Status of Vermont Nursing Home Residents: Results of a Pilot Survey." Bureau of Economic and Behavioral Research, American Dental Association, Chicago, Illinois, January, 1981.

National Center for Health Services Research, National Health Care Expenditures Study. Dental Services: Use Expenditures and Sources of Payment. DHHS - Publication No. (PHS) 82-3319, Washington, D.C., October, 1982.

National Center for Health Statistics. Edentulous Persons in the U.S. Series 10, 89. Washington, D.C., June, 1974a.

National Center for Health Statistics. Comparison of Percent Distribution of Adults of Periodontal Disease According to Sex and Age. Series 10, 89. Washington, D.C., June, 1974b.

National Center for Health Statistics. Basic Data on Dental Examination Findings of Persons 1-74 Years. US 1971-74. Health and Nutrition Examination Survey (HANES). Vital and Health Statistics Series II, No. 24, Washington, D.C., 1979.

Page, W.F. "Why Veterans Choose Veterans Administration Hospitalization: A Multivariate Model." Medical Care, 20(3), pp. 308-320, March, 1982.

Redig, D., Snyder, M., Nevitt, G. and Tocchini, J. "Expanded Duty Dental Auxiliaries in Four Private Dental Offices: The First Year's Experience." Journal of the American Dental Association, 88, p. 969, 1974.

Reinhalter, N. "The Problem of Massachusetts Nursing Homes in Delivering Oral and Dental Care." Unpublished data, 1975.

Soricelli, D. "Implementation of the Delivery of Dental Services by Auxiliaries: The Philadelphia Experience." American Journal of Public Health, 62, p. 1077, 1972.

Stamm, J.W. and Banting, D.W. "Comparison of Root Caries Prevalence in Adults with Lifelong Residence in Fluoridated and Non-Fluoridated Communities." Journal of Dental Research, 59, Special Issue A:405, 1980.

405

Sumney, D.L., Jordan, H.V. and Englander, H.R. "The Prevalence of Root Surface Caries in Selected Populations." Journal of Periodontology, 44, pp. 500–504, 1973.

U.S. Department of Health, Education and Welfare. Public Health Service. Cancer Incidence and Mortality in the United States, 1973–77. SEER-NIH Publ. No. 81 (2330). National Cancer Institute Monograph No. 57. Bethesda: Public Health Service, 1981.

U.S. Veterans Administration. The Aging Veteran, Present and Future Medical Needs. Washington, D.C., 1977.

U.S. Veterans Administration. 1979 National Survey of Veterans, Summary Report. Washington, D.C., 1979.

U.S. Veterans Administration. Department of Medicine and Surgery, Dentistry Manual M-4, Washington, D.C., 1980.

U.S. Veterans Administration. Health Care of the Aging Veteran: A Report of the Geriatrics and Gerontology Advisory Committee. Washington, D.C., April, 1983a.

U.S. Veterans Administration. Office of Dentistry. AMIS Report. Washington, D.C., June 30, 1983b.

U.S. Veterans Administration. Caring for the Older Veteran. Report of the Veterans Administration Special Medical Advisory Group, Task Force on the Geriatric Plan. Washington, D.C., July, 1983c.

U.S. Veterans Administration. Office of Dentistry. Task Force Report on the Utilization of Expanded Function Dental Auxiliaries in the Veterans Administration Dental Service. Washington, D.C., July, 1983d.

Wan, T.T.H. and Odell, D.G. "Factors Affecting the Use of Social and Health Services among the Elderly." Aging and Society, 1(1), pp. 95–114, 1981.

Westcott, W., Starcke, E. and Shannon, I. "Chemical Protection against Post-Irradiation Dental Caries." Oral Surgery, 40, pp. 709–719, 1975.

Wolford, W. Indian Health Service, Albuquerque, New Mexico, personal communication, 1983.

Yellowitz, J.A., Katz, R.A., Portnoy, R. and Smith, B. "The Minnesota Dental Insurance Program for Senior Citizens: Two Year Results for the Utilization of Dental Services." Journal of the American Dental Association, 104, p. 453, 1982.

12. Improving Care of the Older Veteran: Issues and Options

Mark Schlesinger
Terrie Wetle, Ph.D.
James H. Morse, M.D.

Introduction

The Veterans Administration health care system is facing a period of substantial change. The "aging" of the
veteran population is expected to alter the amount and
type of care required by veterans. To meet the needs of
the elder veteran, it may prove necessary to alter the
ways in which the VA delivers health care.

The changes in the health care needs that result from
an aging population are quite complex, touching every institution in the VA system. The nature of this change
differs by institution. For example, age-related influences on outpatient care may be very different from those
affecting inpatient care; the interactions between the VA
and non-VA care systems may be different for nursing homes
than for hospitals. Adapting to such complicated changes
in health care demands represents a substantial challenge.

In the accompanying chapters, the authors developed
sets of specific proposals which would enable the VA to
adapt to these changing needs. Taken together, these outline a fairly comprehensive set of options for the VA
health care system. To effectively respond to the substantial changes facing it, however, the VA requires more

409

than a set of options. These options must be integrated into a coherent strategy for response. This integration must:

- Identify common themes among the individual options since these themes represent factors most broadly affecting the VA;

- Identify conflicts among the individual options, since a number of goals may not be mutually compatable;

- Reflect the basic mandate under which the VA health care system operates, since reforms which conflict with that mandate will prove difficult to implement; and

- Set priorities among the reforms available to the VA, since many require additional resources to be implemented.

This chapter does not develop a comprehensive strategy of change; rather it outlines the issues relevant to the development of such a strategy. More specifically, the discussion is divided into three parts. The first describes in broad terms the challenge facing the VA as it attempts to adapt to the needs of an older veteran population within the constraints and expectations of Congress and veterans groups. The second section reviews and consolidates the options available to the VA, as identified in the accompanying chapters. The third briefly describes issues associated with the implementation of these options, including a description of barriers to change within and outside the VA.

I. The Challenge for the Veterans Administration

A. The VA's Mandate

The mandate for the VA's health care system has been defined and modified by a series of Acts of Congress. These Congressional dictates have at times been quite explicit; at other times somewhat ambiguous. Taken together, they define a mandate with three major elements:

1. The VA is to provide comprehensive health care to veterans of a quality equivalent to that available through the general health care system. This aspect of the man-

410

date has evolved over time. The VA was designed as a system to deliver specialized health care. The current emphasis on the quality of care developed following World War II, prompting the VA to affiliate with academic medical centers (Thompson, 1981). These same concerns, spurred by pressures from other parts of the federal government, have led to the development of a more comprehensive set of services, including outpatient clinics and facilities for long term care.

2. <u>Access to health care under VA auspices is in the form of a "quasi-entitlement."</u> Veteran status entitles an individual to seek care from the VA. It does not, however, guarantee that the veteran will actually receive care -- the VA is constrained to provide only as much treatment as can be financed within a predetermined budget. Because the VA cannot provide service to all veterans who might seek care, access to care is determined by a set of priorities. Current priorities in part reflect a sense of obligation (e.g., the presence of a service-connected disability). Other priorities are based on measures of need, such as the veteran's ability to pay for health care from other sources.

3. <u>The VA health care system is to be supported exclusively by prospective budgeting rather than fee-based revenues.</u> In part this is intended to avoid barriers to using the VA based on financial considerations. Although the VA has periodically sought to decentralize the administration of its health care system, current financing arrangements serve to centralize lines of authority in the VA by making programs dependent on a centrally determined budget for their funding (Sapolsky, 1977).

The nature of the VA mandate has led the VA health care system to develop in particular ways. The emphasis on quality, and subsequent affiliation with academic medical centers, has produced a system which is predominantly oriented to acute care hospitals and the physicians practicing within them (Sapolsky, 1977). This is reflected in the delivery of long term care to veterans. Ninety percent of veterans entering nursing homes under VA auspices pass through a VA medical center (VAMC)(VA, 1983c); physicians play a far more important role on the teams of hospital based home care (HBHC) programs than they do in comparable home care programs outside the VA.[1] The home care delivered under VA auspices is explicitly restricted

411

to not include any non-medical support services (VA, 1983c).

Similarly, the VA health care system has been shaped by the emphasis on eligibility and the limitation that programs be financed exclusively through a central VA budget. Entitlements allow veterans to switch with relative ease between the VA system and non-VA systems. This reduces the ability of the VA to provide continuity of care and may reduce incentives for the VA to develop preventive care programs, since many of the expected benefits of such programs may be more likely felt by non-VA providers than by providers within the VA system. The emphasis on central budgeting means that VAMCs have limited incentives and perhaps limited capacity to cooperate and collaborate with other providers in the community. It may also encourage an emphasis on institutional care, since facilities and filled beds are more visible to Congress than are outpatient programs (Lindsay, 1975).

The ambiguity of the VA's current mandate also serves to create tensions within the health care system. First, priorities for access based on need may conflict with those based on obligation. Second, the desire to deliver comprehensive care to some veterans may imply, given a limited budget, that the VA is unable to provide even minimal care for other veterans. Third, it remains unclear whether the VA has a mandate to provide comprehensive care, as opposed to ensuring that veterans receive that care from some source. Currently the VA falls somewhere between; some care delivered under its auspices is provided through contracts with private or other public agencies. Conversely, there exists no mechanism within the VA to ensure that elder veterans who are eligible for health care benefits receive comprehensive care from any source.[2]

These ambiguities led different groups -- veterans interest groups, oversight committees, Congressional subcommittees, and VA administrators -- to develop divergent expectations regarding the role which the VA is to play in the care of the elder veteran. This chapter assumes that strategies for reform within the VA should be based on an interpretation of the mandate which holds that (1) the VA should ensure that veterans receive comprehensive health care, but need not necessarily provide that care directly, and (2) that need should play the primary role in the allocation of care. The discussion of implementation which follows, however, reflects the possibility that particular

412

interest groups may interpret the VA's mandate in different ways.

B. Changing Demands for Care under VA Auspices

The aging of the veteran population is expected to increase the amount and alter the nature of care demanded from the VA. These changes will be largely outside the control of the VA, and include age-related changes in health and help-seeking behavior, changes in the socio-economic status of elder veterans and fluctuation in the availability of services in the general health care system (see Table 1). The challenge for the VA is to adapt to these changes within the constraints of its mandate. The problem facing the VA can be divided into three parts:

- The demand for outpatient and inpatient care is likely to increase, although the VA budget is likely to remain relatively fixed.

- There will be a shift in the nature of demand toward care of chronic illness, toward need for social services coordinated with health care, and toward a different "style" of help-seeking behavior and utilization of VA facilities.

- There is likely to be considerable variation in the quantity and types of demand for VA services, both over time and from one geographic region to another.

1. Increases in Demand for Care

Age-related increases in utilization will affect the entire VA health care system. Hospital admissions are expected to increase by some 30% by the year 2000 (Seitz, 1981). Outpatient utilization is expected to increase at a slightly less rapid rate (VA, 1983a), but the number of nursing home beds provided under VA auspices is conservatively projected to rise by at least 80% during the same period (Bresler and Mort, 1982). Given the nature of funding for the VA, there is no guarantee that the budget for care will expand at an equivalent rate.

2. Changes in the Nature of Demand for Care

The nature of the use of VA services is likely to shift because 1) older veterans tend to require a differ-

413

Table 1

CHANGING DEMANDS FOR CARE AND ISSUES
FACING THE VA HEALTH CARE SYSTEM

Type of Change in the Need or Demand for Care	Potential Problems Facing the VA
I. Increased Demand for Care	
	• Limited capacity for adjustment in VA budget • Access to non-VA services • Limited involvement in non-VA planning processes
II. Changes in the Nature of Demands	
1. Increased Geriatric Care	• Focus of VAMCs on non-geriatric care • Personnel who lack geriatric interest or expertise
2. Increased Demand for Chronic Care	• Focus of VAMCs on acute care • Separation of health and social programs
3. Continuity of Care	• Full continuum of care not available • Use of VA and non-VA services by eligible veterans • Sporadic contact of veterans with VA health care system
4. Behaviors of Older Veterans	• Late and underreporting of symptoms • Inexperience with health care system

Type of Change in the Need or Demand for Care	Potential Problems Facing the VA
III. Variations in Demand for VA Care	
1. Changes over Time	• Limited involvement in planning processes of other federal agencies • Lack of information regarding future demand • Focus on institutional care provided in VA facilities
2. Geographic Variation	• Limited involvement in local planning efforts • Local data availability

ent set of services than do their younger counterparts, and 2) older patients are more likely to suffer from chronic conditions which require the delivery of a health and social services package (Mac Adam and Piktialis, 1984). To meet these needs, a health care delivery system must provide some continuity of care and a broad set of services delivered by a variety of medical and non-medical professionals (Besdine, et al., 1984). The need for continuity presents problems for the VA health care system as it is currently organized. Only 10% of veterans over the age of 65 consider the VA their regular source of care and approximately 66% of the elder veterans who receive care under VA auspices in any one year also receive care from other sources (Schlesinger, et al., 1984). Veterans without service-connected disabilities are not authorized to receive the outpatient care required for continuity of treatment unless at risk of hospitalization. Continuity of care can therefore be provided entirely within the VA system for only a small fraction of older veterans.

The elder veterans using VA health care facilities may seek treatment in a different manner than do their younger counterparts. The aging of the veteran population may thus lead to a shift in the delivery of health care which departs from what is currently perceived as the VA's "mission." Hospital care has been sought in large part by veterans with below average income, limited insurance, or by those veterans who are otherwise lacking easy access to non-VA facilities (Page, 1982; Schlesinger, et al., 1984). Elder veterans receiving treatment at VA outpatient clinics or nursing homes, in contrast, are often not those with the fewest financial resources (Schlesinger, et al., 1984). As the VA increases the delivery of long term care, therefore, it may serve less as a provider of last resort for veterans unable to receive services elsewhere.

Older veterans are likely to seek care in a different manner than younger veterans. Evidence indicates that older patients tend to underreport symptoms, considering them a natural consequence of aging (Besdine, et al., 1984). This suggests that a system which actively assesses health care needs would lead to higher quality care and reduction in demands for care that result from the failure to treat conditions at an early stage. The current system operated by the VA does not seem well-equipped to deal with this underreporting behavior. There exists little in the way of systematic comprehensive health care assessment even for those veterans who do seek care from VA facilities.[3] Perhaps more importantly, only 7% of all elder veterans have any contact with the VA health care system in the course of a year (Schlesinger, et al., 1984). Case-finding programs could address some of these problems. Such programs, however, are likely to further stimulate demand for care under VA auspices, exacerbating problems created by budget constraints (Mac Adam and Piktialis, 1984).

3. Variability in Demand for Care

Service utilization by elder veterans is likely to be highly variable in three ways. First, the demand for care is likely to vary over time. Much of this variation will be difficult to predict because it is influenced by alterations in coverage by Medicare or Medicaid or changes in the availability of non-VA health care facilities. This variation, though not totally predictable, will have significant consequences for the VA health care system. Only 10% of eligible elder veterans now use VA facilities. Even if a relatively small fraction of the eligible population shifted into the VA health care system, it would represent a significant increase in the amount of care demanded from VA facilities. If, for example, in response

416

to increased co-payments under Medicare, as few as 10% of elder veterans ceased to use a private physician as a regular source of care, the VA could anticipate an increase of roughly 15,000 veterans seeking hospitalization and 40,000 requesting outpatient care (Schlesinger, et al., 1984).

Second, there may be significant geographic variation in the demand for care from the VA. Long term care outside the VA is funded principally through Medicaid. The generosity of Medicaid programs varies greatly from one state to the next, and it is quite possible that some states will, in the near future, adopt policies which explicitly channel eligible veterans into the VA system, rather than pay for them under Medicaid auspices (Black, 1981). Estimates of the number of Medicaid eligible elder veterans suggest that the adoption of such channeling policies would quadruple the demand for nursing home care provided by the VA (Schlesinger, et al., 1984).

Third, some variation in the health care required by elder veterans is quite predictable. The projected increases in care required by the World War II and Korean War cohorts will be followed in subsequent decades by a sharp decline in the need for long term care. Unless there is proper planning, the passing of this "age bulge" may leave the VA with a system of over expanded and underutilized facilities.

The challenge currently facing the VA can thus be attributed to three types of changes in health care needs and demands that accompany an aging veteran population. The discussion above, although far from exhaustive, has sketched some of the potential problems facing the VA as it attempts to adapt to a changing patient mix. These are summarized in Table 1. For each of these changes, the VA has two basic strategies of response. It can either:

- Control the demand for VA health care by influencing the actions of veterans or by diverting them to the general health care system, or

- Increase the VA's capacity to adapt to these changes, either by modifying the mix of services or by changing administrative procedures.

417

In the next section of this chapter, specific options developed in the accompanying chapters are classified by the type of problem they are designed to meet.

II. The VA and the Elder Veteran: Options for Change

The options developed in the preceding chapters address the problems of increased demand for care, the changing nature of demand for care, and variability in demand for care as the population of veterans ages. Table 2 arrays the options as they relate to each of these categories and provides the number of the chapter in which the option is developed. Because of the broad range of programs and client populations addressed in these options, they do not conveniently "fit" into any single system of classification. The classification system in Table 2 is provided to facilitate analysis of the options as a package of reforms.

Review of the options illuminates a number of cross cutting issues. The first is the interrelationship between the VA and non-VA health care systems. Although it is clear that factors in one system influence behaviors in the other, there is also evidence of many barriers to closer coordination among the many components of the VA and non-VA care systems. Many options directly address these barriers. The second cross cutting issue relates to the problem of targeting geriatric services. This involves questions of eligibility as well as problems of developing "needs-based" service provision.

The third cross cutting issue relates to whether the VA will provide services directly, will contract with community agencies to provide services or will enter into one of a variety of "sharing" relationships with community agencies in order to obtain services required by older veterans. Options are provided which address each of these models.

Finally, there is an apparent need to educate staff and older veterans regarding a number of topics including disease and old age, eligibility for VA services, and the community service system. Health services research to evaluate and study the provision of care to older veterans is also needed.

The options in the accompanying chapters were based on the assumption that there should not be fundamental changes in the mandate under which the VA operates. Major changes in this mandate can be adopted only with considerable political difficulty and in many cases large administrative costs. Some of the options described, however, require alterations in the mandate. The first section of this chapter divided the mandate for the VA health care system into three parts: (1) the delivery of comprehensive, high-quality care, (2) the definition of access as a "quasi-entitlement," and (3) the restriction of funding care solely through a centrally determined budget. It is recognized that modifications could be made to any of these three elements in efforts to better provide care for elder veterans.

A. A Shift Away from Comprehensive Care

The VA appears to have a comparative advantage in the delivery of particular types of services. As a large, centralized health care system, the VA holds the potential to develop many sorts of system-wide innovations which are increasingly recognized as assets in the general health care system (Brown, 1981; Vladeck, 1981). As a system which has closely integrated its long term care and acute facilities (VA, 1983a), the VA has a substantial advantage over other providers in developing such innovations as teaching nursing homes or geriatric psychiatric units.

At the same time, it must be recognized that the prevailing incentives within the VA health care system may at times represent liabilities. The strong physician-orientation within the VA, while providing a safeguard on quality of medical care, often lacks an orientation toward community based long term care, and may contribute to the cost of care. Costs in the VA's hospital based home care program, for example, average more than twice the rate paid by Medicare for home health care.[4] It is likely that many veterans could be well-served by less intensive and less expensive care.

Similarly, the advantages of a large-scale system are sometimes offset by the liabilities of reduced program flexibility and accompanying increases in costs. Both construction and operating costs in VA nursing homes, for example, are considerably higher than in facilities operated by either state government or private corporations (GAO, 1981). The VA might be able to increase flexibility and reduce costs by shifting to a mode in which provision of needed service was ensured (but not necessarily delivered) by the VA. This could be accomplished through either a

Table 2 (cont.)
OPTIONS FOR MEETING THE NEEDS OF OLDER VETERANS

II. Changes in Nature of Demand (cont.)   Chapter #

    a. Future care providers
      1) VA serves as training site   1
    b. Current care providers
      1) In-service training   1
      2) VA serves as model for comprehensive care   1
      3) VA develops and disseminates geriatric
         information   1
  2. Comprehensive functional assessment   1,5

B. Chronic Care   1,5,6
1. Develop non-institutional alternatives   1,5,6,8

C. Continuity of Care   1,5,6
1. Comprehensive functional assessment   1
2. Surveillance program for high risk elders   1
3. Case management   1,5,6
   a. VA as case manager   5,6
   b. VA contracts for case managers   5,6
   c. VA cooperates in case management   5,6

D. Changing demands/behavior of older veterans
1. Health promotion/health education   1
   a. Change knowledge and beliefs
      about disease and age   1
   b. Increase knowledge of self-care   1
   c. Instruct veteran regarding use
      of health system   1

III. Variations in Demand

A. Planning process
1. VA plans to meet changes in demand   5,6
2. Identify non-VA strategies which will
   alter demand for VA   5,6

B. Coordination with community services
1. Preferred provider arrangements   5,6
2. Contracts to increase flexibility   5,6

C. Health services research to better predict demand   1

supplemental insurance plan or by the VA acting as case manager and financial intermediary for care delivered by other providers.

B. Changes in Eligibility

A second set of potential changes in the mandate involves alteration of the eligibility priorities. Some options have suggested provision of benefits and services to non-veteran spouses and family members. Others have suggested targeting of services based on need and risk factors. These changes would require a re-examination of the current priorities. Alternatively, the notion of free access might be altered. Veterans wishing care from the VA could be required to agree to a "lock-in" period, during which they would seek care only under VA auspices. This would facilitate the VA's efforts to ensure continuity of care for these veterans. It would also lay the groundwork for developing more innovative methods of linking the financing and administration of care within the VA. This "locked-in" population could be used to establish a network of pre-paid care similar to health maintenance organizations. Incentives within such a network might work to limit unnecessary utilization (Luft, 1981), particularly of acute hospital care, which is likely to be a major problem for the VA as age-related increases in hospitalization appear over the next twenty years (Seitz, 1981).

C. Changes in Financing

Eliminating the restriction on charging fees for care within the VA would open several additional options for coping with age-related shifts in demand. Co-payments on a sliding scale could be introduced both to limit unnecessary use of VA facilities and to redirect demand for particular services to non-VA providers. Establishing the appropriate information systems to permit billing to third-party insurers, though costly, might encourage sharing agreements involving VA and non-VA patients and would make individual VAMCs less dependent on the central budgeting process.[5] A change in the formula used for determining regional or facility budgets which places greater emphasis on non-institutional services is another method of changing financial incentives. Full consideration of changes of this magnitude, however, is neither within the scope of this chapter nor a focus of this project. They are raised as examples of the broad array of options facing the VA.

III. Implementing Change within the VA

In the preceding pages and accompanying chapters we have developed a large set of options for the VA. Identifying options for reform can be helpful, but implementing those options may present considerable problems. Some of these barriers result from the costs of new programs in a period when Congress seems disinclined to increase spending for social services. Other barriers are political. The extent of political opposition will depend in part on the nature of the option. Options which add to the set of services offered under VA auspices are likely to engender very little resistance, while those that favor specialization are likely to create concern. Reforms which alter the basic mandate under which the VA health care system operates are likely to create the most opposition, particularly those that limit the freedom of choice currently available to veterans (Thompson, 1981).

It is not the intent of this chapter to explore in detail either these or other problems of implementation. It is important to recognize, however, that implementing many of the options described above requires that the VA confront a number of administrative issues. More specifically, there are four administrative problems which must be dealt with, to at least some extent, to develop an effective strategy for meeting the changing needs now facing the VA. These are:

- The difficulty in targeting programs to particular subpopulations of elder veterans,

- The unresolved tension between the use of obligation and need as criteria for access to care,

- The limitations which exist on the ability of the VA to integrate its service delivery system with non-VA providers, and

- The difficulties of creating incentives for providers within the VA system to act in ways consistent with system-wide goals.

A. Targeting Programs

Several of the options identified are beneficial to the VA only if programs can be directed to a particular set of elder veterans. Expanding services to the spouses of older

423

veterans, for example, will increase the costs of those programs. It will decrease overall costs for the VA only if (a) these services allow the veteran's spouse to remain living at home, and (b) this leads to reduced need for health care or lower rates of institutionalization under VA auspices (Wetle and Evans, 1984). The more precisely one can target services to couples who respond in these ways, the more desirable this option appears for the VA. Similarly, case management tends to reduce costs of care for many of those at risk of institutionalization, but often increases the overall costs of care because it leads to the identification of previously undetected illness (Mac Adam and Piktialis, 1984). Case management reduces overall costs only if it can be directed to those who are most "at risk" for intensive utilization patterns.

In practice it has proven difficult to successfully target programs in this manner. For this reason, most of the first generation case management programs led to increased health care costs in the community (Stasson and Holakan, 1981; U.S. DHHS, 1981). Similarly, many of the supported housing programs designed to serve the impaired elderly in fact benefited elders who were not impaired (U.S. DHEW, 1978). Targeting problems occurred for two reasons. First, it is difficult to predict which elders are at highest risk for particular outcomes. Second, when instruments do exist to measure targeting criteria, their use is often expensive or impractical.

Under these conditions, it is often most feasible to direct programs to individuals based on readily observable characteristics. These characteristics are often poor proxies, however, for the factors one would ideally use as targeting criteria. Two types of errors can be introduced by using proxies. First the "wrong" individuals may be included, or second, individuals who should receive treatment may be excluded from the program. The extent of these two errors defines the "target efficiency" of a program.

The need to target programs was recognized in the report of the Special Medical Advisory Group (SMAG) to the Task Force on the VA Geriatric Plan (1983). This group advocated multi-stage targeting criteria in which priority for treatment was based on service-connected (SC) disabilities, age (with priority given those over the age of 75) and payment of VA pension. These lead to a ranking of elder veterans as portrayed in Figure 1.

424

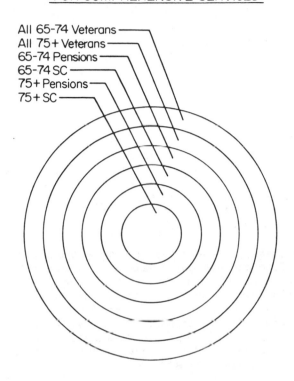

Figure 1
PRIORITIES RECOMMENDED IN SMAG REPORT
FOR COMPREHENSIVE SERVICES

All 65-74 Veterans
All 75+ Veterans
65-74 Pensions
65-74 SC
75+ Pensions
75+ SC

Source: Veterans Administration

Although the SMAG report is important in its recognition of the need for targeting, the proposed criteria are
subject to challenge. Part of this challenge could be on
legal grounds, since the pension criteria essentially create a means test for service to elder veterans. This
would seem to be in conflict with the provisions of P.L.
91-50 which specifically exempt veterans over the age of
65 from means testing to determine eligibility for care
under VA auspices. It could also be argued that the SMAG
criteria have a relatively low target efficiency. Only
30% of elder veterans with service-connected disabilities
reported considering the VA as their regular source of
care; only 40% reported using VA health care facilities
during the previous year.[6] Case-finding programs directed at all veterans with service-connected disabilities

would likely draw into the VA system a large number of veterans who had previously been using other sources of care.

Any criteria will be imperfect. The important questions are: 1) whether it is possible to develop easily obtained measures which make targeting of specific programs effective, and 2) the extent to which these criteria are compatible with existing eligibility criteria.

B. Eligibility and Access

A number of the options identified above involved the VA delivery of care to non-veterans. Some proposals call for the VA to extend services to spouses, others suggest sharing programs in which the VA would serve some non-veterans in exchange for the treatment of veterans in community facilities. Other options require more extensive contracting with non-VA providers.

Each of these proposals has a common theme, the shift of patients from one system to another. These reforms may lead to important benefits for the VA system and the health of elder veterans. To implement the proposals, however, it will be necessary to carefully resolve questions of eligibility and access. More specifically, it is important to deal with two problems: the ineligibility of non-veterans for care under VA auspices and the eligibility of veterans in non-VA settings.

Currently, non-veterans served under sharing agreements are officially accorded the lowest priority for outpatient care and rank just above patients requesting discretionary transfers for inpatient care (SMAG, 1983). If VA facilities are operating with sufficient excess capacity, this represents no serious barrier to sharing programs. Age-related increases in utilization by veterans are likely, however, to strain the capacity of VA services. Under such conditions, sharing agreements will not appear attractive to non-VA providers, since they would have little guarantee that their patients would be expeditiously served. Official priorities also create a dilemma for certain proposals to serve non-veterans. It has been argued, for instance, that the VA could benefit from home health services which simultaneously served the elder veteran and spouse. This creates difficult problems for determining the priorities for care. Would eligibility requirements, for example, mandate delivering care to the

426

spouse of a veteran with service-connected disabilities before serving a veteran without a service-connected disability? It is assumed that the benefits of serving the spouse flow both to the veteran and to the system, but such a change would require that in some circumstances a non-veteran receive a higher effective priority than a veteran.

Somewhat different eligibility issues arise when veterans are served in non-VA settings. It appears unlikely that many community providers would be willing to enforce eligibility rankings which distinguish veterans with service-connected disabilities from those who do not have them. This is particularly true for programs funded under Title III of the Older Americans Act, which are legally constrained in the use of eligibility criteria for access. Thus, if the VA expands its use of contracting and sharing arrangements, maintenance of VA priorities will require careful negotiation.

C. Integrating VA and Non-VA Service Systems

A number of the options identified are based on closer collaboration between VA and non-VA providers. Benefits are foreseen from collaboration in planning (Mac Adam and Piktialis, 1984) as well as in the provision of services (Besdine, et al., 1984; Mac Adam and Piktialis, 1984; Baug, et al., 1984). Again, although these benefits may be very real, it is important to recognize that obtaining them may entail substantial costs.

The principle barriers to collaboration in planning stem from the fragmented nature of the non-VA long term care system. The number of agencies involved in long term care planning may in itself make collaboration a daunting proposition. In Massachusetts, for example, planning for extended care is distributed among the Departments of Elder Affairs, Public Health, Public Welfare, Mental Health and Social Services, the Massachusetts Commission for the Blind, the Rate Setting Commission, the Commission on Administration and Finance, and the system of local health planning agencies. The situation is further complicated by the divergent objectives of those agencies. In their review of planning for extended care in New England, Wennberg and Gittleson (1981) noted that "the many studies and white papers notwithstanding, there is usually disagreement within state government as to the preferred direction for long term care policy" (pp. 187-188).

427

Under these circumstances, it may be more practical to develop planning agreements with particular sets of provider agencies. The delivery of care within the VA is likely to be more sensitive to the availability of certain types of non-VA services than for others. It may thus make sense to coordinate planning only for those services most affecting the VA. This sort of "target planning" clearly suffers from the liability of not being comprehensive, but the complication of more comprehensive planning may make such planning not feasible.

The second source of interaction between VA and non-VA agencies involves contracting and sharing agreements. As noted above, the VA may have difficulty incorporating existing eligibility requirements into such agreements. In addition, the VA may face serious problems monitoring the quality of care delivered in non-VA settings. The VA's experience in monitoring other providers has met with mixed results. On one hand, its ability to select community nursing homes to provide care to veterans has been praised (National Academy of Sciences, 1977); on the other hand, its attempts to monitor performance of the relatively small (41 facilities) state nursing home program has been soundly criticized (GAO, 1981). The more extensively the VA seeks to use community based providers, the more difficult it may become to select only those agencies that can assuredly provide high quality care (Smith, 1981).

D. Reforms and Internal Incentives

One of the clearest lessons from the experience of non-VA health planning programs over the past decade is that the best intentioned and most carefully designed programs will not significantly alter the delivery of health care unless they provide the appropriate incentives to the providers of care. It has often been argued that the incentives which prevail in the VA lead to excessive lengths of stay and over-emphasis on inpatient at the expense of outpatient care (Sapolsky, 1977; Lindsay, 1975). Other incentives which may lead to undesirable practices also exist, but are less widely recognized. The open nature of the VA health care system provides few incentives for the delivery of preventive care, since benefits of reduced utilization are shared with non-VA providers. The separation of pension and health care programs in the VA creates no incentives to integrate benefits to control overall costs of the two programs.

428

These incentives can be changed in various ways. Centralized budgeting could be continued, but formulas for allocating funds to VAMCs altered to encourage the delivery of non-institutional care. Alternatively, programmatic changes, such as short term "lock-in" for veterans using the VA system could be implemented. Each of these might well eliminate a number of undesirable incentives which currently exist in the VA system. They would do little, though, to change the incentives facing the individual providers of care who make many of the decisions which affect the delivery of care.

The behavior of providers could be altered in several ways. First, financial incentives could be changed. Payment to providers in VA settings could be linked to patient treatment along the model of a number of non-VA physician capitation plans. This might prove difficult to implement without some sort of lock-in for veterans using the system, but the existing VA information system, if sufficiently automated, could be sufficient to operate such a system. A second approach would base providers' compensation on incentive payments designed to encourage specific sorts of treatment (Eisenberg and Williams, 1981). Alternatively, education programs -- like those proposed to improve the quality of care for veterans -- could be expanded to sensitize providers to the cost implications of their decisions (Lawrence, 1981). Studies of such programs in VA and non-VA settings suggest that all three methods could have at least some impact on the delivery of care with the VA (Eisenberg and Williams, 1981; Eisenberg, 1977).

Conclusion

The VA health care system faces major changes as the veteran population ages. These changes are wide-reaching, affecting every program within the VA. Without central guidance, individual programs will adapt to this changing demand. Such piecemeal adaptation is likely, however, to be incomplete and to miss opportunities for system-wide reform which could both improve the quality and reduce the costs of care under VA auspices. One of the VA's greatest strengths lies in its potential to react as a system, to develop a set of incentives and practices which ensure continuity of care for the elder veteran. To do this, however, it may be necessary to consider strategies of reform which are as far-reaching as the age-related changes which have prompted the need for reform.

1. Not only must physicians periodically assess patients to receive VA HBHC benefits, but doctors make almost 10% of the home visits authorized under the VA HBHC program (Goldman, 1980).

2. Experiments with case management and integration with a network of community health and social service providers, such as that at the Loma Linda VAMC, represent a step in this direction.

3. Geriatric evaluation units have, however, been established at a small number of VAMCs (VA, 1983b).

4. The VA's hospital based home care program had an average cost of almost $60 per visit in 1977, compared to a national average for Medicare of $25 per visit (Callahan, 1981). Although some of this difference may have reflected a concentration of patients with greater impairments in the VA program, it seems unlikely that such differences in case mix could account for cost differences of this size. The active participation of physicians is also a contributing factor.

5. It was estimated at recent Congressional hearings that the cost of processing claims for reimbursement by third party insurers would be about 1-3% of the revenues generated by a health care program (U.S. Senate Committee on Veterans Affairs, 1980).

6. This information was calculated from data found in the 1979 National Survey of Veterans: Summary Report (Hammond, 1980).

REFERENCES

Bang, A., Morse, J. and Campion, E. "Transition of VA Acute Care Hospitals into Acute and Long Term Care." Chapter 4 in this book.

Besdine, R., Levkoff, S. and Wetle, T. "Health and Illness Behaviors in Elder Veterans." Chapter 1 in this book.

Black, G. "Pennsylvania Department of Aging Perspective: Planning Services for Aging Veterans and Their Spouses." Paper presented at Seventh National Association of Social Workers Professional Symposium, "Social Work Practice in a Turbulent World," Philadelphia, November, 1981.

Bresler, J. and Mort, E. Nursing Home Care Needs of Veterans in 1990. Veterans Administration Office of Program Analysis and Development, Washington, D.C., July, 1982.

Brown, M. "Multihospital Systems: Trends, Issues and Prospects." In Multihospital Systems: Policy Issues for the Future, Bisbee, G. (Ed.). The Hospital Research and Educational Trust, Chicago, 1981.

Callahan, W. Medicare: Use of Home Health Services, 1977. Health Care Financing Administration, Publication No. 03064, Baltimore, Maryland, January, 1981.

Eisenberg, J. "An Educational Program to Modify Laboratory Use by House Staff." Journal of Medical Education, 52, pp. 578-581, July, 1977.

Eisenberg, J. and Williams, S. "Cost Containment and Changing Physician Practice Behavior: Can the Fox Learn to Guard the Chicken Coop?" Journal of the American Medical Association, 246(19), pp. 2195-2201, 1981.

General Accounting Office. State Veterans' Homes: Opportunities to Reduce VA and State Costs and Improve Program Management. HRD-82-7, Washington, D.C., October 22, 1981.

Goldman, R. Extended Care Letter: Hospital Based Home Care (HBHC) Survey Results FY 1977 and FY 1979. Veterans Administration, Washington, D.C., June 2, 1980.

431

Hammond, D. 1979 National Survey of Veterans: Summary Report. Veterans Administration, Reports and Statistics Service of the Office of the Comptroller, Washington, D.C., December, 1980.

Lawrence, R. "The Role of Physician Education in Cost Containment." Journal of Medical Education, 56, pp. 504-511, June, 1981.

Lindsay, C. Veterans Administration Hospitals. American Enterprise Institute for Public Policy Research, Washington, D.C., 1975.

Luft, H. Health Maintenance Organizations: Dimensions of Performance. New York: John Wiley and Sons, 1981.

Mac Adam, M. and Piktialis, D. "Mechanisms of Access and Coordination." Chapter 6 in this book.

National Academy of Sciences. Health Care for American Veterans. Washington, D.C.: National Academy of Sciences, 1977.

Page, W. "Why Veterans Choose Veterans Administration Hospitalization: A Multivariate Model." Medical Care, 20 (3), pp. 308-320, March, 1982.

Sapolsky, H. "America's Socialized Medicine: The Allocation of Resources within the Veterans' Health Care System." Public Policy, 25(3), pp. 359-382, Summer, 1977.

Schlesinger, M., Moran, A. and Zangwill, L. "Utilization of the VA by Elder Veterans: An Empirical Analysis." Chapter 10 in this book.

Seitz, L. The Impact upon the VA Health Care Delivery System of Treating a Higher Proportion of Older Veterans. Veterans Administration, HSIS Report No. 81-8, Washington, D.C., October, 1981.

Smith, D. Long Term Care in Transition. Ann Arbor, Michigan: Aupha Press, 1981.

Special Medical Advisory Group, Task Force on the VA Geriatric Plan. Caring for the Older Veteran. Veterans Administration, Washington, D.C., July 18, 1983.

Stasson, M. and Holakan, J. Long Term Care Demonstration Projects: A Review of Recent Evaluations. Working Paper 1227-2. The Urban Institute, Washington, D.C., February, 1981.

Thompson, F. Health Policy and Bureaucracy. Cambridge, Massachusetts: The MIT Press, 1981.

U.S. Department of Health and Human Services. A Comparative Study of Long Term Care Demonstrations. Human Services Monograph Series, Project SHARE, Washington, D.C., 1981.

U.S. Department of Health Education and Welfare, Federal Council on Aging. Public Policy and the Frail Elderly. DHEW Publication No. (OHDS) 79-20959, Washington, D.C., December, 1978.

U.S. Senate Committee on Veterans Affairs, "Hearing on Health Insurance Reimbursement" (September 19, 1979). Washington, D.C.: U.S. Government Printing Office, 1980.

U.S. Veterans Administration. Health Care of the Aging Veteran: A Report of the Geriatrics and Gerontology Advisory Committee. Washington, D.C., April, 1983a.

U.S. Veterans Administration, Geriatric Department of Medicine and Surgery Liaison Coordinating Committee. Patient Treatment and Program Developments in the Care of the Aging Veteran. Washington, D.C., July 15, 1983b.

U.S. Veterans Administration. VA Manual, M1, Part I, Chapter 30, Washington, D.C., 1983c.

Vladeck, B. "Multihospital Systems and the Public Interest." In Multihospital Systems: Policy Issues for the Future, Bisbee, G. (Ed.). Chicago: The Hospital Research and Educational Trust, 1981.

Wennberg, J. and Gittleson, A. Health Planning and Regulation: The New England Experience. DHHS Publication No. (HRA) 81-14008. Washington, D.C.: U.S. Government Printing Office, March, 1981.

Wetle, T. and Evans, L. "Serving the Family of the Elder Veteran." Chapter 8 in this book.

INDEX

ACCESS (New York), 108-110, 118, 121

Adult Day Care (see Adult Day Health Care)

Adult Day Health Care, 46, 59, 67, 96-104, 105, 134, 162, 163, 170, 184, 192, 193, 240, 241, 246

Aid and Attendance, 147, 192, 241-242

Alternative Health Services Project (Georgia), 110-112, 120, 121

American Hospital Association (AHA), 76, 355

Area Agency on Aging (AAA), 141, 142-143, 165, 166, 179, 180, 188

Attitudes, 1-3, 11-13, 15, 19-25, 27-28, 66, 75, 83, 86, 205-230, 359, 377, 392, 393, 399

California In-Home Supportive Service, 236

Cash Grants (see Support for Family Caregivers)

Case Coordination (see Case Management)

Case Management, 83, 109, 110, 114, 115, 122, 123, 124, 125, 126, 127, 128, 129, 130, 131, 132, 134, 137, 138, 139-142, 143, 144, 147, 150, 160, 165, 167, 179, 183, 184, 185, 189, 394, 395, 421, 424, 430

CHAMPVA (See Civilian Health and Medical Program)

Channeling (see National Long Term Care Channeling Project)

Chronic Disease, 5, 8-11, 13, 21, 23, 24, 25, 28, 159-171, 344, 370, 375, 413, 415

Civilian Health and Medical Program (CHAMPVA), 44, 247

Clinical Decisions, 209-211, 212-213, 221-228

437

Hospital Based Home Care, 56, 64, 76, 134, 143, 161, 162, 167, 170, 187, 192, 193, 237–238, 241, 378, 396, 400, 419, 430

Hospital Utilization, 40–41, 44, 69–70, 102, 141, 241, 245–246, 273–274, 321–367

Hospitals, 41, 69–92, 109, 121, 134, 146, 150, 151, 160–162, 164, 181, 183, 192, 237, 241, 245, 246, 248, 261–320, 321–367, 370, 398

Illness Behavior, 1–33, 261–320, 330, 321–367, 376–379, 321–367, 376–379, 394–395, 414, 416

In-Service Training, 21–22, 421

Long Term Care, 69–88, 93–157, 158–203, 261–320, 321–367, 409–433

   Access, 85, 128, 132, 136, 159–203, 321–367, 409–433

   Coordination, 20, 321–322, 413, 418, 420–421

Long Term Care Gerontology Center, 22, 167, 181, 190

Long Term Care Services, (see individual listings - Adult Day Health Care, Community Nursing Home, Domiciliary, Geriatric Evaluation Units, Geriatric Research Education and Clinical Centers, Hospice, Hospital Based Home Care, Nursing Home, Residential Care Home Program, Respite Care, State Home Program, State Nursing Home)

Long Term Care Targeting (see Targeting)

MEDIPP (see Medical District Initiated Program Planning)

Medicaid, 39, 49, 59, 75, 78–80, 84, 87, 98, 112–113, 151, 191, 236, 266, 276, 278, 280, 282, 284, 292, 329, 322, 352, 384, 416–417

Medical District Initiated Program Planning (MEDIPP), 138, 162, 167, 177, 179–181, 183, 185

Medicare, 39, 49, 59, 75, 82, 84–85, 87, 95, 112–113, 124, 236, 247, 262, 276, 278, 280, 282, 284, 292, 329, 330, 331, 332, 349, 352, 384, 416–417, 419, 430

Presentation of Disease (see Illness Behavior)

Prevention, 19, 129, 374, 377, 379–380, 396–398, 400, 412, 420, 428

Residential Care, 134–135, 163, 170, 183, 187, 192, 241, 248

Residential Care Home Program, 45, 57, 134–135, 163–170, 183, 187, 192

Respite Care, 98, 109, 135, 142, 184–185, 238, 241, 242, 243, 245–246

S/HMO (see Social/Health Maintenance Organization)

SSI (see Supplemental Security Income)

Screening, 86, 395

Section 222, 96–105, 121

Self-Evaluation of Health, 11–12

Service-Connected Disability (see Eligibility)

Service Providers (see Attitudes)

Social/Health Maintenance Organization (S/HMO), 87, 94, 130–132, 145, 159

Social Work Service, 134, 140, 149, 179, 182–183, 185, 187, 190

SMAG (see Special Medical Advisory Group)

Special Medical Advisory Group (SMAG), 324–325, 424, 425

Spinal Cord Injury Units, 143, 179, 183

State Domiciliary Housing (VA), 44, 77–78

State Home Program (VA), 43, 54, 181–182, 342, 356

State Nursing Home (VA), 44, 54, 77, 161, 181, 192, 428

Supplemental Security Income (SSI), 113, 191